VENTRICULAR ASSIST DEVICES

Edited by **Jeffrey H. Shuhaiber**

Ventricular Assist Devices
Edited by Jeffrey H. Shuhaiber

Published by InTech

Janeza Trdine 9, 51000 Rijeka, Croatia

Publishing Process Manager Ana Nikolic

Technical Editor Teodora Smiljanic

Cover Designer InTech Design Team

Additional hard copies can be obtained from orders@intechopen.com

Ventricular Assist Devices, Edited by Jeffrey H. Shuhaiber
p. cm.
ISBN 978-953-307-164-0

Meet the editor

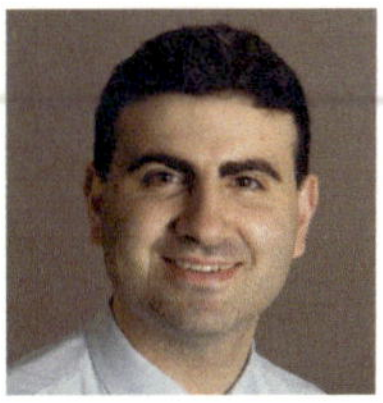

Dr. Shuhaiber, MD, is cardiothoracic and transplant surgeon at University of Cincinnati and Cincinnati Children Hospital. Dr. Shuhaiber joined the staff in 2009. He had previously been chief resident of Cardiac Surgery at Children's Hospital in Boston at Harvard Medical School. Dr. Shuhaiber completed his medical school training in England at Kings College London and undertook fellowships in USA and England. Dr. Shuhaiber's research goal is to orderly adjust risk outcomes following cardiac surgery both in children and adults. Study endpoints have included mortality, morbidity and qualitative improvement initiatives. His interests include temporal relationships of complications following surgery. Results of these clinical research studies have led to controlled studies of which have had important impacts on outcomes following transplantation and ventricular assist devices. He is member of a number of professional societies and has more than 50 original publications as well as several book chapters. He is active in the clinical field and mentors a number of students both from medicine and engineering.

Contents

Preface

Ventricular assist devices are here to stay and will stand the test of time. The imaginative frontier is a reality with multiple venues for active clinical, basic and translational research. Clinically applicable assist devices for short-, intermediate- and long-term support have improved significantly in the last ten years. Current devices are downsizing with enhanced durability and reliability. The associated complication burden including thomboembolism and hemolysis remain a limitation that is not insurmountable in the near future. Patient selection and technical surgical performance are the key aspects to successful surgical outcome following device insertion. The assist devices will continue adding a large number of years of life to humans globally and empower the medical society to optimize heart failure therapy. While expensive and cumbersome task, the foundation provided in this book reflects a contemporary product of original research from a multitude of different experts in the field. The book has been organized into parts reflecting the process by which the caring physician is involved. Part 1 identifies contemporary indications for device placement, part 2 reviews the role of echocardiographic imaging for ventricular assist device and mycoarium, part 3 identifies current cellular research prior and following assist device support, part 4 reviews the various types of devices available and their efficacy both with regard to short term and long term outcomes, part 5 reviews the three major complications following device insertion; infection, stroke and arrythmias, part 6 reflects some thoughts on managing these patients following hospital discharge and part 7 provides most recent research on patients who had assist device explanted following heart transplantation.

We hope this cumulative international effort provides the necessary tools for both the novice as well as the active practitioner aiming to change the outcome of these complex patients.

Jeffrey H. Shuhaiber
Boston, Massachusetts 2011

Part 1

Indication for Ventricular Assist Device

1

Indications for Ventricle Assist Devices

Guillermo Reyes and Sara Badia
Hospital Universitario La Princesa, Madrid
Spain

1. Introduction

Despite widespread use of evidence-based therapies the morbidity and mortality of heart failure has not changed, and it remains the most common hospital discharge diagnosis for patients older than 65 years old of age. Approximately 5 million patients in the United States of America have cardiac failure, and over 550,000 patients are diagnosed with heart failure for the first time each year (Levy et al, 2002; Hunt et al, 2005). The European Society of Cardiology represents countries with a population of more than 900 million, and in their last guidelines they reported that there are at least 15 million patients suffering this disease in those 51 countries (Dickstein et al, 2008). Heart failure is primarily a condition of the elderly (Kannel & Belanger, 1991), and thus the widely recognized "aging of the population" also contributes to the increasing incidence of heart disease. The incidence of cardiac failure approaches 10 per 1,000 population after age 65 years, and approximately about 80% of patients hospitalized with heart failure are older than 65 years old (Masoudi & Havranek, 2002).

There are several reasons that may explain why the prevalence of heart failure is increasing: ageing of the population, the success in prolonging survival in coronary patients, and the success in postponing coronary events by effective prevention in those patients at high risk or those patients who have already survived a first event (secondary prevention) (Senni et al, 1999). Advances in medical therapy have resulted in improved survival in patients with moderate and severe heart failure, but the prognosis for end-stage heart failure patients still remains poor. The conclusion of all these aspects is that there is a change in the demographics of heart failure patients in recent years, and an increased survival of older patients with heart disease.

At present time, cardiac transplantation remains the gold standard of cardiac replacement therapy. However, the supply of donor hearts is limited and therefore is not an option for many patients because of age and other comorbid conditions. Alternative forms of cardiac replacement therapy are being investigating. This includes cell therapy, xenotransplantation, ventricle assist devices implantation and total artificial heart.

Although initially the indications for heart mechanical assistance are similar to those developed in the1960s for the use of intra-aortic balloon pumps the indications have developed into more complex cases which must be considered. Ventricle assist devices are more and more reliable and its size is becoming smaller with the passing of time, improving patient's outcomes.

2. Cardiac transplantation: where we are and what can we expect

The first human cardiac transplant was performed by Dr. Barnard in Cape Town in South Africa in 1967. With the development of immunosuppression, orthotopic cardiac transplantation, what exists today, is a highly successful procedure for the treatment of end-stage heart disease. Over time, survival of patients undergoing orthotopic heart transplantation has improved significantly, mainly due to a reduction in rejection rates, better prevention and treatment of opportunistic infections and defined management protocols (Taylor D et al, 2008).
Indications for cardiac transplantation at the present time include patients with severe heart failure symptoms, a poor prognosis, and with no alternative form of treatment (class of recommendation I, level of evidence C). Contraindications to heart transplantation are: current alcohol and/or drug abuse, lack of proper cooperation, serious mental disease not properly controlled, treated cancer with remission and, 5 years follow-up, systemic disease with multiorgan involvement, active infection, significant renal failure (creatinine clearance <50 mL/min), irreversible high pulmonary vascular resistance (6–8 Wood units and mean transpulmonary gradient >15 mmHg), recent thromboembolic complications, unhealed peptic ulcer, evidence of significant liver impairment, or other serious co-morbidities with a poor prognosis. Patients must be well informed, motivated, emotionally stable, and capable of complying with intensive medical treatment.
According to the registry of the International Society for Heart and Lung Transplantation reported in 2008 (Taylor D et al, 2008) the one-year survival after primary orthotopic cardiac transplantations has increased from 79% between 1982 and 1991, to 82% between 1992 and 2001, and to 86% between 2002 and 2005 ($p<0.0001$). However, long-term mortality has not changed and in fact the overall survival patterns remain largely unchanged with a steep fall in survival up to 6 months and linear decrement in survival thereafter, at approximately 3.5% per year (figure 1)
Some factors need to be in consideration, as they are changing the demographics of heart transplantation. The primary cardiac transplantation has shifted in the last years towards a

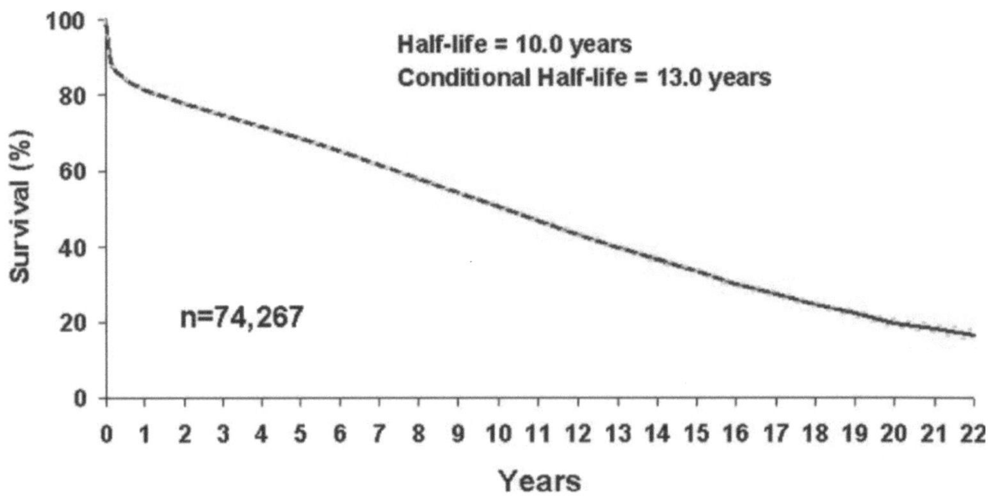

Fig. 1. Kaplan-Meier survival for all cardiac transplants (1/1982-6/2006) (Taylor D et al, 2008)

slight predominance of patients with nonischemic cardiomyopathy (50%) vs. ischemic (34%). It is a fact that the relative contribution of patients with ischemic cardiomyopathy has declined over the last decade. Also the age of donors and recipients has increased in the past 20 years. Almost 25% of cardiac transplant patient recipients in the last years were over the age of 60 years, with a relative fall in the number of recipients aged 40-49 years. Also at the present time the number of transplants being performed worldwide is far outnumbered by the number of potential candidates, as donor hearts are a very limited resource. These aspects are essential in the understanding of patient outcomes and they explain why other alternatives to heart transplantation should be investigated in an effort to offer alternative therapies to those patients suffering severe heart failure.

The need for those alternative therapies include the lack of cardiac donors, long cardiac transplantation waiting list, patients with any contraindication to cardiac transplantation (definitive or temporal) and patients requiring more time for the heart to recover.

The use of ventricle assist devices has acquired an important role in the management of end-stage heart failure and it is very likely that its importance will increase with time. Historically, the development of cardiopulmonary bypass technology in the fifties was the achievement that really started the development of more permanent means of mechanical cardiac support. Technological progress has allowed the design and production of smaller devices that have bridged patients towards recovery and transplantation.

In this chapter we will review the indications of ventricle assist devices implantation. We will star giving some general indications that every patient should follow from a theoretical point of view. Then we will divide the indications in three different groups: 1) bridge to transplantation, 2) bridge to recovery and 3) destination therapy.

We will also discuss when it is required to use a short term ventricle assist device, a long ventricle assist devices and the total artificial heart. Finally we will review in the literature when it is necessary to have a right ventricle assist device especially when a left ventricle assist device is already implanted.

The authors would like to remark that this chapter is a compilation of the literature regarding ventricle assist device therapy. Therefore each patient must be considered as a particular case and there are no strict rules or guidelines to be followed.

3. General indications for ventricle assist device implantation

The general rule is simple: ventricle assist devices are used when the heart is incapable of maintaining its function. Therefore, the organism is in danger or is going to be in danger because cardiac output is not enough to maintain vital organ flow. Cardiac dysfunction may be caused in an acute fashion, like in a cardiogenic shock caused by an extensive myocardiac infarction or after a major cardiac surgery when a patient is not able to weaned from the heart-lung machine. Also, cardiac failure may be a consequence of a chronic condition like in the ischemic chronic heart disease or in patients with dilatated myocardiopathy.

There are some registries that compile from different centers the indications for a ventricle assist devices implantation. These registries are a good resource of information about what the indications of ventricle assist device are. One of the databases is the Interagency Registry for Mechanical Assisted Circulatory Support (INTERMACS), which is an audited registry for patients who receive a mechanical circulatory support device to treat advanced medically refractory heart failure. From June 2006 to December 2007, a total of 75 institutions in the United States of America prospectively entered 420 patients. Most of the patients (n=336) had a mechanical circulatory support device implanted for the indication of bridge to transplantation. The indication of destination therapy was applied in 63 patients whereas the rest of patients received a ventricle assist device as a bridge to recovery (Holman et al, 2009). This perfectly describes what the indications in the clinical practice are at the present time. Several aspects must be considered for indicating a ventricle assist device:

3.1 Clinical status

Patients requiring a ventricle assist device suffer severe heart failure acutely or chronically. When cardiac failure has been caused acutely, the patient is in cardiogenic shock. This may be from different causes: extensive acute myocardial infarction (Killip IV), mechanical complications after an infarction (papillary muscle rupture, interventricular septal rupture), patients that cannot be weaned from the cardiopulmonary bypass machine, acute myocarditis and others. It should be noticed that the use of ventricle assist device in the setting of cardiogenic shock must be contemplated when the use of inotropes and intra-aortic ballon pump is not enough to maintain an adequate cardiac output and there is a risk of death or other organ failure. Also, there should be no other options such as major cardiac surgery or other surgical options that may reverse the status of the patient.
However, although ventricle assist devices are not the first treatment option in this type of situation, their implantation should not be delayed. Most cardiologist and cardiac surgeons agree to implant a ventricle assist device in patients with severe heart failure, despite intra-aortic balloon pump or inotropic support with unstable hemodynamics, and with early signs of end-organ dysfunction (Osaki et al, 2009). In the last years, there has been an attempt to prevent deterioration of the ventricle assist device candidate's condition. Actually, whenever possible some co-morbid conditions should be nullified by a period of therapy prior to implant. Some examples are renal dysfunction, localized infection or severe pulmonary edema, which can be reversed with medical therapy prior to a mechanical device implantation. Every patient should be in the best clinical position, considering that these patients are in a really bad clinical status, avoiding the implantation in pre-mortem conditions. This rule should also be applied in those patients with end-stage chronic cardiac dysfunction. Mechanical device implantation should be kept in mind before other organs deteriorate. This will definitely improve clinical outcomes. Other clinical conditions that may indicate the use of some mechanical support are intractable arrhythmias and intractable angina not responsive to medical therapy or revascularization procedures in patients with poor left ventricle function.

3.2 Hemodynamic parameters

A hemodynamic study may be required in some situations to assure that cardiac function is severely deteriorated. Table 1 summarizes hemodynamic data that represent severe left and right ventricle dysfunction.

4. Ventricle assist device as bridge to transplantation

As we have previously descibed in the introduction section, orthotopic cardiac transplantation is the gold standard for treating end-stage heart failure. The International Society for Heart and Lung Transplantation (ISHLT) has reported outcome data on transplant recipients for more than 25 years with data that includes more than 74,000 patients (Taylor et al, 2008).

Left ventricle assist device	Right ventricle assist device	Biventricular ventricle assist device
Systolic blood pressure <90mmHg	Right atria pressure > 20mmHg	Right atria pressure > 20mmHg
Left atria pressure > 20mmHg	Left atria pressure < 15mmHg	Left atria pressure > 20mmHg
Systemic vascular resistance >2,100 dynes-sec/cm	No tricuspid regurgitation	No tricuspid regurgitation
Urine output <20mL/h		Inability to maintain left ventricle assist device flow >2.0L/min/m^2 with right atrial pressure >20mmHg

Table 1. Haemodynamic indications for circulatory assist device

This registry includes data mainly from USA and European countries. We see from those reports that primary indications for cardiac transplantation has changed with an increase of patients with nonischemic cardiomyopathy and less ischemic patients. In addition, the age of donors and recipients has been increasing in the last 20 years, especially in Europe. It is clear that heart donors are a limited resource and some patients die while awaiting cardiac transplantation due to that lack of donors. Actually, in the last two decades, decreasing numbers of organ donors have led to longer waiting times for cardiac transplantation and subsequently increasing mortality. Other patients´ statuses may worsen while waiting and they may need some kind of cardiac circulatory support in order to maintain vital blood flow and preserve organ systems like kidney, hepatic, or brain function.

Therefore, we can summarize that ventricle assist device as a bridge to transplantation is indicated in those patients that are candidates for cardiac transplantation and need some cardiac support while they are waiting for the heart. This indication includes a wide spectrum of patients. On one side, we may have patients that suffer an acute event (postinfarction cardiogenic shock, postcardiotomy) which leads them into an irreversible severe heart failure that requires urgent cardiac transplantation. Until a donor is found, cardiac mechanical support is necessary to save patients life and to preserve their vital organs. As we will see later, organ failure is associated with a worse prognosis after heart transplantation. On the other side, there are patients that are awaiting cardiac transplantation and whose conditions become refractory to medical therapy.

At present time, ventricle assist devices are an important tool in the management of this kind of patient (Frazier at al, 2001; Miller et al, 2007; Russo et al, 2009). Also, in the last decade, the number of heart transplant recipients supported by ventricle assist devices at the time of transplantation has more than doubled to over 400 per year in the USA (Taylor DO et al, 2008) as well as in European countries. This clearly reflects the need of mechanical circulatory support in patients awaiting transplantation. Also as previously described, if we consider some registries as the INTERMACS, bridge to transplantation is by far, the most frequent indication for a ventricle assist device implantation (Holman et al, 2009).

There are some questions that should be answered regarding mechanical circulatory support as a bridge to transplantation.

1. Does the use of a ventricle assist device as a bridge to transplantation affect the outcome of patients when compared to those patients who receive transplants without the need of mechanical assistance?
2. When should one implant a mechanical device in a patient awaiting cardiac transplantation?
3. What kind of device should be implanted?

Although several studies have demonstrated the benefits of ventricle assist devices in the pretransplant period, findings from studies analyzed the impact of mechanical circulatory support on posttransplant outcomes have conflicted. The majority of studies have concluded that short term, but not long term, survival is diminished in recipients bridge with a mechanical device (Taylor DO et al, 2008; Cleveland JC et al, 2008). However, there are some reports that do not confirm these findings. In a recently published study (Osaki et al, 2009) Osaki et al compared patients´ outcomes undergoing cardiac transplantation with and without the use of a ventricle assist device. They also divided patients in two different time groups as an attempt to analyze both, the experience of the group and the improvement of devices technology. A total of 531 consecutive heart transplant recipients in a 17 years period were included. They concluded that post-transplant survival has improved in the last years. Actually in their study, outcomes for orthotopic heart transplantation after bridge to transplantation have become equivalent to that of orthotopic heart transplantation without ventricle assist device. The data suggest that advances in device technology and multidisciplinary programs, have improved survival and allowed bridges to transplantation candidates to have an outcome equivalent to that of non-ventricle assist device in recent times (Figure 2).

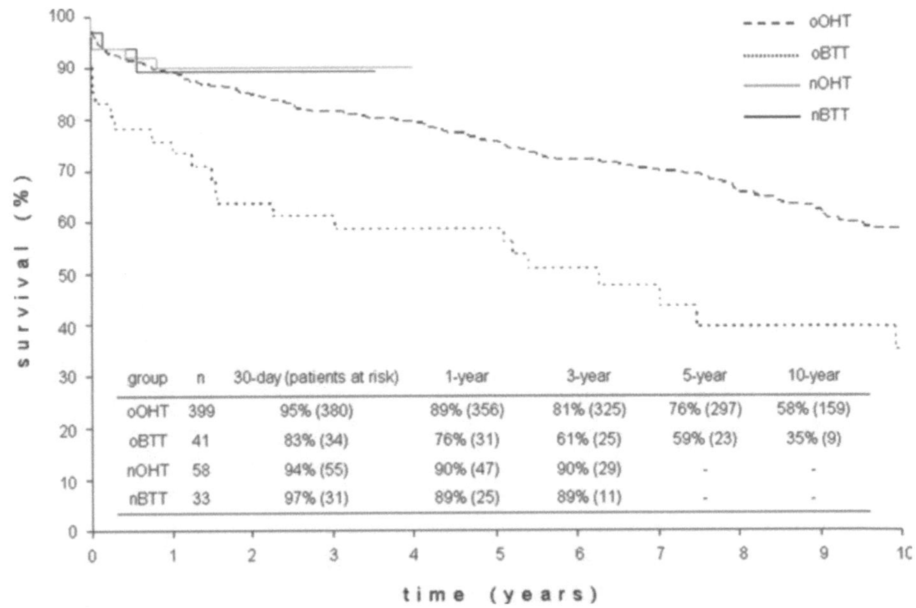

Fig. 2. Post-transplant survival by Kaplan–Meier analysis. oOHT, old orthotopic heart transplant (January 1990 to July 2003); nOHT, new orthotopic heart transplant (August 2003 to August 2007); oBTT, old bridge to transplant (January 1990 to July 2003); nBTT, new bridge to transplant (August 2003 to August 2007).

In that study, multivariate analysis revealed that diabetes and biventricular (but no univentricular) support were the only independent predictors of post-transplant mortality. These findings have been confirmed by other groups (Russo et al, 2009). In the study published by Russo et al, they included more than 10,000 heart transplantation recipients from the United Network for Organ Sharing in a seven-year period. They concluded that the use of implantable left ventricle assist devices (both intracorporeal and extracorporeal devices) as bridges to transplantation are not associated with diminished posttransplant survival. However, an increase in 90-day mortality was seen in patients bridged with extracorporeal devices.

These findings suggest that more than 80% of well-selected patients implanted with intracorporeal devices as a bridge to transplantation are successfully transplanted, providing additional evidence that a more aggressive use of implantable devices may benefit candidates whose condition is refractory to medical management. Outcomes seem to be better when implantable device support is implemented before patients clinical status deteriorates badly. The findings further suggest that a more aggressive use of implantable support may benefit candidates who are likely to face long waiting times as candidates with higher body mass index or blood type O. The fact that patient survival is diminished in patients with extracorporeal devices may suggests that in some cases, candidates supported by an extracorporeal device may benefit from further optimization before transplantation, and that this type of devices may be best used as a bridge to an implantable device especially in those patients that may have long waiting times.

As it has been suggested in other studies (Cleveland et al, 2008), the general perception among most cardiac transplantation centres is that explantation of a ventricle assist device confers a more technically challenging operation and therefore, might adversely affect survival not in medium term but in a short term. In the Cleveland group experience, one year survival was similar in those recipients receiving a heart transplantation with or without a mechanical circulatory support. However, when they analyzed patients who died after transplantation, most of the ventricle assist device group died within 30 days of transplant. In contrast, only a minority of patients without a mechanical assist device died within those thirty days.

This may reflect an inherent complexity and higher risk operation that occurs in the explantation of a ventricle device.

It is essential to have a good knowledge of the heart transplantation situation in every country. There are some countries such as Spain, where there is a high prevalence of donors and where the waiting times are not to long. Short term extracorporeal devices may be used as they are less expensive and very simple to use. Good results can be achieved this way (Reyes et al, 2007). In other countries like Germany or the USA where the waiting times are much longer, long term assistance may be a better option (Korfer et al, 1999).

5. Ventricle assist device as bridge to recovery

Ventricle assist devices have been successfully implanted in patients who are expected to recover sufficient myocardial function and it is not expected that they will need a cardiac transplantation. In this type of patient a short-term bridge to recovery device may be a good option as these devices are less expensive and very easy to use (Samuels et al, 2005; Nicolini & Gherti, 2009). The most frequent clinical settings in which a mechanical circulatory support may be needed are described below:

5.1 Post-cardiotomy

Patients with compromised left ventricle function who have undergone long operations may need a ventricle assist device because the severity of the postoperative circulatory shock. It is estimated that about 5% of patients undergoing coronary or valve cardiac procedures will have some degree of postcardiotomy cardiogenic shock (Pae et al, 1992). Short term mechanical support as bridge to recovery has been successfully used in patients who are expected to recover sufficient myocardial function. Since the ABIOMED system was approved by the Food and Drug Administration in 1992, it has become the second most commonly used mechanical support device for patients with post-cardiotomy ventricular dysfunction after the intra-aortic balloon pump with excellent rates of myocardial recovery and device removal after short-term support (Morgan et al, 2004). We highly recommend the early implantation of mechanical circulatory assistance in this clinical setting to provide mechanical unloading of the ventricle and rapid restoration of normal end-organ perfusion in order to improve survival rates.

In those patients in whom a high risk of cardiac failure is anticipated (severely impaired ventricular function undergoing high risk cardiac procedures) transplant evaluation should be initiated preoperatively and the procedure performed with a ventricle assist device back up. If needed it, mechanical support may be used as bridge to recovery or bridge to transplantation.

5.2 Post acute myocardial infarction shock

Despite the advances in the management of cardiogenic shock secondary to acute myocardial infarction, the prognosis is still poor with mortality rates as high as 70% (Goldberg RJ et al, 1999). There are some aspects that must be considered in this clinical setting. One of the surgical dilemmas, when implanting an LVAD into a patient with an acute anterior wall myocardial infarction, is the safety of apical cannulation in the presence of acutely infarcted apical myocardium, which is typically necrotic and friable. Ventricular disruption and bleeding from the cannulation site are major concerns with lethal consequences. Although left atrial cannulation is an option, it is suboptimal as it affords inadequate left ventricular decompression and limits LVAD inflow. Furthermore, left atrial cannulation has been shown to have independent risk factors for the development of left ventricular thrombus and stroke. There are some surgical techniques that should be considered. Some authors have maintained that left ventricle devices can be safely implanted into acutely infarcted, friable myocardium by modifying their surgical technique. This involves placing cannulation sutures through the full thickness of the infarcted ventricular myocardium and reinforcing their suture line with pericardium or Teflon felt (Park SJ et al, 2000; Chen et al, 1999). Other technique used in patients with cardiogenic shock and with extensive anterior wall infarcts, consists of securing the cannula with interrupted, pledgeted, horizontal mattress sutures through the full-thickness of the infarcted myocardium. If significant bleeding is observed, additional sutures and/or haemostatic products can be applied to the cannulation site (Leshnower et al, 2005).

It is important to highlight that patients with ventricle assist devices due to cardiogenic shock after an acute myocardial infarction may follow different outcomes. In this situation there should be flexibility to the treatment algorithm that these patients may follow. Mechanical circulatory system may be used as a bridge to recovery, a bridge to bridge (to other long term assist device system) or as a bridge to transplant. Also, some authors consider that the use of a biventricular assist device is important in these patients

(Leshnower et al, 2005). This must be taken in consideration in right ventricular heart failure, intractable arrhytmias and in the presence of shock with multisystem organ failure. Recently, some authors consider that less invasive percutaneous ventricular assist devices may be helpful in the decision making of the treatment as they are less expensive and sternotomy is not required, which may helps subsequent transplantation or surgically ventricle assist device insertion (Brinkman et al, 2010).

5.3 Myocarditis

Myocarditis may cause severe cardiac failure, sometimes very acutely. It is believed that almost every infectious agent can cause myocarditis (bacterias, virus, spiroquetas, mycotic infections, parasital agents, ricketsias). Also there may be immunologic causes as the so call giant cells myocarditis in which, apart from inmunosupresor therapy, ventricle assist device may be needed. These patients trend to be younger (many of them children) and it is characterized by an unpredictable clinical course. Actually it remains a real challenge to determine which group of patients will recover and which will require mechanical support or heart transplantation (Houel R et al, 1999). As myocarditis is an inflammatory process that affects the whole myocardium (both the right and left ventricle) it is frequent that biventricular support is required (Grinda JM et al, 2004). As we have previously said it is important anticipate the prognosis of the patient in order to convert a short-term assist device into a long term assist device or cardiac transplantation in those patients in which an optimal recovery is not expected.

6. Destination therapy

Ventricle assist device as a destination therapy has some aspects that may concern cardiologists and cardiac surgeons. It is necessary to know how the mechanical devices may affect survival rates compared with alternative treatment strategies, the durability of the devices, and its safety profile. Also we must take into account the quality of life of these patients and if the up-front costs of implantation may be offset by the long-term benefits of the patients.

The *R*andomized *E*valuation of *M*echanical *A*ssistance for the *T*reatment of *C*ongestive *H*eart Failure (REMATCH) trial is a multicentered study supported by the National Heart, Lung, and Blood Institute. It compares long-term implantation of left ventricular assist devices with optimal medical management for patients with end-stage heart failure who require, but do not qualify to receive cardiac transplantation. This trial demonstrated that the implantation of left-ventricular assist devices decreased the 1-year mortality by a third (from 75% down to 51%) and the two year survival rate was 29% for left ventricle assist device patients versus 13% for medical patients (95% CL; 5%-22%), representing a 48 percent reduction in the risk of death from any cause, compared with the optimal medical therapy.

The survival advantage was associated with a considerable improvement in the quality of life and functional status of these patients, as compared with their medical counterparts (Rose et al., 1999). The MLHF scores, (Minnesota Living with Heart Failure questionnaire) for left ventricle assist device patients were 75.1 (0 being the best – 105 the worst). The REMATCH trial demonstrated that is superior to any available medical therapy in patients with end-stage heart failure who are not eligible for transplantation (Lietz & Miller, 2005). The Thoratec HeartMate was subsequently approved in 2003, by the Food and Drug Administration (FDA), for long-term support of this kind of patient.

The next logical step for expanding the indications for mechanical circulatory assistance would be to use the left ventricle assist device as an alternative to cardiac transplantation. However, heart transplantation cannot serve the estimated 30,000-60,000 people who die of heart failure in the US each year and could be candidates for heart transplantation or some form of mechanical circulatory support. More than 40% of the patients waited more than 1 year for a cardiac transplantation, and the waiting time is increasing every year. In 1995, the average waiting time for cardiac transplantation was over 200 days (Penningtonet al., 1999), but the average national waiting time in 2003 for a heart was 230 days (UNOS/OPTN Annual Report 2003). Each year, approximately 4000 new patients are added to the waiting list for cardiac transplant, and about 28,000-30,000 are apparently not considered viable candidates to be placed on the list. About 50%of the patients not included in the waiting list (13,000) would be candidates for a permanent ventricular assist device. An important deterrent to being listed may be advanced age.
The most obvious advantage of these mechanical device systems over transplantation would be their immediate availability. They could be placed in UNOS status II rather than UNOS status I hospital-bound patients. Table 2 shows the indications and characteristics of the total artificial heart.

<table>
<tr><th>Total artificial heart</th><th>Characteristics</th><th>Use</th><th>Cost</th></tr>
<tr><td>Abiomed Total Artificial Heart</td><td rowspan="2">Is inserted orthotopically; this procedure is accompanied by removal of the patient's own ventricles</td><td>TAH is currently undergoing clinical trials</td><td rowspan="2">The cost of these devices is likely to be quite high, but may not be very different from the cost of heart transplantation, therapy and immunosuppression.</td></tr>
<tr><td>CardioWest device</td><td>Pneumatic TAH that has been used investigationally as a bridge to transplantation</td></tr>
</table>

Table 2. Indications and characteristics of the total artificial heart. TAH: Total artificial heart.

6.1 Exercise capacity

An important determinant of quality of life in cardiac transplant recipients and left ventricle assist device recipients is exercise capacity.
Studies in cardiac transplant recipients demonstrate that, at rest, they have an increased heart rate, increased blood pressure, and low normal cardiac output. During exercise, peak heart rate, stroke volume, cardiac output, peak power output, pulse pressure, heart rate reserve, total VO2, and absolute VO2 at ventilatory threshold are all less than normal. Their exercise capacity may increase with time up to 5 years and may improve with an increase in muscle mass and lean body weight. Autonomic reenervation may actually increase the peak heart rate during exercise, although this is quite controversial. Recent studies suggest that cavo-caval anastomosis may increase atrial emptying, resulting in better functional capacity. While some individual patients with cardiac transplantation function well, most patients have important physiological limitations.
The exercise capacity of patients with implantable mechanical cardiac devices is based on the results obtained during the use like bridge to transplant, it is apparent that improvement

in exercise tolerance occurs. Maximum VO2 is a well-characterized indicator of functional status and prognosis in patients with advanced heart failure.

Peak oxygen consumption with upright treadmill exercise increased from 10 to 14 mL O2/kg/min in a group of patients supported for a mean of 50 days after left ventricle assist device implantation. Pennington et al remarked that many postoperative studies suggest that the native left ventricle may contribute to this function during exercise by actively filling the left ventricle assist device, which reduces filling time and overcomes inflowing cannula impedance. It may also augment total cardiac output with parallel ejection out of the native aortic valve and reduce ventricular interaction-related changes in functional right ventricular diastolic compliance.

It is clear that exercise capacity increases during the first several months after ventricle assist device insertion because patients have improved organ function, reducing pulmonary edema and pulmonary artery resistance. These changes significantly augment right ventricular function, which also usually improves with time.

It is anticipated that patients with long-term left ventricle assist devices will achieve reasonably high levels of exercise capacity and they will not be limited by activities of daily living. Whether they will be able to participate in athletic events and vigorous work is not entirely clear, but seems feasible (Pennington et al., 1999).

6.2 Psychological factors

A common sensation between the patients with left ventricle assist devices is that of being machine-dependent. It is important to indicate a definitive cardiac assist device in very strongly motivated patients which may need to be prepared from a psychological point of view. A positive psychological feature is the fact that left ventricle assist device insertion does not require removal of the natural heart, which might be able to temporarily support the circulation, or recover sufficiently to allow for device removal.

Quality of life may be reasonably satisfactory. Despite externalized battery sources, these patients are capable of recovering their daily activities, even returning to work. Although patients are capable of concealing external batteries so that it is not so obvious that they are supported mechanically, they cannot forget that they are dependent on the device. This factor may be resolved with new more modern devices that can be completely implanted inside the pericardium or the peritoneum. Presuming the availability of a safe and effective, totally implantable, electrically driven, left ventricle assist devices prompts a comparison with the current strategy of cardiac transplantation as a universal therapy for patients with severe heart failure.

6.3 Economical factors

It is very important to be aware of the cost of the implantation of definitive mechanical devices. Since there are limited resources availables, it is necessary to demonstrate that they are economically feasible. The average total cost to insert a left ventricle assist device in the REMATCH patient population was $210,187 which includes a $60,000 charge for the device. When implantation hospitalization costs are compared between hospital survivors and nonsurvivors, the mean costs increase from $159,271 ± 106,423 to $315,015 ± 278,713.

Sepsis, pump housing infection, and perioperative bleeding are the major drivers of implantation cost, established by regression modeling. In the patients who survived the procedure, bypass time, perioperative bleeding, and late bleeding were the drivers of cost.

The average annual readmission cost per patient for the overall cohort was $105,326, the cost of which was considerably influenced by device reliability (Oz et al, 2003).

In a recent study published by the Institute of Medicine, cost effectiveness was measured by the relationship of costs to quality-adjusted life years (QALYs). It was estimated that the cost per quality-adjusted life years in dollars for hemodialysis was $50,000, for two-vessel coronary artery bypass grafting, $34,000, and for a total artificial heart for 2 years, approximately $105,000.

The cost calculation of quality-adjusted life years for left ventricle assist devices was not calculated, but it was estimated that it would be significantly less than that for a total artificial heart.

If the devices can be relatively problem free and not require multiple readmissions for replacement of parts or devices, employers may be receptive to these patients returning to work. It is not known whether the relatively low reemployment percentage for cardiac transplant patients is related to their need to continue to take expensive medications or other medical problems.

It is possible that within four years, one could return to society with an income greater in value than the investment if the individual earns an annual salary of $40,000 per year. However, by Poirier's estimation, circulatory support systems represented a potential to increase our gross national product, leading to a higher standard of living.

The current generation of pumps continue to undergo incremental improvement. These devices exhibit smaller and more flexible drivelines or use a totally implantable design that eliminates a major gateway for infection. They are being introduced in clinical trials that may more fundamentally address the device´s shortcomings observed in the REMATCH study.

7. Short, long and intermediate ventricle assists devices

We can divide the ventricle assist devices according to its capacity to be used as support during a short, long, or intermediate time, depending on the requirements of patients. The following tables describe the indications and the more notable characteristics of the different kinds of ventricular assist devices.

7.1 Intermediate ventricle assist devices

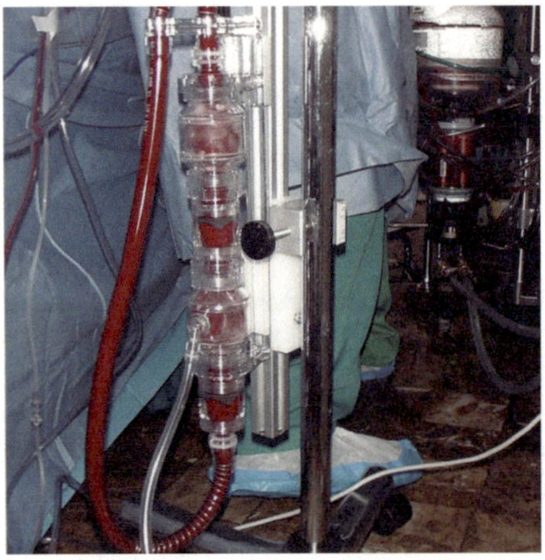

Fig. 3. ABIOMED BVS 5000 blood pump.

Intermediate term devices	Indications	Versions	Use	Advantages
Thoratec VAD	Bridge to transplantation Bridge to recovery	Thoratec Paracorporeal ventricular Assist Device (PVAD) Thoratec Implantable Ventricular Assist Device (IVAD)	RVAD LVAD BiVAD	The device uses suction drainage with pulsatile flow. Each ventricle costs approximately $50,000 but can be maintained with minimal personnel PVAD has supported patients for up to 3.3 years
Abiomed AB 5000				It is compatible with the cannulae for the Abiomed BVS 5000 support system

Table 3. Intermediate ventricle assist devices: Indications and characteristics. Intermediate term devices can be thought of as the true "bridges" to transplantation. They are intended to be removed during transplantation and are not designed for constant, permanent support.

7.2 Short ventricle assists devices

Short term VAD	Specific indications	Common indications	Use	Insertion	Limitation
Centrifugal pumps: • Bio-Medicus • Sarns	Patients who cannot be weaned from cardiopulmonary bypass. Patients who are awaiting cardiac transplantation.	VAD/cardiac transplant backup in patients undergoing high risk surgical procedures Patients with unanticipated post-operative cardiac dysfunction who required mechanical support with VAD support of the right ventricles or less commonly both ventricles. Post-operative cardiogenic shock.	RVAD LVAD BiVAD	Sternotomy Percutaneously (in the catheterization laboratory)	Non-pulsatil flow The devices are traumatic to blood, causing hemolysis. Patients are unable to ambulate or exercise with the device in place.
Extracorporeal pump: • Abiomed biventricular system (BVS 5000) • AB5000	It allows recovery of end organs and is approved for postcardiotomy use. Patients with potentially reversible heart failure. Donor heart dysfunction following transplantation.		RVAD LVAD BiVAD	Sternotomy	The devices are more expensive than centrifugal pumps, but can be maintained with minimal personnel.
Axial flow pumps: Impella microaxial flow device	Postcardiotomy failure			Sternotomy Percutaneously	Nonpulsatile flow. Moderate degree of hemolysis and thrombocytopenia.
Percutaneous left atrial-to-femoral-arterial VAD: Tandem Heart™	Stabilization until recovery of jeopardized myocardium. Bridge to definite surgical treatment.			Percutaneously	Complications such as severe bleeding and acute limb ischemia are more common

Table 4. Intermediate ventricle assist devices: Indications and characteristics.

7.3 Long ventricle assists devices

Long term devices	Indications	Versions	Use	Advantages	Disadvantages
Novacor device	Replacement therapy for patients with heart failure		LVAD		Requires normal native aortic valve
HeartMate I (pulsatil flow)	Bridge to transplantation. Destination therapy.	HeartMate I is a paracorporeal device that comes in two versions: implantable pneumatic (IP) and vented-electric (XVE) versions	XVE only in a LVAD	Anticoagulation with warfarin not required. Low thromboembolic rate. Outpatient support appears to be cost-effective Improvement in renal function and reduction in pulmonary hypertension prior to transplantation. Improvement in hemodynamic measurements at rest and during exercise and exercise capacity	Expensive device
HeartMate II		Smaller devices and greater durability		Improvements in NYHA functional class, six minute walk, and quality of life	
Axial-flow impeller pumps	Bridge to myocyte recovery. Transplantation Long-term support	Jarvik 2000 pump DeBakey pump	RVAD	Small size Low noise Absence of a compliance chamber. The device is practically encapsulated by the native myocardium, reducing the risk of infection around the device. Quality of life improved significantly	
Centrifugal continuous flow pumps	Undergoing a clinical trial as a bridge to transplantation in the US.	Ventrocor VentrAssist LVAD. Heartware HVAD. Terrumo Duraheart.		Energetically more efficient Lower tolerances so manufacturing is easier and they are less prone to thrombosis They are potential very durable (>10 year life-span) Fits in the pericardial space.	

Table 5. Long ventricle assist devices: Indications and characteristics.

8. Biventricular assist device: why and when should it be implanted?

It is well described in the literature that between 15-25% of patients with a left ventricle assist device will develop a right heart failure, even in those patients with a good preoperative right cardiac function. Severe right ventricle failure, requiring insertion of a right ventricles assist device, has been proved to negatively affect a successful bridge to transplant, increase device-related morbidity, prolong hospital length of stay, and increase total hospital cost (Slater JP et al, 1996; Karavan et al, 2002). This can be explained with the following:

1. Pre-existing right ventricle dysfunction. This dysfunction may be latent secondary to the augmented preload presented to the right side following left mechanical device implantation.
2. Interventricular septal shifting movement. The mechanical unloading of the left ventricle may displace the interventricular septum which may contribute to impaired right-sided function.
3. Other perioperative conditions as ischemia, myocardial stunning, embolism or arrythmias.

It is essential to anticipate which patients will develop right side heart failure, however, this may be a difficult task. Several papers have reported preoperative risk factors for development of right ventricle failure in patients with implantable left ventricle assist devices. A study from Ochiai and colleagues (Ochiai et al, 2002) reported in a large number of patients that preoperative circulatory support, female gender, and non-ischemic etiology of heart failure were significant predictors of right ventricle failure. Other risk factors that have been related with the need of right circulatory support are low pulmonary artery pressure, low right ventricle stroke work index, preoperative ventilation and higher left ventricle assist device scores (Fukamachi et al, 1999, Morgan et al, 2004).

Apart from the difficult task of anticipating which patient will require a right ventricle assist device, another important problem is the difficulty associated with anticipating when it is the right moment to implant a right ventricle device. It is important to note that while optimal timing of right ventricle assist device insertion for severe right ventricle failure after left ventricle assist device implantation has yet to be clearly defined, a low threshold for early right ventricle assist device insertion may be preferable to subsequent development of multisystem organ failure that could potentially develop with a more conservative approach.

Some studies describe that patients with an implantable left ventricle assist device and with a prompt right ventricle assist device insertion (within 24 hours) have a better outcome than patients in which the right mechanical device was inserted after the first 24 hours (Morgan et al, 2004). In general, it is believed that right ventricle assist device insertion should be performed early after the development of severe right ventricle failure after left ventricle assist device implantation, and that right ventricle assist device support should be continued for an adequate duration to allow for right ventricle recovery or until transplantation. It is essential that while on RVAD support, opportunities to maximally improve the patient's hemodynamic status and fluid balance, such as the use of continuous veno-venous hemofiltration and dialysis, should be pursued.

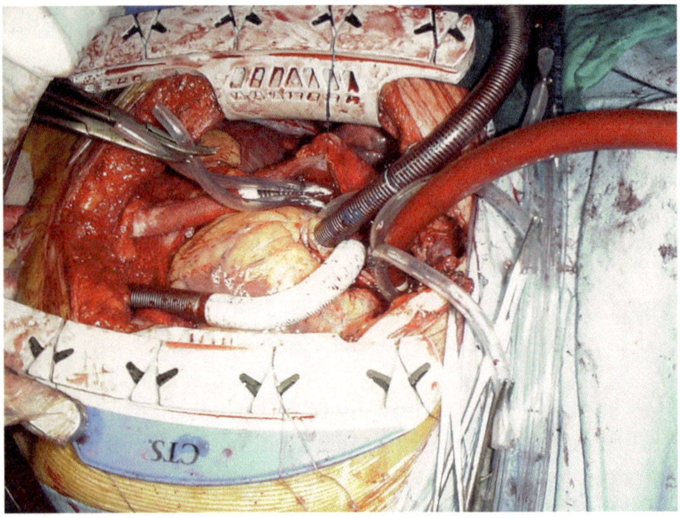

Fig. 4. Biventricular assist device. Cannula implantation.

9. Conclusions

Heart transplantation is the gold standard therapy for end stage heart failure disease. However, there is a lack of donors and some patients have some kind of contraindications.

Ventricle assist devices can be used in different clinical situations. The most common indication nowadays is bridge to transplantation. As more experience and more modern devices are available, better the outcomes. Patients being transplanted with a mechanical device can have as good results as patients without a ventricle device.

In some cases an external cardiac support is required while the heart recovers from an acute event. Ventricle assist devices can also be used as a bridge to recovery with excellent results using a short term ventricle device. In patients awaiting a transplantation or with a contraindication for transplantation a long term cardiac device or the total artificial heart are very good options in which a high quality of life can be expected.

It is important not to delay ventricle device implantation till there is a severe multi-organ dysfunction. Patients need to be in the best clinical status when receiving a mechanical cardiac support. Biventricular assist devices should be kept in mind as right ventricle failure can happen after a left ventricle device implantation.

10. Acknowledgement

Authors would like to thank Dr. Duarte, Dr. Cañizo and Dr. Nuche for their contribution and development of the ventricle cardiac devices in Spain. Also we would like to thank our National Cardiovascular Society for being interested in creating special groups focusing in cardiac mechanical devices.

11. References

Amir, O.; Aravot, D. & Pizov, R. (2007). Permanent left ventricular assist device for end-stage heart failure: first successful implantation of the axial flow HeartMate II rotary pump as destination therapy for heart failure in Israel. *Isr Med Assoc J.* 9(12), (Dec 2007) 887-8.

Barker, LE. (1991). The total artificial heart. *AACN Clin Issues Crit Care Nurs.* 2(3), (Aug 1991) 587-97.

Brinkman, WT.; Rosenthal, JE. & Eichhorn, E. (2009). Role of a percutaneous ventricular assist device in decision making for a cardiac transplant program. *Ann Thorac Surg.* 88(5), (Nov 2009) 1462-6.

Chen, EA.; Patel-Raman, SM. & O'Callaghan, K. (2009). FDA's perspectives on cardiovascular devices. *J Cardiovasc Transl Res.* 2(2), (Jun 2009)143-6. Epub 2009 Mar 10.

Chen, JM.; DeRose, JJ. & Slater, JP. (1999). Improved survival rates support left ventricular assist device implantation early after myocardial infarction. *J Am Coll Cardiol* . 33, (1999) 1903– 8.

Cleveland, JC Jr.; Grover, FL. & Fullerton. (2008). Left ventricular assist device as bridge to transplantation does not adversely affect one-year heart transplantation survival. *J Thorac Cardiovasc Surg.* 136, (2008) 774-7.

Copeland, JG.; Arabia, FA. & Tsau, PH. (2003). Total artificial hearts: bridge to transplantation. *Cardiol Clin.* 21(1), (Feb 2003) 101-13.

De Paulis, R.; Riebman, JB. & Deleuze, P. (1987). The total artificial heart: indications and preliminary results. *J Card Surg.* 2(2), (Jun 1987) 275-81.

Donald, S.; Esmore, F. & David, K. First Clinical Implant of the VentrAssist Left Ventricular Assist System as Destination Therapy for End-Stage Heart Failure. The *Journal of Heart and Lung Transplantation.* 24(8).

Douglas, L.; Mann & James, T. (1998) Left Ventricular Assist Devices and the Failing Heart : A Bridge to Recovery, a Permanent Assist Device, or a Bridge Too Far? *Circulation.* 98(1998) 2367-2369.

Esmore, DS.; Kaye, D. & Salamonsen, R. (2005). First clinical implant of the VentrAssist left ventricular assist system as destination therapy for end-stage heart failure. *J Heart Lung Transplant.* 24(8), (Aug 2005) 1150-4.

Fang, JC. (2009). Rise of the machines--left ventricular assist devices as permanent therapy for advanced heart failure. *N Engl J Med.* 3;361(23) (Decm 2009) 2282-5. Epub 2009 Nov 17.

Frazier, OH.; Rose, EA. & Oz, MC. (2001). Multicenter clinical evaluation of the HeartMate vented electric left ventricular assist system in patients awaiting heart transplantation. . *J Thorac Cardiovasc Surg.* 112, (2001) 1186-95.

Frazier, OH.; Shah, NA. & Myers, TJ. (2004). Use of the Flowmaker (Jarvik 2000) left ventricular assist device for destination therapy and bridging to transplantation. *Cardiology.* 101(1-3), (2004) 111-6.

Fukamachi, K.; McCarthy, PM. & Smedira, NG. (1999). Preoperative risk factors for right ventricular failure after implantable left ventricular assist device insertion. *Ann Thorac Surg.* 68, (1999) 2181–4.

Goldberg, RJ.; Samad, NA. & Yarzebski, J. (1999). Temporal trends in cardiogenic shock complicating acute myocardial infarction. *N Engl J Med.* 340, (1999) 1162– 8.

Gordan, S.; Cristian, R. & Nadia, G. (2009). The Impella® LP 5.0 as a bridge to long-term circulatory support. *Interact CardioVasc Thorac Surg*. 8, (2009) 682-683; originally published online Mar 2, 2009.

Grindal, JM.; Chevalier, P. & D´Attellis. (2004). Fulminant myocarditis in adults and children:bi.ventricular assist device for recovery. *Eur J cardiothorac Surg*. 26 (2004) 1169.

Hernandez, AF.; Grab, JD. & Gammie, JS. (2007). A decade of short-term outcomes in post cardiac surgery ventricular assist device implantation: data from the Society of Thoracic Surgeons' National Cardiac Database. *Circulation*. 116, (2007) 606.

Hernandez, AF.; Shea, A. & Milano, C. (2008). Long-term Outcomes and Costs of Ventricular Assist Devices Among Medicare Beneficiaries. *JAMA*, 300(20), (2008) 2398-2406.

Hill, JG.; Bruhn, PS. & Cohen, SE. (1992). Emergent applications of cardiopulmonary support: A multiinstitutional experience. *Ann Thorac Surg*. 54, (1992) 699.

Holman, WL.; Kormos, RL. & Naftel, DC. (2009). Predictors of death and transplant in patients with a mechanical circulatory support device: a multi-institutional study. *J Heart Lung Transplant*. 28(1), (Jan 2009) 44-50.

Houel, R.; Vermes, E. & Tixier, DB.(1999). Myocardial recovery after mechanical circulatory support for acute myocarditis: is sustained recivery predictable? *Ann Thorac Surg*. 68, (1999) 2177.

Hunt, SA.; Abraham, WT. & Chin, MH.;American College of Cardiology; American Heart Association Task Force on Practice Guidelines; American College of Chest Physicians; International Society for Heart and Lung Transplantation; Heart Rhythm Society. ACC/AHA 2005 Guideline Update for the Diagnosis and Management of Chronic Heart Failure in the Adult: a report of the American College of Cardiology/American Heart Association Task Force on Practice Guidelines. *Circulation*. 20;112(12), (Sept 2005) 154-235.

Hutchinson, J.; Scott, DA. & Clegg, AJ. (2008). Cost-effectiveness of left ventricular-assist devices in end-stage heart failure. *Expert Rev Cardiovasc Ther*. 6(2), (Feb 2008) 175-85.

Jonathan, EE.; Yager, MD. & Michael, FG. Left ventricular assist devices as destination therapy for end-stage heart failure. *American Heart Journal*. 148(2).

Jurmann, MJ.; Weng, Y. & Drews, T. (2004). Permanent mechanical circulatory support in patients of advanced age. *Eur J Cardiothorac Surg*. 25(4), (Apr 2004) 610-618.

Jurmann, MJ.; Siniawski, H. & Erb, M. (2004). Initial experience with miniature axial flow ventricular assist devices for postcardiotomy heart failure. *Ann Thorac Surg*. 77, (2004) 1642.

Kannel, WB. & Belanger, AJ. (1991). Epidemiology of heart failure. *Am Heart J*. 121, (1991) 951-7.

Kato, S.; Morimoto, Sm. & Hiramitsu, S. (1999). Use of percutaneous cardiopulmonary support of patients with fulminant myocarditis and cardiogenic shock for improving prognosis. *Am J Cardiol*. 83, (1999) 623.

Kavarana, MN.; Pessin-Minsley, MS. & Urtecho, J. (2002). Right ventricular dysfunction and organ failure in left ventricular assist device recipients: a continuing problem. *Ann Thorac Surg*. 73 (2002) 745–50.

Kenneth, D.; Alain CS. & Gerasimos F. (2008). ESC Guidelines for the diagnosis and treatment of acute and chronic heart failure 2008. *Eur Heart J.* 29 (2008) 2388-442

Kherani, AR.; Garrido, MJ. & Cheema, FH. (2003). Nontransplant surgical options for congestive heart failure. *Congest Heart Fail.* 9(1), (Jan-Feb 2003) 17-24.

Korfer, R.; El-Banayosy, A. & Arusoglu, L. (1999). Minami K, Breymann T, Seifert D, et al. Temporary pulsatile ventricular assist devices and biventricular assist devices. *Ann Thorac Surg.* 68, (1999) 678-83.

Leshnower, B.; Gleason, T. & O'Hara, M. (2006). Safety and Efficacy of Left Ventricular Assist Device Support in Postmyocardial Infarction Cardiogenic Shock. *Ann Thorac Surg.* 81 (2006) 1365–71.

Levy, D.; Kenchaiah, S. & Larson, MG. (2002). Long-term trends in the incidence of and survival with heart failure. *N Engl J Med.* 347 (2002) 1397–402.

Lietz, K. & Miller, LW. Will left-ventricular assist device therapy replace heart transplantation in the foreseeable future? *Current Opinion in Cardiology.* 20 (2), (March 2005) 132-137 Heart transplantation.

Macris, MP. (1995). Permanent mechanical replacement of the left ventricle. *Cardiol Clin.* 13(1), (Feb 1995) 111-20.

Mann, DL. & Willerson, JT. (1998). Left ventricular assist devices and the failing heart: a bridge to recovery, a permanent assist device, or a bridge too far? *Circulation.* 98(22), (Dec 1998) 2367-9.

Marelli, D. & Shemin, RJ. (2007). Post-cardiac surgery mechanical support: a tool for decision making. *Circulation.* 116, (2007) 586.

Martínez, MV.; Fraile, JR. & Gómez-Arnau, J. (1989). Artificial heart. Management and clinical utilization. *Rev Esp Anestesiol Reanim..* 36(4), (Jul-Aug 1989) 213-8.

Masoudi, FA.; Havranek, EP. & Krumholz, HM. (2002). The burden of chronic congestive heart failure in older persons: magnitude and implications for policy and research. *Heart Fail Rev.* 7, (2002) 9-16.

McCarthy, PM.; Schmitt, SK. & Vargo, RL. (1996). Implantable LVAD infections: implications for permanent use of the device. *Ann Thorac Surg.* 61(1), (Jan 1996) 359-65; discussion 372-3.

McCarthy, PM.; Young, JB. & Smedira, NG. (1997). Permanent mechanical circulatory support with an implantable left ventricular assist device. *Ann Thorac Surg.* 63(5), (May 1997) 1458-61.

Mehmet, C.; Oz, A. & Gelijn, C. (2003). Left Ventricular Assist Devices as Permanent Heart Failure Therapy The Price of Progress. *Annals of Surgery.* 238 (4), (2003) 577-585.

Millere, LW.; Pagani, FD. & Russell, SD. (2007). Use of a continuos –flow device in patients awaiting list transplantation. HeartMate II Clinical Investigators. *N Engl J Med.* 357, (2007) 885-96.

Morgan, J.; John, R. & Lee, B. (2004). Is severe right ventricular failure in left ventricular assist device recipients a risk factor for unsuccessful bridging to transplant and post-transplant mortality. *Ann Thorac Surg.* 77, (2004) 859-863.

Morgan, JA.; Stewart, AS. & Lee, BJ. (2004). Role of the Abiomed BVS 5000 device for short-term support and bridge to transplantation. *ASAIO J.* 50, (2004) 360-3.

Moritz, A.; Wolner, E. & Nose, Y. (1988). Clinical use of the artificial heart, indications and results. *Wien Klin Wochenschr.* 100(6), (Mar 1988) 161-7.

Navia, JL.; McCarthy, PM. & Hoercher, KJ. (2002). Do left ventricular assist device (LVAD) bridge-to-transplantation outcomes predict the results of permanent LVAD implantation? *Ann Thorac Surg.* 74(6), (Dec 2002) 2051-62.

Nicolini, F. & Gherti, T. Alternatives to transplantation in the surgical therapy for heart failure. *Eur J Cardiothorac Surg.* 35, (2009) 214-228

Ochiai, Y.; McCarthy, PM. & Smedira, NG. (2002). Predictors of severe right ventricular failure after implantable left ventricular assist device insertion: analysis of 245 patients. *Circulation.* 106(Suppl 1), (2002) I198–202.

Osaki, S.; Edwards, NM. & Johnson, MR. (2009). (2009). Improved survival after heart transplantation in patients with bridge to transplant in the recent era: a 17-year single-center experience. *J Heart Lung Transplant.* 28(6), (Jun 2009) 591-7.

Oz, MC.; Gelijns, AC. & Miller, L. (2003). Left ventricular assist devices as permanent heart failure therapy: the price of progress. *Ann Surg.* 238(4), (Oct 2003) 577-83.

Pae, WE.; Miller, CA. & Matthews, Y. (1992). Ventricular assist devices for postcardiotomy cardiogenic shock. A combined registry experience. *J Thorac Cardiovasc.* 104, (1992) 541.

Pal, JD.; Piacentino, V. & Cuevas, AD. (2009). Impact of left ventricular assist device bridging on posttransplant outcomes. *Ann Thorac Surg.* 88(5), (Nov 2009) 1457-61.

Park, SJ.; Nguyen, DQ. & Bank, AJ. (2000). Left ventricular assist device bridge therapy for acute myocardial infarction. *Ann Thorac Surg.* 69, (2000) 1146 -51.

Park, SJ.; Tector, A. & Piccioni, W. (2005). Left ventricular assist devices as destination therapy: A new look at survival. *J Thorac Cardiovasc Surg.* 129, (2005) 9-17.

Pennington, DG.; Oaks, TE. & Lohmann, DP. (1999). Permanent ventricular assist device support versus cardiac transplantation. *Ann Thorac Surg.* 68(2), (Aug 1999) 729-33.

Raman, J. & Jeevanadam, V. (2004). Destination therapy with ventricular assist devices. *Cardiology.* 101(1-3), (2004) 104-10.

Reilly, MP.; Wiegers, SE. & Cucchiara, AJ. (2000). Frequency, risk factors, and clinical outcomes of left ventricular assist device-associated ventricular thrombus. *Am J Cardiol.* 86, (2000) 1156.

Reul, H. & Akdis, M. Temporary or permanent support and replacement of cardiac function. *Expert Rev Med Devices.* 1(2), (Nov 2004) 215-27.

Reyes, G.; Fernández-Yáñez, J. & Rodríguez-Abella, H. (2007). "Asistencia ventricular mecánica como puente al trasplante" *Rev Esp Cardiol.* 60(1), (2007) 72-5.

Rose, EA.; Gelijns, AC. & Moskowitz, AJ. (2001). Randomized Evaluation of Mechanical Assistance for the Treatment of Congestive Heart Failure (REMATCH) Study Group. Long-term mechanical left ventricular assistance for end-stage heart failure. *N Engl J Med.* 345(20), (Nov 2001) 1435-43.

Russo, MJ.; Hong, KN. & Davies, RR. (2009). Posttransplant survival is not diminished in heart transplant recipients bridged with implantable left ventricular assist devices. *J Thorac Cardiovasc Surg.* 138(6), (Dec 2009) 1425-32.

Samoukovic, G.; Rosu, C. & Giannetti, N. (2009). The Impella LP 5.0 as a bridge to long-term circulatory support. *Interact Cardiovasc Thorac Surg*. 8(6), (Jun 2009) 682-3. Epub 2009 Mar 2.

Samuels, LE.; Holmes, EC. & Garwood, P. (2005). Initial experience with the Abiomed AB 5000 ventricle assist device system. *Ann Thorac Surg*. 80, (2005) 309-12

Senni, M.; Tribouilloy, CM. & Rodeheffer, RJ. (1999). Congestive heart failure in the community: trends in incidence and survival in a 10-year period. *Arch Intern Med*. 159, (1999) 29–34.

Shams, OF. & Ventura, HO. (2008). Device therapy for heart failure: when and for whom? *Am J Cardiovasc Drugs*. 8(3), (2008) 147-53.

Shawl, FA.; Domanski, MJ. & Hernandez, TJ. (1989). Emergency percutaneous cardiopulmonary bypass support in cardiogenic shock from acute myocardial infarction. *Am J Cardiol*. 64, (1989) 967.

Shumakov, V.; Zimin, N. & Kazakov, E. (1991). Clinical indications for the use of the "Poisk-IOM" total artificial heart: the experience of 13 implantations in humans. *Artif Organs*. 15(5), (Oct 1991) 372-5.

Siegenthaler, MP.; Brehm, K. & Strecker, T. (2004). The Impella Recover microaxial left ventricular assist device reduces mortality for postcardiotomy failure: A three-center experience. *J Thorac Cardiovasc Surg* 127, (2004) 812.

Slater, JP.; Rose, EA. & Levin, HR. (1996). Low thromboembolic risk without anticoagulation using advanced-design left ventricular assist devices. *Ann Thorac Surg*. 62, (1996) 1321–8

Stevenson, LW. (2004). Left Ventricular Assist Devices as Destination Therapy for End-stage Heart Failure. *Curr Treat Options Cardiovasc Med*. 6(6), (Dec 2004) 471-479.

Tang, DG.; Oyer, PE. & Mallidi, HR. Ventricular assist devices: history, patient selection, and timing of therapy. *J Cardiovasc Transl Res*. 2(2), (Jun 2009) 159-67. Epub 2009 Mar 19.

Taylor, DO.; Edwards, LB. & Aurora, P. (2008). Registry of the International Society for Heart and Lung Transplantation: twenty-fifth official adult heart transplant report—2008. *J Heart Lung Transplant*. 27, (2008) 943-56.

Teirstein, PS.; Vogel, RA. & Dorros, G. (1993). Prophylactic versus standby cardiopulmonary support for high risk percutaneous transluminal coronary angioplasty. *J Am Coll Cardiol*. 21, (1993) 590.

Thiele, H.; Lauer, B. & Hambrecht, R. (2001). Reversal of cardiogenic shock by percutaneous left atrial-to-femoral arterial bypass assistance. *Circulation*. 104, (2001) 2917.

Thiele, H.; Sick, P. & Boudriot, E. (2005). Randomized comparison of intra-aortic balloon support with a percutaneous left ventricular assist device in patients with revascularized acute myocardial infarction complicated by cardiogenic shock. *Eur Heart J*. 26, (2005) 1276.

Vogel, RA.; Shawl, FA. & Tommaso, CL. (1990). Initial report of the National Registry of Elective Cardiopulmonary Bypass Supported Coronary Angioplasty. *J Am Coll Cardiol*. 15, (1990) 23.

Weitkemper, HH.; El-Banayosy, A. & Arusoglu, L. (2004). Mechanical circulatory support: reality and dreams experience of a single center. *J Extra Corpor Technol.* 36(2), (Jun 2004) 169-73.

Wilson, SR.; Givertz, MM. & Stewart, GC. (2009). Ventricular assist devices the challenges of outpatient management. *J Am Coll Cardiol.* 54(18), (Oct 2009) 1647-59.

Part 2

Imaging and Ventricular Assist Device

2

Echocardiographic Evaluation of Ventricular Assist Devices

Dr David Platts MBBS MD FRACP FCSANZ FESC
University of Queensland
Australia

1. Introduction

Ventricular assist devices (VAD) are used to treat selected patients with severe heart failure and their role in this field is expanding. Indications for VAD insertion include bridge to transplant, bridge to decision, bridge to recovery and destination therapy. Due to their complicated mechanical structure and function and interaction with complex patients, echocardiography plays a key role in managing patients supported with a VAD. Echocardiography is integral in four areas; pre-operative assessment of potential candidates, guidance during VAD insertion, detection of complications and monitoring for cardiac recovery. Transthoracic echocardiography is the initial imaging modality used. However, trans-oesophageal echocardiography is usually required for a more detailed cardiac examination. Intracardiac echocardiography (ICE), contrast enhanced echocardiography and epicardial echocardiography may used in specific cases.

2. Pre-operative assessment

During the selection process of suitable patients for a VAD, existing cardiac anatomy and function can significantly influence the surgical approach, choice of assist device and cannula placement. Echocardiography is optimally placed to evaluate all these variables. Native valve dysfunction may be present which can significantly affect haemodynamic support. Of particular importance is aortic regurgitation (and pulmonary regurgitation if an RVAD is required). The presence of a prosthetic valve is also a key variable affecting management of these patients. Due to the high risk of prosthetic valve thrombosis following a VAD insertion, a prosthetic mechanical valve may need to be changed over to a biological valve during VAD insertion to overcome this. The presence of intracardiac thrombus affects VAD inflow cannula positioning. Patients with severe left ventricular dysfunction may have an apical LV thrombus which the implanting surgeon will need to be aware of prior to considering any apical cannula insertion. Echocardiography is also used to assess for any intracardiac shunts, such as a patent foramen ovale or an atrial or ventricular septal defect. Assessment of the ascending aorta for atherosclerotic disease is required to help guide placement of the VAD outflow cannula. Right ventricular assessment prior to LVAD insertion is of fundamental importance to help determine whether RVAD insertion is required concurrently with an LVAD.

Ventricular Function

Echocardiography is the investigation of choice to assess right and left ventricular function prior to VAD insertion. The left ventricular ejection fraction (LVEF) is usually significantly reduced prior to LVAD insertion. Severe reduction is classified as a LVEF of less than 25%. This is typically assessed with transthoracic echocardiography, with Simpson's biplane method a common technique utilised to calculate the LVEF (1). In those patients with sub-optimal TTE images, which can account for up to 25% of patients in the critical care complex (2-5), contrast enhanced TTE can be utilised to improve calculation of the LVEF (6-9). Additionally, these patients usually undergo trans-oesophageal echocardiography, enabling improved visualisation of the endocardial border, to assess the LVEF. Coincident with LV systolic dysfunction, is the presence of diastolic dysfunction. There are numerous parameters used in echocardiography to evaluate for this. Routine measures include mitral valve inflow pulse wave Doppler, pulmonary vein flow Doppler, and mitral annular tissue Doppler velocities (usually septal and lateral annular velocities) (10). Whilst these measures may not directly influence VAD insertion, they do provide robust data on the severity of ventricular dysfunction and help predict prognosis (11).

Once left ventricular systolic function has been assessed, echocardiography is then used to determine left ventricular morphology and to evaluate for the presence of any ventricular thrombus. These points are pertinent because if a ventricular cannula is being considered, a ventriculotomy will be required and this often occurs in the region where there may be abnormal ventricular morphology or a ventricular apical thrombus. LV apical thrombi may be difficult to detect, especially if they are small or laminar. Due to imaging orientation and scan planes, transoesophageal echocardiography may not detect LV apical thrombi and transthoracic echocardiography can have a higher diagnostic yield. However, this can be related to image quality and contrast enhancement may be required to further assess for apical thrombi (12-16). Additionally, apical trabeculation (often seen in dilated cardiomyopathy) is a common mimicker of LV apical thrombi. These can be distinguished from one another using contrast enhanced TTE. However, delayed enhancement cardiac MRI is considered as the "gold standard" for detection of LV apical thrombi, particularly if they are small and laminar (17, 18).

Assessment of right ventricular function peri-operatively is of key importance when deciding on mechanical support. Adequate right ventricular function is not only required for adequate filling and function of an LVAD but RV dysfunction may occur following implantation of an LVAD. Up to one third of patients that have an LVAD may also require an RVAD (19-21). However, the incidence of RV dysfunction following LVAD insertion may be lower in the newer continuous flow pumps as compared to pulsatile pumps (22). The interaction between an LVAD and native right ventricle is complex. The insertion of an LVAD may result in improvement of RV systolic function or it may result in reduction in RV systolic function. It is difficult to predict prior to insertion how an LVAD will influence RV systolic function and this is an area requiring further research. Echocardiographic parameters that have been used to help predict RV dysfunction following LVAD insertion include right ventricular dilatation, right ventricular fractional area change of less than 20% and evidence of poor right ventricular performance, measured by right ventricular stoke work index and ability to generate an adequate right ventricular systolic pressure. Additionally, newer parameters such as echocardiographic derived pulmonary vascular resistance (PVR) may be of benefit in assessing the right ventricle and pulmonary haemodynamics following LVAD insertion (23).

Cardiac Shunts

Assessment for cardiac shunting prior to VAD insertion is performed to evaluate the risk of significant right to left shunting and to determine the risk of paradoxical embolisation. These shunts may be at two levels, atrial or ventricular. A ventricular shunt occurs if there is a ventricular septal defect and these may occur following an acute myocardial infarction. It is important to detect these prior to VAD insertion, as they would require closure (usually with a pericardial patch) at the time of VAD insertion. A more frequent cardiac shunt is at the atrial level, due to either a patent foramen ovale (PFO) or atrial septal defect (ASD). Both these defects have the risk of intracardiac shunting which may cause hypoxia or paradoxical emboli. A PFO or ASD can usually be accurately detected and assessed using transoesophageal echocardiography, with direct visualisation of the defect on 2D imaging and detection of flow direction using colour Doppler imaging. However, an atrial shunt is a function of the pressure differential between the right and left atria and this can be a dynamic parameter. A PFO with right to left shunting may not become apparent until after LVAD insertion, which may reduce left heart pressures and hence promote right to left shunting, particularly in the setting of pulmonary hypertension, which is relatively common in this group of patients (24, 25).

Assessment of the Ascending Aorta

The outflow cannula of an LVAD device is usually attached to the ascending aorta in as end to side anastomosis. As such, any pathology that may be present within the ascending aorta needs to evaluated using transoesophageal echocardiography. The two main abnormalities that impact on LVAD insertion are aneurysmal dilatation of the ascending aorta and atherosclerotic disease. If there is significant dilatation of the ascending aorta (>45 mm) detected at the time of LVAD insertion, the ascending aorta is usually replaced with a Dacron graft and the LVAD cannula attached in an end to side manner to the graft. Transoesophageal echocardiography is well placed to assess for atherosclerotic disease in the ascending aorta (26). The images acquired help determine optimal siting of the outflow cannula anastomosis to the aorta. Epi-aortic echocardiography, using high frequency transducers, provide aortic images with very high spatial resolution, that can help locate and grade the severity of aortic atherosclerotic disease (27).

Assessment of Native Cardiac Valves

Echocardiography is fundamental in the assessment of native valvular structure and function prior to insertion of a VAD. Dysfunction of all four cardiac valves can have an impact of management of patients at the time of VAD insertion.

Mitral regurgitation is commonly associated with end stage heart failure. The mechanism for this is often multi-factorial, with annular dilatation and leaflet restriction due to dilation and impairment (remodelling) of the left ventricle common mediators of this valve disorder. With adequate unloading of the ventricle post LVAD insertion, there is often improvement in the degree of mitral regurgitation. Typically no specific intervention is required for mitral regurgitation at the time of VAD insertion. However, some authors recommend a modified mitral valve repair at the time of LVAD insertion (28). The rationale for this is that with pulsatile LVADs, as VAD flow is asynchronous to ventricular contraction, some VAD output may flow retrograde across an open mitral valve, resulting in pulmonary venous congestion. The presence of haemodynamically significant mitral stenosis at the time of LVAD insertion usually results in surgical correction at the same time, via either a commisurotomy of mitral valve replacement, using a tissue mitral valve (28).

Pulmonary valve disorders may also impact patient management at the time of VAD insertion, although haemodynamically significant pulmonary valve dysfunction is rare. However competence of the pulmonary valve is of key importance if an RVAD is being inserted with an end to side anastomosis onto the pulmonary artery. Haemodynamically significant pulmonary stenosis would also require surgical intervention or a valvuloplasty at the time of VAD insertion.

Aortic valvular dysfunction is clinically important in the setting of VAD insertion. Uncorrected aortic regurgitation has a negative impact on forward flow provided by an LVAD due to regurgitation of VAD flow back into the left ventricular cavity. This then results in a short length loop circuit. It is generally recommended that moderate and greater levels of severity of aortic regurgitation should be corrected at the time of VAD insertion (29). However, questions still remain as to which intervention is most appropriate. This choice in part depends upon whether recovery is expected or not and whether a continuous or pulsatile device is being considered. Options include over-sewing the valve, repairing the valve and replacing the valve (28, 29). Aortic stenosis is usually not of such clinical significance compared to aortic regurgitation. However in continuous flow devices, depending upon the configuration, aortic stenosis may limit forward flow and may need surgical replacement at the time of VAD insertion (19).

Tricuspid regurgitation is a relatively common condition in patients being assessed for mechanical support. This is typically due to right heart failure secondary to chronic elevation of the pulmonary pressures due to left heart failure. There are numerous complex factors that can influence the degree of tricuspid regurgitation post LVAD insertion. The decision to correct tricuspid regurgitation at the time of VAD insertion is a complex one. If significant tricuspid regurgitation is present and it is expected that improvement (via annuloplasty or repair but not replacement due to the risk of valve thrombosis) of this would result in improved RV function, then intervention on the tricuspid valve may be warranted (19, 28).

<u>Assessment of Prosthetic Cardiac Valves</u>

Patients with prosthetic valves in situ who are being considered for VAD represent a complex group in terms of their management. The key issue here is the risk of prosthetic valve thrombosis (with resultant embolisation) due to low flow states across the valve in the setting of a mechanically supported circulation. This may occur with both biological and mechanical valves, though the risk is likely to be higher with mechanical valves. If a mechanical valve is in situ at the time of VAD insertion, one approach is to remove the mechanical valve and insert a biological one instead. Another approach is to over-sew the valve completely with a Dacron patch (if it is in the aortic position). Current practice varies between institutions and there is a paucity of data to guide the clinician as to the optimal approach in this situation (28, 30, 31).

3. Guidance during VAD insertion

Echocardiography is fundamental to accurate insertion of a VAD. Intra-operative transoesophageal echocardiography is routinely performed to guide the surgical team in numerous aspects to this procedure. The key components in this evaluation are assessment of satisfactory cannulae anatomic positioning within the cardiac chambers, determination of adequate flows within the cannulae using Doppler imaging, obtaining adequate chamber decompression and excluding the presence of air within the circuit.

Cannulae that drain blood out of the heart and into the VAD can be defined as inflow cannulae (to the VAD) or access cannulae. They can be located either within the atrium or within the left ventricle. There are several anatomic and physiological parameters that will decide on atrial or ventricular cannulation. For example, the presence of a large region apical infarction would preclude satisfactory apical cannulation and a left atrial cannula would be inserted. Intra-operative transoesophageal echocardiography is used to help guide and optimise atrial and ventricular cannulation. Regardless of the location, it has to be ensured that unobstructed blood flow can be achieved into these cannulae. If placed in the left ventricle, imaging is required to ensure that the mitral valvular or sub-valvular apparatus does not interfere with adequate cannulae flow. Additionally, transoesophageal echocardiography is used to exclude the cannulae being placed into the left ventricular outflow tract, left atrium or directly against a left ventricular wall which my interfere with cannulae flow. The advent of real time three dimensional echocardiography can help in the rapid, multi-planar spatial assessment/orientation of the VAD cannulae in relation to the left ventricular structures (32). Figure 1 demonstrates 2D, simultaneous biplane and 3D transoesophageal echocardiographic images of a left ventricular cannula. If placed within the left atrium, echocardiography is also used to optimise cannulae positioning. It assists the implanting surgeon by providing real time feedback as to location in relation to surrounding structures such as the mitral valve, pulmonary veins and inter-atrial septum. If inserted into the right atrium, it provides information as to cannulae positioning in relation to the inferior vena cave, superior vena cave, tricuspid valve and the inter-atrial septum. As with ventricular insertion, optimal atrial cannulae positioning is one where it is anatomically removed from surrounding structures and where there is satisfactory flows into the cannula.

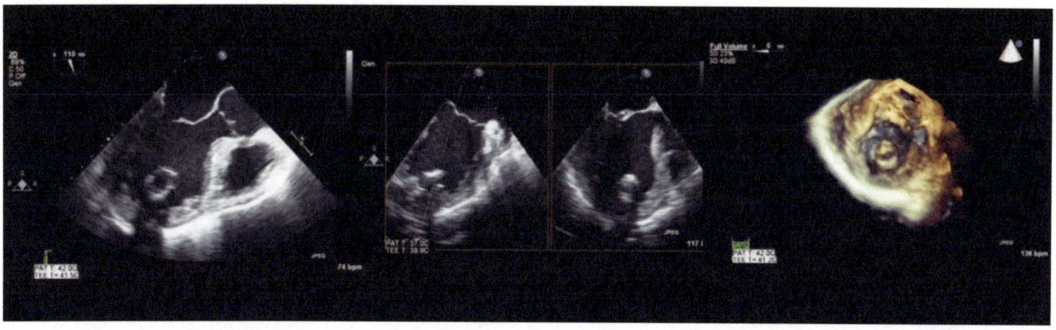

Fig. 1. 2D, simultaneous biplane and 3D transoesophageal echocardiographic images of a left ventricular cannula.

Cannulae that return blood to the native circulation and flow away from the VAD can be defined as outflow (out from the VAD) or return cannulae. These cannulae are usually fashioned as an end to side anastomosis to either the ascending aorta or pulmonary artery. Conventional transoesophageal echocardiographic views are used to image the ascending aorta (for LVAD outflow) and main pulmonary artery (for RVAD outflow).
Following assessment of satisfactory cannulae anatomic positioning, Doppler imaging (both colour Doppler and spectral Doppler) is used to determine adequate flows into and out of the cannulae. Colour Doppler imaging can assess for satisfactory flow into and out of a cannula, as well as determine whether any part of the cannula is obstructed. Cannulae usually have a large end orifice and multiple side holes. Colour Doppler helps to assess

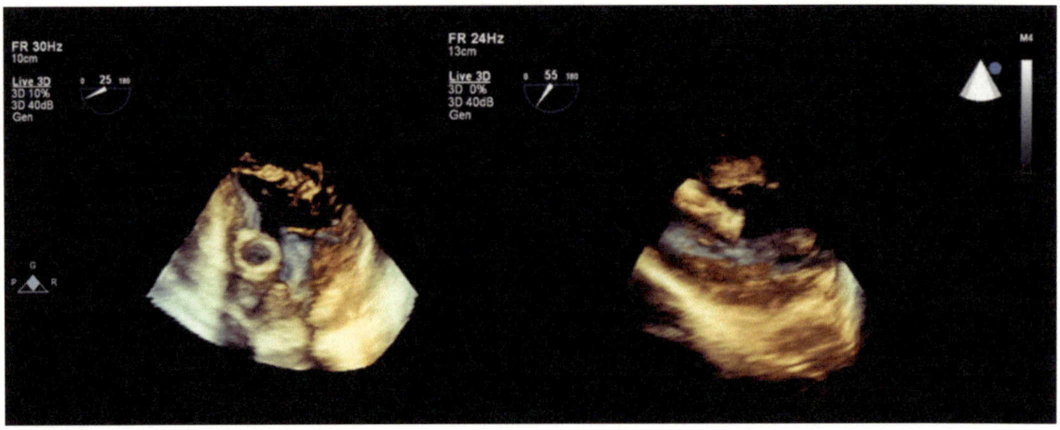

Fig. 2. Live 3D transoesophageal echocardiographic images of a left ventricular VAD cannula

flow into these parts of the cannula. Continuous wave Doppler can then be used if the ultrasound bean can be aligned with the flow. The type of signal obtained (both for colour and spectral Doppler) is dependent upon which type of VAD device is inserted. A pulsatile device will result in an intermittent flow profile (usually asynchronous with the ECG rhythm) whilst a continuous flow pump will provide a lower velocity continuous signal. However, there may be a degree of pulsatility to the continuous flow outflow signal due to variation in filling if there is native heart contraction as well. There is a paucity of data that has been published regarding normal reference ranges for VAD cannulae Doppler flow assessment. Obtaining baseline haemodynamic data can help in the serial evaluation of cannulae flow. The actual velocities obtained can vary depending upon the cannulae diameter, preload, afterload and contribution of native cardiac function. Inflow velocities into a VAD cannula are usually below around 2 metres/second (33). Velocities above this usually indicate pathology within or around the inflow cannula, such as partial obstruction with a thrombus or impingement from a surrounding structure such as a papillary muscle or atrial wall.

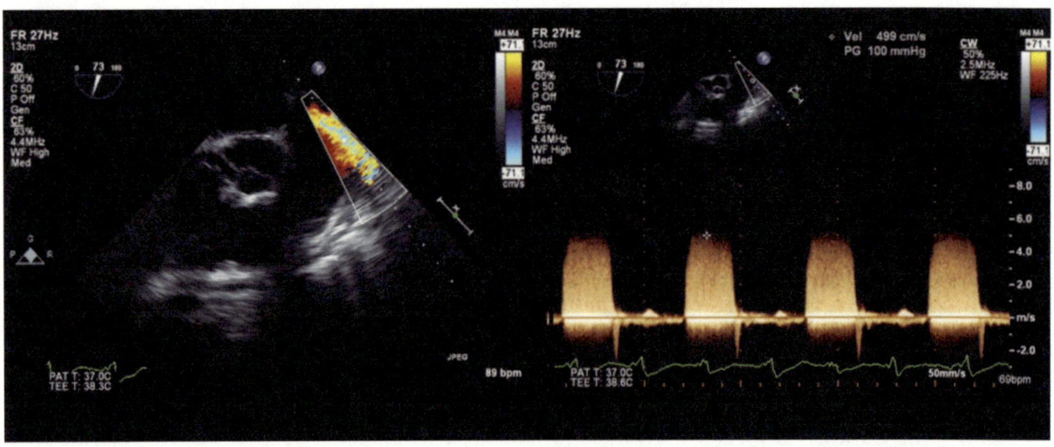

Fig. 3. Colour Doppler (left) and continuous wave Doppler (right) imaging of an RVAD outflow anastomosis onto the main pulmonary artery

Doppler imaging of the outflow cannulae is also important. It enables assessment of satisfactory flow out of the VAD. Due to the higher velocities present, continuous wave spectral Doppler is often needed to interrogate these flows. Again the normal velocities can vary depending upon the type of pump used and the loading conditions. Outflow from a continuous flow device has a continuous flow pattern with a flow velocity of usually less than 2 metres/second (34). Outflows from a pulsatile pump can be higher, with velocities up to 4 metres/second for an Abiomed AB5000 being normal (35). However, outflow velocities of 2 metres/second are normal for the Heartmate VE or Heartmate XVE. The outflow velocities were lower in those patients who had inflow valve regurgitation (36). Higher flows than this usually indicate obstruction within the outflow cannula, usually by a thrombus. Additionally, external compression or kinking of the cannula can also cause an increased velocity detected on spectral Doppler imaging. This may occasionally be detected with transoesophageal echocardiography by careful and thorough evaluation of the cannulae as they course through the mediastinum.

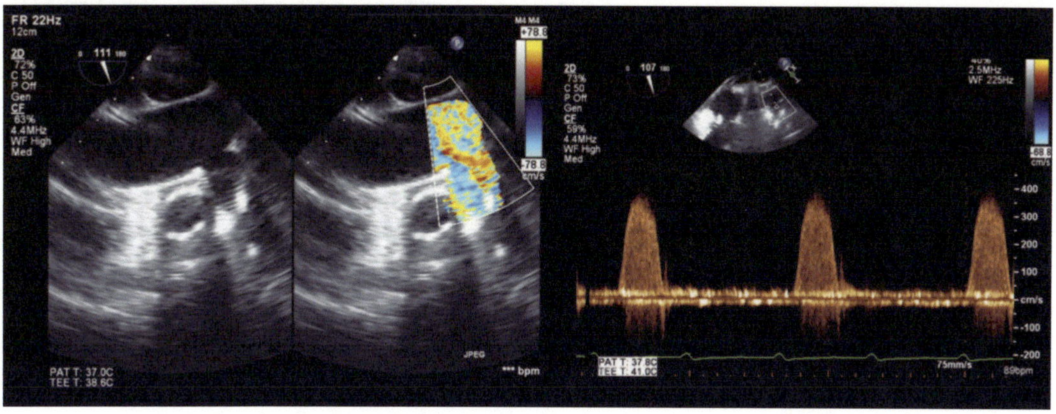

Fig. 4. Simultaneous biplane transoesophageal echocardiogram with colour Doppler (left) and spectral Doppler (right) image of an LVAD outflow anastomosis onto the ascending aorta.

During insertion and initiation of VAD support, de-airing of the circuit is of crucial importance. Air can enter the circulation and circuit form numerous sources, including inadequate priming of the pump and lines, from the bypass pump or from entrainment around the cannulae insertion. Systemic air embolisation from any of these sources can result in significant morbidity or mortality. Echocardiography is usually able to detect the presence of air within the circulation. This can be manifest as either a small amount of bubbles or in the worse case, an air lock within the heart or circuit. A large collection of air has the appearance of a localised echo-intense region (32).

4. Detection of complications

VAD complications have a significant impact on both the morbidity and mortality of these complex patients. Echocardiography plays a fundamental role in determining the presence of these complications. Bleeding (cardiac tamponade), thrombus formation (both intra-cardiac and intra-device/cannulae), infection (cannulae endocarditis), aortic dissection and air entrainment/embolisation are significant complications that can be detected using

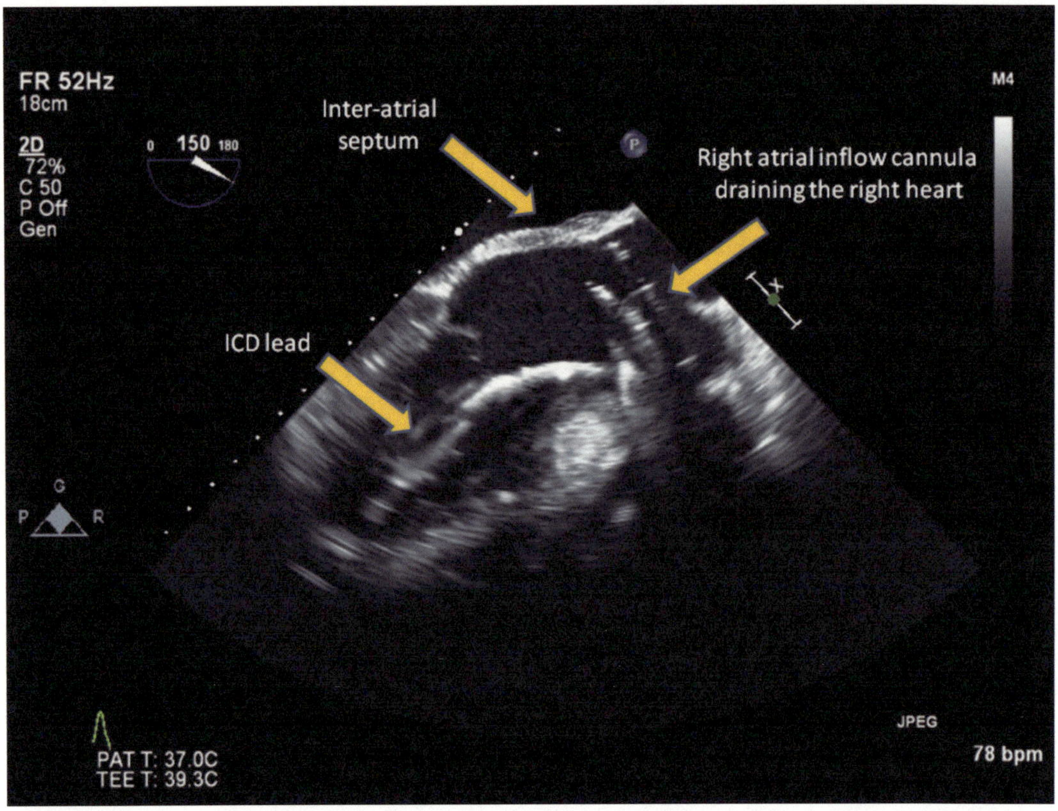

Fig. 5. Right atrial cannula draining the right heart

echocardiography. Sub-optimal VAD function can also be determined with echocardiography by determining volume status and cannula obstruction due to "suck-down" or opposition of the cannulae against other cardiac structures.

Post operative bleeding is very common in these patients, particularly in the early post operative period (first 24-48 hours). So much so that systemic anti-coagulation is usually withheld in this early period. However, significant bleeding may also occur at a later stage (37, 38). Factors which promote bleeding include recent cardiopulmonary bypass, critical illness, thrombocytopenia (both from consumption and heparin induced thrombocytopenia) and transfusion associated coagulopathy. However, the incidence of bleeding can vary and may relate to the type of device being inserted, level of illness prior to insertion, surgical experience and peri-operative management. In the REMATCH trial, which studied a pulsatile device, the frequency of bleeding was quoted at 42% at 6 months (39). In a recently published trial, compared pulsatile versus continuous flow VADs (40), bleeding requiring surgery occurred in 30% with continuous flow pumps and 15% with pulsatile pumps (p=ns). Bleeding requiring transfusion occurred in 81% with a continuous flow VAD and in 76% with a pulsatile VAD (p=0.06).

Bleeding can cause cardiac tamponade which will result in haemodynamic instability. In VAD supported patients, tamponade is often difficult to diagnose with TTE and a transesophageal echocardiogram is usually required to confirm diagnosis. Even with a TOE,

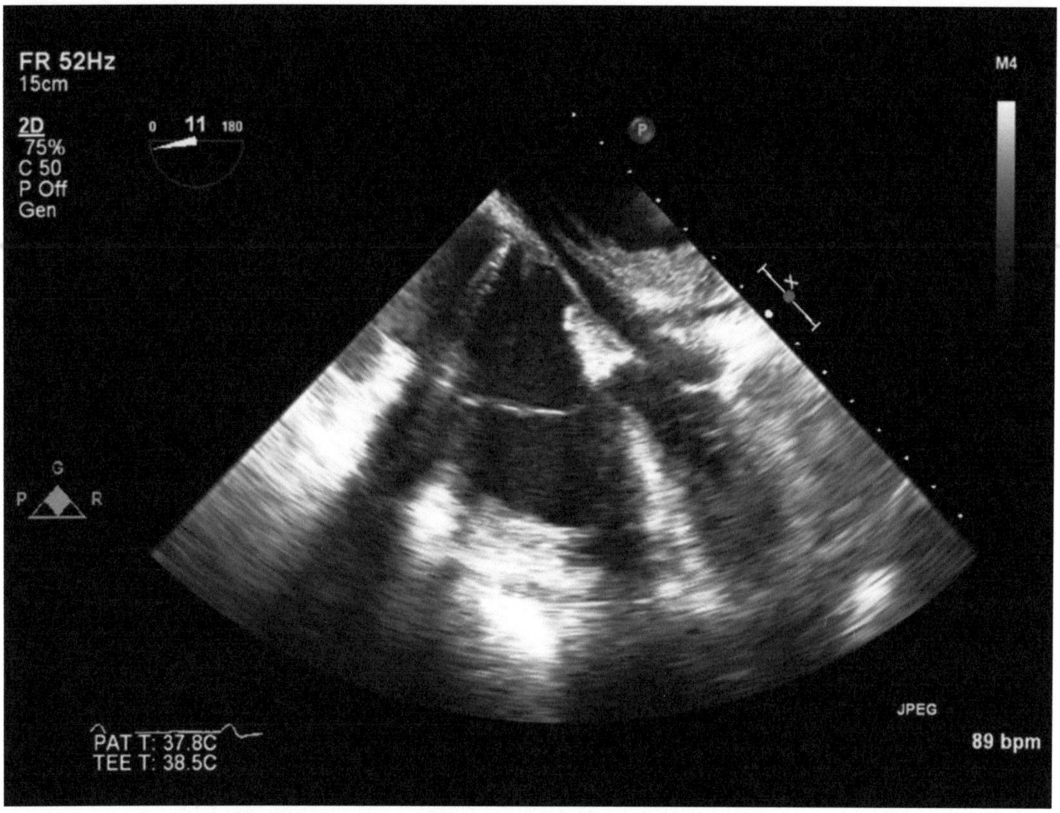

Fig. 6. Left heart compression from a large pericardial haematoma

a pericardial collection may be difficult to assess, especially if it is localised. Additionally, small volume collections can have significant consequences if they are in a critical location, such as around the atria which may limit flow into a VAD cannula. Classic echocardiographic features of tamponade may be absent in patients supported by a VAD. Clues to tamponade include haemodynamic instability (especially early post operatively) with chamber compression or compression limiting flow around a cannula. Diffuse bleeding may result in a generalised mediastinal haematoma which can also result in significant cardiac compression. Due to the these often being more anterior in location, these can be difficult to diagnose on transoesophageal echocardiography and a TTE may be helpful in this circumstance.

VAD associated thrombosis is another serious complication with significant morbidity and mortality. Thrombus formation may occur within the cardiac chambers themselves, within the cannulae or actually within the pump chamber. As for bleeding, the incidence of thrombus formation can vary. In patients with a left atrial cannula, left ventricular thrombus is more likely to occur due to a relative 'bypassing " of the left ventricle in the circuit (41). Bleeding has also been found to be a predictor of thrombus formation (41). Transoesophageal echocardiography usually enables detection of cardiac chamber thrombus formation. It can also detect thrombus around the tips or just within the cannulae. Echocardiography does not directly visualise intra-cannulae or intra-device thrombus formation, but will provide information to help diagnose this condition. Figure 8 shows a

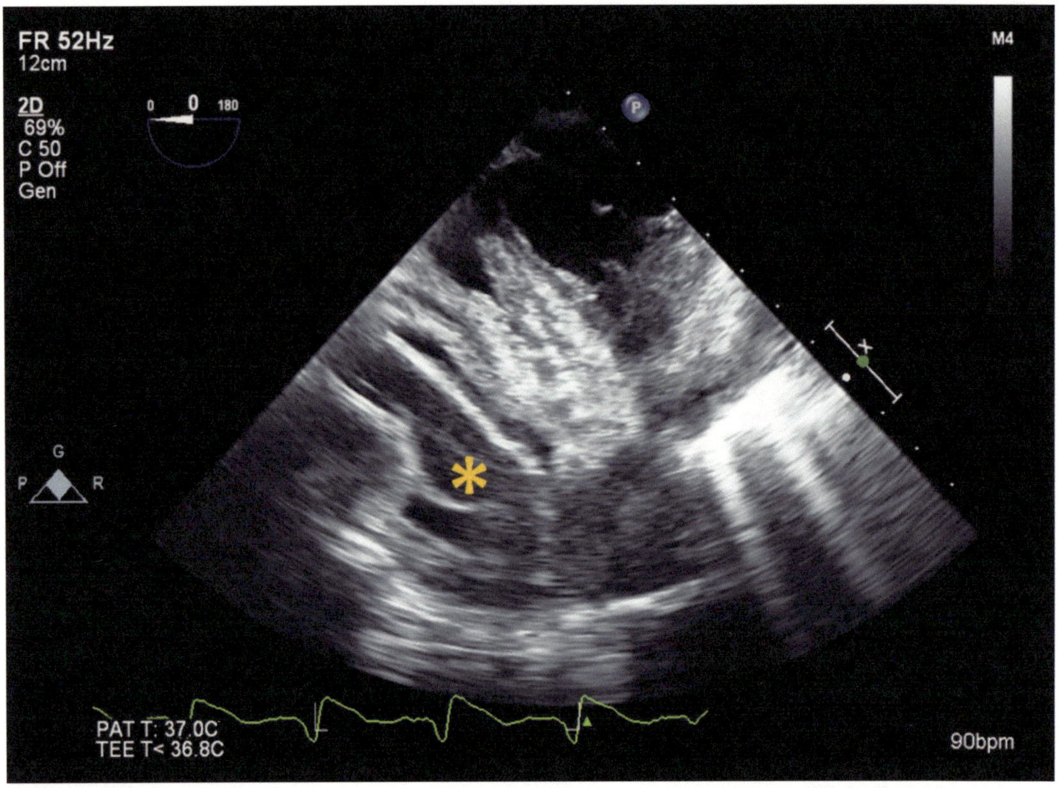

Fig. 7. Right heart compression from a large anterior mediastinal haematoma (marked with a *)

thrombus found within a VAD cannulae following an alarm for low VAD flows. Figure 9 shows a 3D TOE of an apical LV thrombus prior to LVAD insertion. However, intracavity thrombi may be hard to detect with echocardiography, particularly laminar thrombi at the apex of the left ventricle or smaller thrombi around the cardiac insertion points of a cannula. Mobility of a thrombus increases the likelihood of detection using echocardiography when the thrombus is small. Compounding this limitation is the fact that a thrombus does not have to be particularly large to have a significant impact following systemic embolisation. Contrast enhance echocardiography has a role in improving the diagnostic yield of intra-ventricular thrombus detection.

Patients supported by a VAD are at increased risk of infection, including infective endocarditis. The presence of extensive prosthetic material within the mediastinum and heart, along with external drive lines and associated medical issues put these patients at risk of endocarditis. VAD associated infection results in significant morbidity and mortality and poses complex questions regarding appropriate management (42). Due to its greater spatial resolution, transoesophageal echocardiography is usually required to investigate these patients. There are several sites where infection may be present in a patient supported on a VAD (43). Infective material may be visualised around the tip of a cannula, on the native cardiac valves, around the insertion point of the cannulae or focal infective collections around the heart or within the mediastinum. Patients with VADs may also get infections around the drivelines, within the pump pocket or inside the actual pump chamber (44).

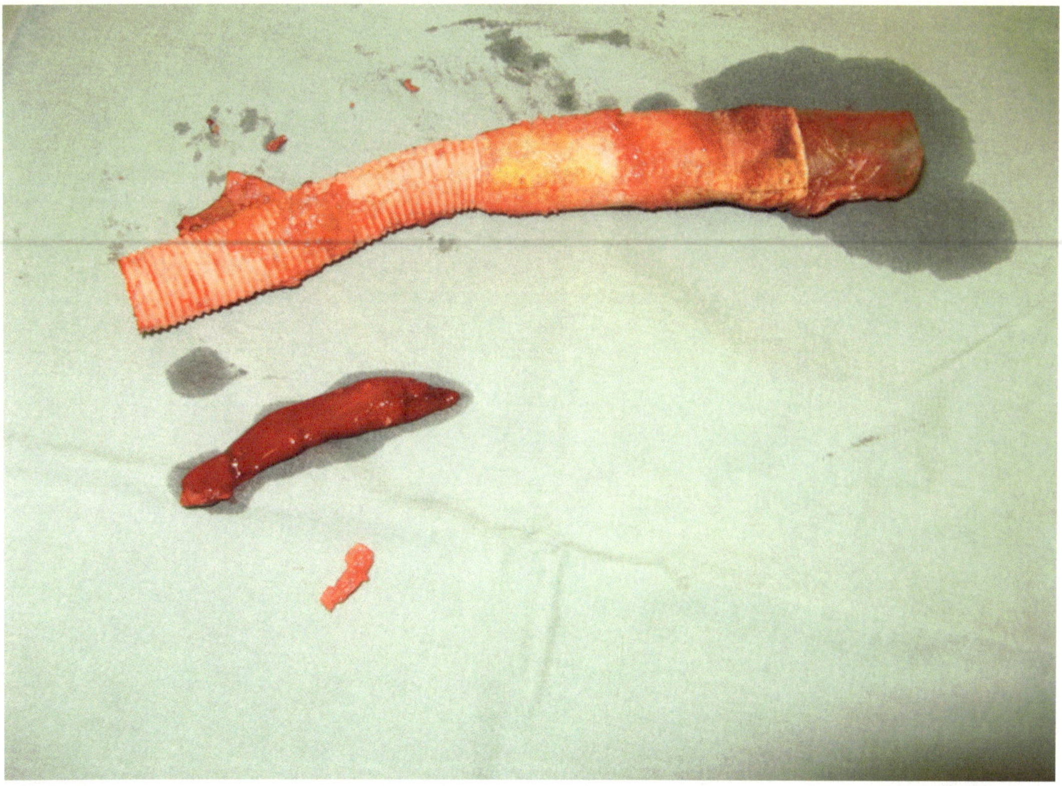

Fig. 8. Thrombus found within a VAD cannulae following an alarm for low VAD flows

The presence of air within a VAD circuit can have significant adverse consequences. Air bubbles can usually be clearly visualised within the circulation using echocardiography. Exclusion of air from the circulation and VAD circuit is an important process during VAD insertion. This is important during VAD cannula anastomosis and removal from cardiopulmonary bypass. Close attention needs to be paid to anstomotic sites for the entry of air. Visualisation of outflow cannula will aid in the detection of any air that has entered the VAD circuit. A confluence of bubbles within a cardiac chamber has the echocardiographic appearance of an echo-dense region, which may initially cause diagnostic confusion unless the operator is aware of this complication and its appearance.

Air embolism is a known risk with VAD use, due to potential anatomic (connection of the circulation to the atmosphere via VAD cannulae or occasionally an open chest) and mechanical (device malfunction) entry points for air entry. However, it is a very rare complication, with only three case reports in the literature of air embolism associated with LVAD use, due to either device malfunction (45), entry of air into the systemic circulation during a pump exchange (46) or systemic air embolization through the left atrial wall cannula site, from an intermittent pleural air leak (47). Figure 10 demonstrates air in the left atrium and left ventricle, after entering around the LA cannula cuff.

Aortic dissection is a recognised but rare complication of VAD insertion (48-50). It usually arises due to the associated shear forces imparted on the ascending aortic wall from a high velocity jet being ejected from an LVAD outflow cannula. Transoesophageal echocardiography is the imaging modality of choice to detect a dissection flap in the

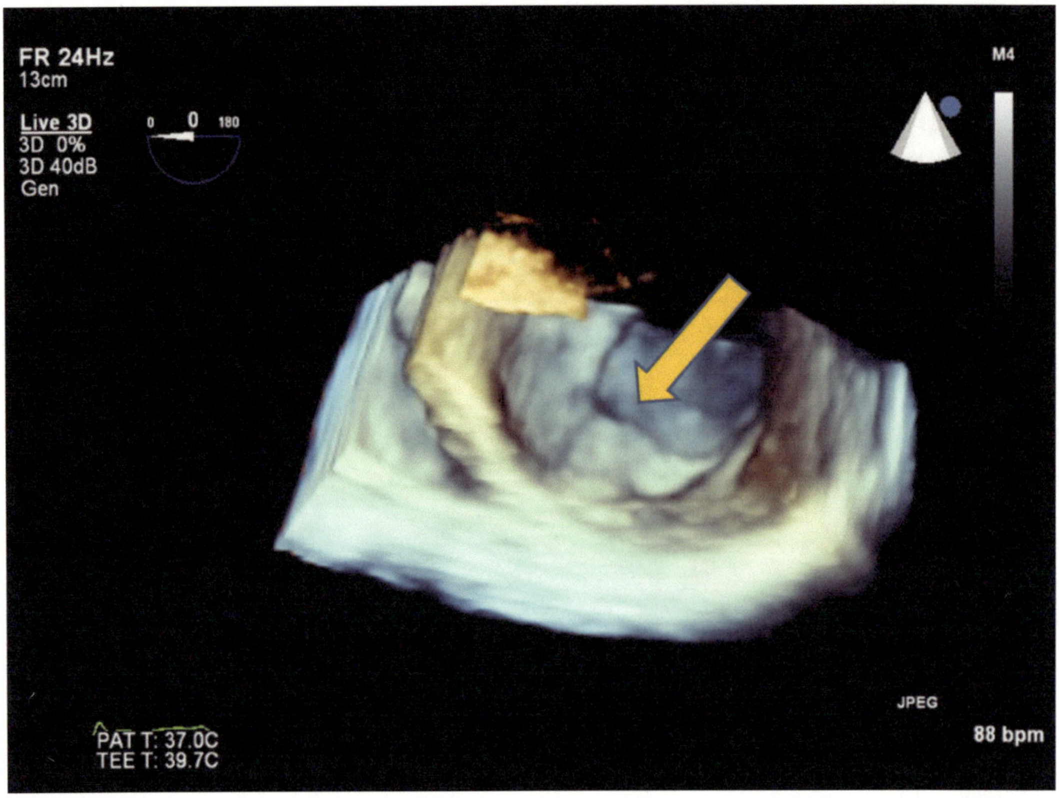

Fig. 9. Real time 3D transoesophageal echocardiogram of a left ventricular apical thrombus (arrow)

ascending aorta in this group of patients. It enables the visualisation of the typical features of aortic dissection, including an intimal flap or tear, identification of the true and false lumen and associated complications.

VAD Weaning and Explantation

VAD explantation may occur following satisfactory recovery of native cardiac function or if cardiac transplantation occurs. Echocardiography is fundamental in the assessment of native cardiac function when determining if there has been any recovery and can the VAD be explanted. However, the decision making process is a complex one and does not get rely on one set of parameters. There is not a consensus as to the best way to assess cardiac recovery during weaning and it is likely multiple parameters from multiple investigative procedures are likely to be required to assess for recovery. There is even less work evaluating weaning of an RVAD and assessing right ventricular recovery following RVAD support.

Multiple clinical, haemodynamic and echocardiographic variables are analysed in an attempt to determine whether recovery has occurred. The likelihood and degree of recovery can also be related to the aetiology and chronicity of the underlying disease process. Due to the left ventricle being in an unloaded state when supported by a VAD, it is usually not possible to accurately assess underlying function unless a challenge/wean of VAD support tis attempted. Numerous protocols are in place during echocardiographic assessment during VAD weaning and these tend to vary between institutions (51-60).

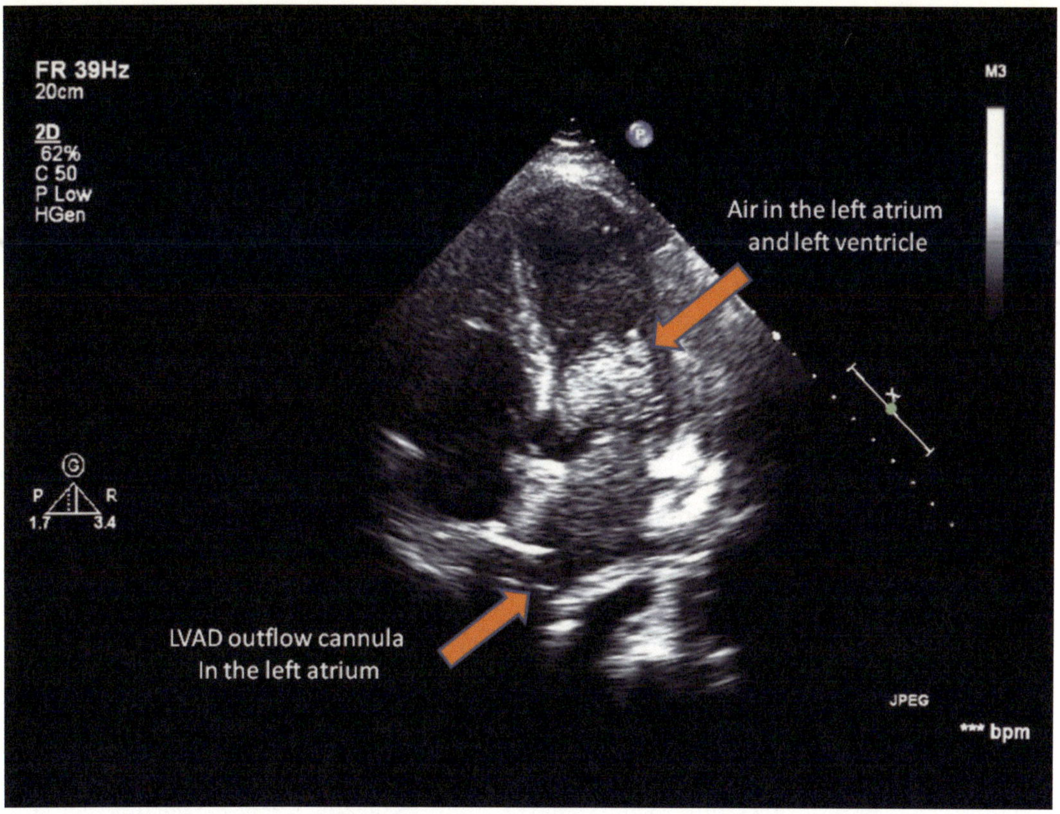

Fig. 10. Air bubbles in the left atrium and left ventricle, after entering around the LA cannula cuff, originating from a pleural tear.

During attempted weaning from a VAD, echocardiographic parameters that can be evaluated to help predict recovery include left ventricular systolic function and ejection fraction, left ventricular end diastolic dimension, left ventricular stoke volume, left ventricular fractional area change, degree of mitral regurgitation and right ventricular size and systolic function. Additionally, dynamic manoeuvres may be applied to elucidate recovery. Kahn et al evaluated the role of using dobutamine stress echocardiography to assess for recovery (56). In this study, 19 patients on VAD support had a dobutamine stress echocardiogram (with a dose increasing from 5 to 40 mcg/kg/min). Echocardiographic parameters assessed included left ventricular end diastolic dimension, left ventricular ejection fraction, along with other invasively derived haemodynamic parameters. Patients had a favourable response to dobutamine stress if the LVEF increased and the LVEDD decreased. 9 patients had a favourable response and underwent explantation with 6 surviving beyond 12 months. Of the 7 unfavourable responders, 2 died and 5 required cardiac transplantation.

Further research is required to ascertain which echocardiographic variables and weaning protocols should be used to determine myocardial recovery during VAD weaning. Additionally, these echocardiographic variables need to be integrated with other clinical and haemodynamic parameters to arrive at a clinically useful paradigm in assessing VAD weaning and cardiac recovery.

Echocardiography and Extra-Corporeal Membranous Oxygenation

Extra-Corporeal Membranous Oxygenation (ECMO) is an increasingly utilised form of short term cardiopulmonary support for either severe pulmonary or cardiac failure. There are two types of ECMO support: VV ECMO - veno-venous for isolated respiratory support and VA ECMO - veno-arterial for haemodynamic support (61). There are also two types of ECMO cannulation, peripheral cannulation and central/surgical cannulation. First successful use of ECMO was in 1971 and it has been more widely available since the 1990s. However, improvements in device design, cannulae, oxygenators and medical management has extended duration of ECMO support from days to several weeks.

VV ECMO is used for respiratory failure. Blood is drained from the venous system, oxygenated and then returned to the venous system. Cannulae are typically placed in the venae cavae and right atrium. They are usually introduced percutaneously via the femoral &/or jugular veins. VV ECMO relies on adequate native cardiac output to maintain circulation. VV ECMO is used for severe acute respiratory failure where typical support measures have been inadequate & adequate cardiac function is anticipated for the duration of therapy. VA ECMO is used to support cardio±respiratory failure (CO up to 5.0L/min) Blood is drained from the venous system, oxygenated and returned to the arterial system. As such, it can provide complete or partial haemodynamic support as well as maintaining oxygenation. Support with VA ECMO can be provided by either central or peripheral cannulation. VA ECMO is indicated for potentially reversible, life-threatening forms of cardiac failure which are unresponsive to conventional therapy and use of a VAD is deemed inappropriate.

Due to the patient population and nature of the therapy, ECMO does have significant complications. However, with increasing experience and technological advances, along with formation of specialist ECMO centres, these are likely to become less common. Common complications include bleeding/coagulopathy, limb ischaemia, sepsis, haemolysis and mechanical failure (oxygenator or cannula/device thrombosis). Echo has a fundamental role in managing patients supported with ECMO. It provides information that determines appropriate patient selection, guides insertion of cannulae, monitors progress, detects complications and helps in determining recovery/weaning of support. Insertion and commencement of ECMO is done with transoesophageal echocardiographic guidance. TOE is indicated at ECMO insertion to exclude new reversible pathology such as pericardial effusion, exclude aortic valve and aortic pathology, help position the cannulae, ensure the heart is adequately decompressed and ensure there is no intra-cardiac thrombus or stasis. Figure 11 demonstrates a 3D transoesophageal colour Doppler image of oxygenated blood being returned to the right atrium. Note also the flow out of the sides holes of the return cannula.

The ICU setting frequently limits satisfactory transthoracic imaging and contrast echocardiography has been shown to improve image quality. However, there is little published work on the role of echocardiographic contrast agent use in those patients supported with non pulsatile ventricular assist devices or ECMO(62) . In patients supported by an ECMO circuit who have non diagnostic transthoracic echocardiographic images, the addition of a microsphere contrast agent can result in obtaining diagnostic images, despite passage of the agent through a mechanical circuit. Figure 12 demonstrate pre and post TTE contrast enhanced images of a ventilated patient in ICU on VA ECMO. The recently published CESAR trial (63) may result in an increased number of patients in ICU supported by ECMO, where contrast enhancement may need to be considered. As such, this technique could be utilized to assess these patients prior to proceeding to more invasive diagnostic strategies.

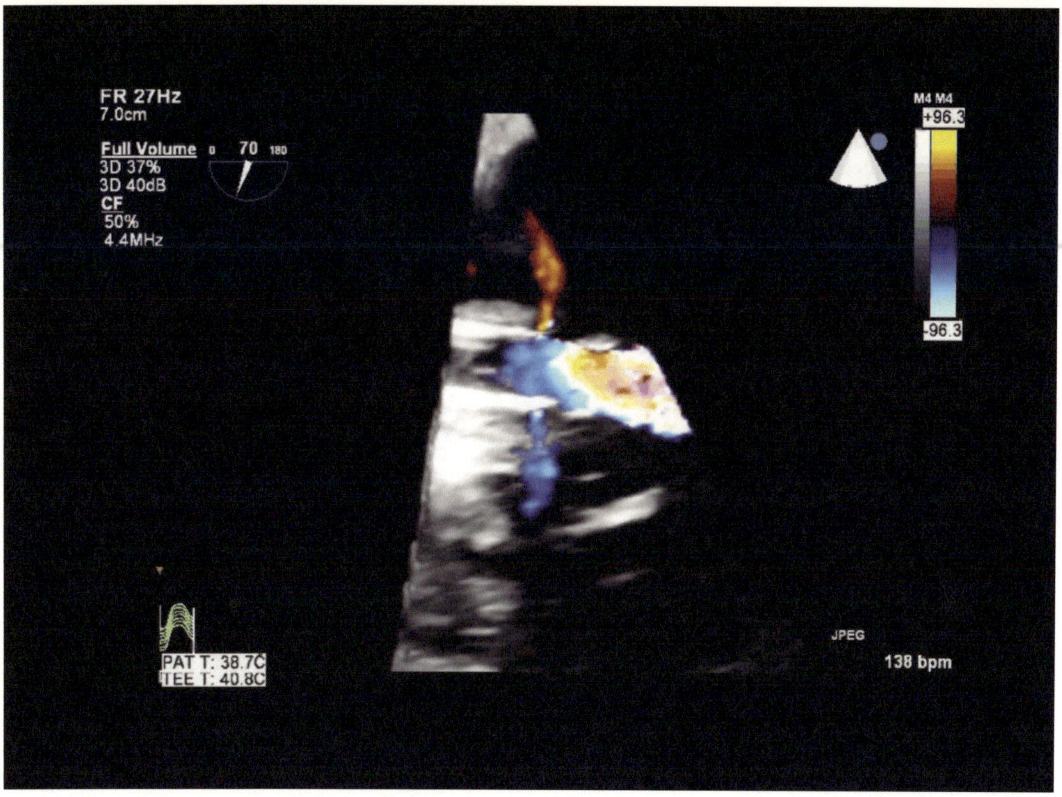

Fig. 11. 3D transoesophageal colour Doppler image of oxygenated blood being returned to the right atrium.

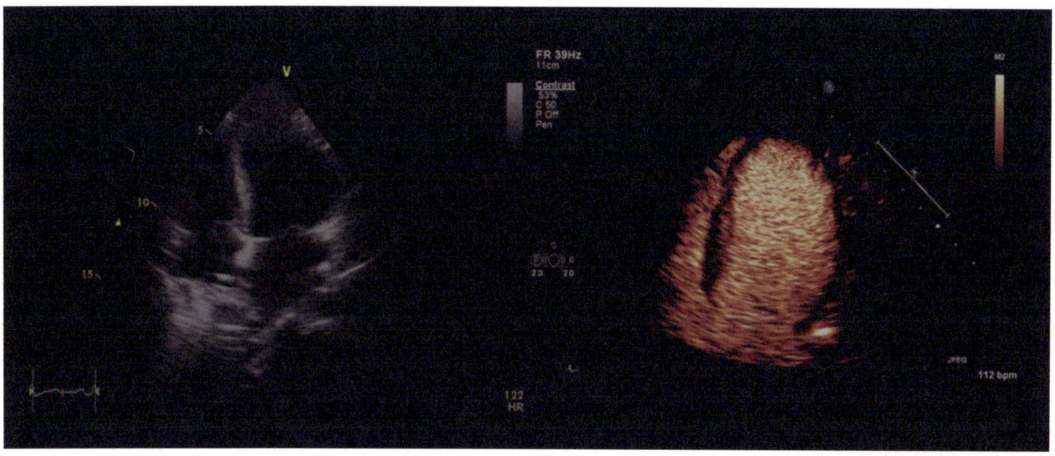

Fig. 12. Pre (left) and post TTE (right) contrast enhanced images o f a ventilated patient in ICU on VA ECMO

5. References

[1] Roberto ML, Michelle B, Richard BD, Frank AF, Elyse F, Patricia AP, et al. Recommendations for Chamber Quantification: A Report from the American Society of Echocardiography's Guidelines and Standards Committee and the Chamber Quantification Writing Group, Developed in Conjunction with the European Association of Echocardiography, a Branch of the European Society of Cardiology. Journal of the American Society of Echocardiography : official publication of the American Society of Echocardiography. 2005;18(12):1440-63.

[2] Cohen JL, Cheirif J, Segar DS, Gillam LD, Gottdiener JS, Hausnerova E, et al. Improved left ventricular endocardial border delineation and opacification with OPTISON (FS069), a new echocardiographic contrast agent: Results of a phase III multicenter trial. J Am Coll Cardiol. 1998 September 1, 1998;32(3):746-52.

[3] Kornbluth M, Liang D, H., Brown P, Gessford E, Schnittger I. Contrast echocardiography is superior to tissue harmonics for assessment of left ventricular function in mechanically ventilated patients. American heart journal. 2000;140(2):291-6.

[4] Reilly JP, Tunick PA, Timmermans RJ, Stein B, Rosenzweig BP, Kronzon I. Contrast echocardiography clarifies uninterpretable wall motion in intensive care unit patients. J Am Coll Cardiol. 2000 February 1, 2000;35(2):485-90.

[5] Daniel G, K. , Chawla M, K., Sawada S, G. , Gradus-Pizlo I, Feigenbaum H, Segar DS. Echocardiographic imaging of technically difficult patients in the intensive care unit: Use of Optison in combination with fundamental and harmonic imaging. Journal of the American Society of Echocardiography : official publication of the American Society of Echocardiography. 2001;14(9):917-20.

[6] Costa JM, Tsutsui JM, Nozawa E, Morhy SS, Andrade JL, Ramires JF, et al. Contrast echocardiography can save nondiagnostic exams in mechanically ventilated patients. Echocardiography. 2005 May;22(5):389-94.

[7] Makaryus A, N. , Zubrow M, E. , Gillam LD, Michelakis N, Phillips L, Ahmed S, et al. Contrast Echocardiography Improves the Diagnostic Yield of Transthoracic Studies Performed in the Intensive Care Setting by Novice Sonographers. Journal of the American Society of Echocardiography : official publication of the American Society of Echocardiography. 2005;18(5):475-80.

[8] Kurt M, Shaikh KA, Peterson L, Kurrelmeyer KM, Shah G, Nagueh SF, et al. Impact of Contrast Echocardiography on Evaluation of Ventricular Function and Clinical Management in a Large Prospective Cohort. J Am Coll Cardiol. 2009 March 3, 2009;53(9):802-10.

[9] Senior R, Becher H, Monaghan M, Agati L, Zamorano J, Vanoverschelde JL, et al. Contrast echocardiography: evidence-based recommendations by European Association of Echocardiography. Eur J Echocardiogr. 2009 March 1, 2009;10(2):194-212.

[10] Quiñones M, A. , Otto C, M., Stoddard M, Waggoner A, Zoghbi W, A. . Recommendations for quantification of Doppler echocardiography: A report from the Doppler quantification task force of the nomenclature and standards committee of the American Society of Echocardiography. Journal of the American Society of Echocardiography : official publication of the American Society of Echocardiography. 2002;15(2):167-84.

[11] Mariell J, Nicholas B, Susan B, Carlo C, Angelika C-J, Thomas D, et al. Optimal Pharmacologic and Non-pharmacologic Management of Cardiac Transplant Candidates: Approaches to Be Considered Prior to Transplant Evaluation: International Society for Heart and Lung Transplantation Guidelines for the Care of

Cardiac Transplant Candidates—2006. The Journal of heart and lung transplantation : the official publication of the International Society for Heart Transplantation. 2006;25(9):1003-23.
[12] Srihari T, Kenneth BS, Julio EP. Improved Echocardiographic Delineation of Left Ventricular Thrombus with the Use of Intravenous Second-Generation Contrast Image Enhancement. Journal of the American Society of Echocardiography : official publication of the American Society of Echocardiography. 1999;12(12):1022-6.
[13] Kirkpatrick J, Wong T, Bednarz J, Spencer K, Sugeng L, Ward R, et al. Differential diagnosis of cardiac masses using contrast echocardiographic perfusion imaging. J Am Coll Cardiol. 2004;43:1412 - 9.
[14] Khouzam RN, D'Cruz IA, Minderman D. Use of Contrast in Distinguishing Apical Mural Thrombus from Its Echocardiographic Simulators. Echocardiography. 2007;24(3):279-83.
[15] Mansencal N, Revault-d'Allonnes L, Pelage J-P, Farcot J-C, Lacombe P, Dubourg O. Usefulness of contrast echocardiography for assessment of intracardiac masses. Archives of Cardiovascular Diseases. 2009;102(3):177-83.
[16] Siebelink H-MJ, Scholte AJHA, Van de Veire NR, Holman ER, Nucifora G, van der Wall EE, et al. Value of contrast echocardiography for left ventricular thrombus detection postinfarction and impact on antithrombotic therapy. Coronary Artery Disease. 2009;20(7):462-6 10.1097/MCA.0b013e328330d58f.
[17] Weinsaft JW, Kim HW, Shah DJ, Klem I, Crowley AL, Brosnan R, et al. Detection of Left Ventricular Thrombus by Delayed-Enhancement Cardiovascular Magnetic Resonance: Prevalence and Markers in Patients With Systolic Dysfunction. J Am Coll Cardiol. 2008 July 8, 2008;52(2):148-57.
[18] Weinsaft JW, Kim RJ, Ross M, Krauser D, Manoushagian S, LaBounty TM, et al. Contrast-Enhanced Anatomic Imaging as Compared to Contrast-Enhanced Tissue Characterization for Detection of Left Ventricular Thrombus. J Am Coll Cardiol Img. 2009 August 1, 2009;2(8):969-79.
[19] Chumnanvej S, Wood MJ, MacGillivray TE, Melo MFV. Perioperative echocardiographic examination for ventricular assist device implantation. Anesthesia & Analgesia. 2007 Sep;105(3):583-601.
[20] Ochiai Y, McCarthy PM, Smedira NG, Banbury MK, Navia JL, Feng J, et al. Predictors of Severe Right Ventricular Failure After Implantable Left Ventricular Assist Device Insertion: Analysis of 245 Patients. Circulation. 2002 September 24, 2002;106(90121):I-198-202.
[21] Farrar DJ, Hill JD, Pennington DG, McBride LR, Holman WL, Kormos RL, et al. Pre operative and postoperative comparison of patients with univentricular and biventricular support with the thoratec ventricular assist device as a bridge to cardiac transplantation. J Thorac Cardiovasc Surg. 1997 January 1, 1997;113(1):202-9.
[22] Kormos RL, Teuteberg JJ, Pagani FD, Russell SD, John R, Miller LW, et al. Right ventricular failure in patients with the HeartMate II continuous-flow left ventricular assist device: Incidence, risk factors, and effect on outcomes. J Thorac Cardiovasc Surg. 2010 May 1, 2010;139(5):1316-24.
[23] Lam KM-T, Ennis S, O'Driscoll G, Solis J, M., MacGillivray TE, Picard M, H. . Observations From Non-Invasive Measures of Right Heart Hemodynamics in Left Ventricular Assist Device Patients. Journal of the American Society of Echocardiography : official publication of the American Society of Echocardiography. 2009;22(9):1055-62.

[24] Kilger E, Strom C, Frey L, Felbinger T, Pichler B, Tichy M, et al. Intermittent atrial level right-to-left shunt with temporary hypoxemia in a patient during support with a left ventricular assist device. Acta Anaesthesiologica Scandinavica. 2000;44(1):125-7.
[25] Baker JE, Stratmann G, Hoopes C, Donateillo R, Tseng E, Russell IA. Profound Hypoxemia Resulting from Shunting Across an Inadvertent Atrial Septal Tear After Left Ventricular Assist Device Placement. Anesthesia & Analgesia. 2004 April 1, 2004;98(4):937-40.
[26] Shanewise J, S., Cheung A, T. , Aronson S, Stewart W, J., Weiss R, L. , Mark J, B. , et al. ASE/SCA Guidelines for Performing a Comprehensive Intraoperative Multiplane Transesophageal Echocardiography Examination: Recommendations of the American Society of Echocardiography Council for Intraoperative Echocardiography and the Society of Cardiovascular Anesthesiologists Task Force for Certification in Perioperative Transesophageal Echocardiography. Journal of the American Society of Echocardiography : official publication of the American Society of Echocardiography. 1999;12(10):884-900.
[27] Glas K, E. , Swaminathan M, Reeves S, T. , Shanewise J, S. , Rubenson D, Smith P, K. , et al. Guidelines for the Performance of a Comprehensive Intraoperative Epiaortic Ultrasonographic Examination: Recommendations of the American Society of Echocardiography and the Society of Cardiovascular Anesthesiologists; Endorsed by the Society of Thoracic Surgeons. Journal of the American Society of Echocardiography : official publication of the American Society of Echocardiography. 2007;20(11):1227-35.
[28] Rao V, Slater JP, Edwards NM, Naka Y, Oz MC. Surgical management of valvular disease in patients requiring left ventricular assist device support. Ann Thorac Surg. 2001 May 1, 2001;71(5):1448-53.
[29] Bryant AS, Holman WL, Nanda NC, Vengala S, Blood MS, Pamboukian SV, et al. Native Aortic Valve Insufficiency in Patients With Left Ventricular Assist Devices. Ann Thorac Surg. 2006 February 1, 2006;81(2):e6-8.
[30] Swartz MT, Lowdermilk GA, Moroney DA, McBride LR. Ventricular assist device support in patients with mechanical heart valves. Ann Thorac Surg. 1999 December 1, 1999;68(6):2248-51.
[31] Barbone A, Rao V, Oz MC, Naka Y. LVAD support in patients with bioprosthetic valves. Ann Thorac Surg. 2002 July 1, 2002;74(1):232-4.
[32] Castillo JG, Anyanwu AC, Adams DH, Nyirenda T, Fischer GW. Real-time 3-dimensional echocardiographic assessment of current continuous-flow rotary left ventricular assist devices. Journal of Cardiothoracic & Vascular Anesthesia. 2009 Oct;23(5):702-10.
[33] Scalia GM, McCarthy PM, Savage RM, Smedira NG, Thomas JD. Clinical utility of echocardiography in the management of implantable ventricular assist devices. Journal of the American Society of Echocardiography. 2000 Aug;13(8):754-63.
[34] Catena E, Milazzo F, Montorsi E, Bruschi G, Cannata A, Russo C, et al. Left Ventricular Support by Axial Flow Pump: The Echocardiographic Approach to Device Malfunction. Journal of the American Society of Echocardiography : official publication of the American Society of Echocardiography. 2005;18(12):1422.e7-.e13.
[35] Abiomed. AB500 Circulatory Support System Operating Room Reference Guide.
[36] Horton SC, Khodaverdian R, Chatelain P, McIntosh ML, Horne BD, Muhlestein JB, et al. Left Ventricular Assist Device Malfunction: An Approach to Diagnosis by Echocardiography. Journal of the American College of Cardiology. 2005;45(9):1435-40.

[37] Smart K, Jett GK. Late tamponade with mechanical circulatory support. Ann Thorac Surg. 1998 December 1, 1998;66(6):2027-8.
[38] Kohmoto T, Oz MC, Naka Y. Late bleeding from right internal mammary artery after heartmate left ventricular assist device implantation. Ann Thorac Surg. 2004 August 1, 2004;78(2):689-91.
[39] Rose EA, Gelijns AC, Moskowitz AJ, Heitjan DF, Stevenson LW, Dembitsky W, et al. Long-Term Use of a Left Ventricular Assist Device for End-Stage Heart Failure. New England Journal of Medicine. 2001;345(20):1435-43.
[40] Slaughter MS, Rogers JG, Milano CA, Russell SD, Conte JV, Feldman D, et al. Advanced Heart Failure Treated with Continuous-Flow Left Ventricular Assist Device. New England Journal of Medicine. 2009;361(23):2241-51.
[41] Reilly MP, Wiegers SE, Cucchiara AJ, O'Hara ML, Plappert TJ, Loh E, et al. Frequency, risk factors, and clinical outcomes of left ventricular assist device-associated ventricular thrombus. The American Journal of Cardiology. 2000;86(10):1156-9.
[42] de Jonge KC, Laube HR, Dohmen PM, Ivancevic V, Konertz WF. Diagnosis and management of left ventricular assist device valve-endocarditis: LVAD valve replacement. Ann Thorac Surg. 2000 October 1, 2000;70(4):1404-5.
[43] Gordon R, J. , Quagliarello B, Lowy F, D. Ventricular assist device-related infections. LANINF. 2006;6(7):426-37.
[44] Baddour LM, Bettmann MA, Bolger AF, Epstein AE, Ferrieri P, Gerber MA, et al. Nonvalvular Cardiovascular Device-Related Infections. Circulation. 2003 October 21, 2003;108(16):2015-31.
[45] Elkind MSVMM, Chin SSMDP, Rose EAM. Massive air embolism with left ventricular assist device. Neurology. 2002;58(11):1694.
[46] Gregoric IDMD, Myers TJBS, Kar BMD, Loyalka PMD, Reverdin SMD, La Francesca SMD, et al. Management of Air Embolism during HeartMate(R) XVE Exchange. Texas Heart Institute Journal. 2007;34(1):19-22.
[47] Platts D, Burstow D, Hamilton-Craig C, Wright G, Thomson B. Systemic Air Embolization Originating from a Pleural Air Leak via a Left Ventricular Assist Device Cannula Anastomosis Site. Journal of the American Society of Echocardiography : official publication of the American Society of Echocardiography. 2010;23(3):341.e1-.e2.
[48] Dworschak M, Wiesinger K, Lorenzl N, Wieselthaler G, Wolner E, Lassnigg A. Late aortic dissection in a patient with a left ventricular assist device. The Japanese Journal of Thoracic and Cardiovascular Surgery. 2001;49(6):395-7.
[49] Naka Y, Edwards NM, Oz MC. Novel technique to repair type A acute aortic dissection in patients with a left ventricular assist device. Ann Thorac Surg. 2001 October 1, 2001;72(4):1403-4.
[50] Lacroix V, d'Udekem Y, Jacquet L, Noirhomme P. Resection of the ascending aorta and aortic valve patch closure for type A aortic dissection after Novacor(R) LVAD insertion. Eur J Cardiothorac Surg. 2003 August 1, 2003;24(2):309-11.
[51] Muller J, Wallukat G, Weng Y-G, Dandel M, Spiegelsberger S, Semrau S, et al. Weaning From Mechanical Cardiac Support in Patients With Idiopathic Dilated Cardiomyopathy. Circulation. 1997 July 15, 1997;96(2):542-9.
[52] Hetzer R, Muller J, Weng Y, Wallukat G, Spiegelsberger S, Loebe M. Cardiac recovery in dilated cardiomyopathy by unloading with a left ventricular assist device. Ann Thorac Surg. 1999 August 1, 1999;68(2):742-9.

[53] Slaughter MS, Silver MA, Farrar DJ, Tatooles AJ, Pappas PS. A new method of monitoring recovery and weaning the thoratec left ventricular assist device. Ann Thorac Surg. 2001 January 1, 2001;71(1):215-8.

[54] Farrar DJ, Holman WR, McBride LR, Kormos RL, Icenogle TB, Hendry PJ, et al. Long-term follow-up of thoratec ventricular assist device bridge-to-recovery patients successfully removed from support after recovery of ventricular function. The Journal of Heart and Lung Transplantation. 2002;21(5):516-21.

[55] Gorcsan J, Severyn D, Murali S, Kormos RL. Non-invasive assessment of myocardial recovery on chronic left ventricular assist device: results associated with successful device removal. The Journal of Heart and Lung Transplantation. 2003;22(12):1304-13.

[56] Khan T, Delgado RM, Radovancevic B, Torre-Amione G, Abrams J, Miller K, et al. Dobutamine stress echocardiography predicts myocardial improvement in patients supported by left ventricular assist devices (LVADs): hemodynamic and histologic evidence of improvement before LVAD explantation. The Journal of Heart and Lung Transplantation. 2003;22(2):137-46.

[57] Liang H, Lin H, Weng Y, Dandel M, Hetzer R. Prediction of cardiac function after weaning from ventricular assist devices. J Thorac Cardiovasc Surg. 2005 December 1, 2005;130(6):1555-60.

[58] Simon MA, Kormos RL, Murali S, Nair P, Heffernan M, Gorcsan J, et al. Myocardial Recovery Using Ventricular Assist Devices: Prevalence, Clinical Characteristics, and Outcomes. Circulation. 2005 August 30, 2005;112(9_suppl):I-32-6.

[59] Osaki S, Sweitzer NK, Rahko PS, Murray MA, Hoffmann JA, Johnson MR, et al. To Explant or Not to Explant: An Invasive and Noninvasive Monitoring Protocol to Determine the Need of Continued Ventricular Assist Device Support. Congestive Heart Failure. 2009;15(2):58-62.

[60] Santelices LC, Wang Y, Severyn D, Druzdzel MJ, Kormos RL, Antaki JF. Development of a Hybrid Decision Support Model for Optimal Ventricular Assist Device Weaning. Ann Thorac Surg. 2010 September 1, 2010;90(3):713-20.

[61] Marasco SF, Lukas G, McDonald M, McMillan J, Ihle B. Review of ECMO (extra corporeal membrane oxygenation) support in critically ill adult patients. Heart, Lung & Circulation. 2008;17 Suppl 4:S41-7.

[62] Platts D, Fraser JF, Mullany D, Burstow D. Left Ventricular Endocardial Definition Enhancement Using Perflutren Microsphere Contrast Echocardiography during Peripheral Venoarterial Extracorporeal Membranous Oxygenation. Echocardiography 2010;27:E112-E114

[63] Peek GJ, Mugford M, Tiruvoipati R, Wilson A, Allen E, Thalanany MM, et al. Efficacy and economic assessment of conventional ventilatory support versus extracorporeal membrane oxygenation for severe adult respiratory failure (CESAR): a multicentre randomised controlled trial. The Lancet. 2009 2009/10/23/;374(9698):1351-63.

Part 3

Translational Research and Ventricular Assist Device

Altered Expression of mRNA and miRNA during Mechanical Support of the Failing Human Heart

Marguérite E.I. Schipper[1], Sjoukje I. Lok[2], Hub Dullens[1], Joyce Van Kuik[1], Frits H.J. Gmelig-Meyling[3], Jaap Lahpor[2], Marc A. Vos[4], Arnoud Van Der Laarse[5], Nicolaas De Jonge[2], Matthijs F.M. Van Oosterhout[1] and Roel A. De Weger[1]
[1]*Depts of Pathology,* [2]*Heart and Lung,* [3]*Immunology, and* [4]*Medical Physiology, University Medical Centre Utrecht, Utrecht*
[5]*Dept of Cardiology, Leiden University Medical Center, Leiden*
The Netherlands

1. Introduction

Remodeling during heart failure is characterized by structural rearrangement of the cardiac ventricular wall architecture. It involves hypertrophy of cardiomyocytes, fibroblast proliferation, and increased deposition of extracellular matrix (ECM) proteins (Brower et al., 2006). Support of the left ventricle with a Left Ventricular Assist Device (LVAD) in patients with end-stage heart failure results in less neurohormonal activation (Estrada-Quintero et al., 1995; Frazier and Myers, 1999; Bruggink et al., 2006a), improvement of the patient's general condition (De Jonge et al., 2001; Grady et al ., 2003), reduction in ventricular diameter (reverse remodeling), and limited recovery of contractile elements in cardiomyocytes (Muller et al., 1997; De Jonge et al., 2002). Furthermore, reduction of ECM volume (Milting et al., 2008; Goldsmith and Borg , 2002; Bruggink et al., 2006b), diminished production of tumor necrosis factor (Thohan et al., 2005; Bruggink et al., 2008), and reduction in brain natriuretic protein serum levels (Bruggink et al., 2006a; Kemperman et al., 2004) have been described during LVAD support. The changes in ECM during this process of reverse remodeling resulted not only in a time-dependent change of type I and type III collagen protein (Goldsmith and Borg, 2002; Stamenkovic, 2003), but also in considerable changes in composition of the basal membrane. These included amongst others reduced collagen type IV content in the cardiomyocyte basal membrane, as a result of increased matrix metalloproteinase activity (Bruggink et al., 2007; Spinale, 2002; Li et al., 2001; Klotz et al., 2005). So, during LVAD support myocardial architecture and composition change at the level of both the cardiomyocytes and the ECM.

The mechanics of the heart require a close interplay between cardiomyocytes and the ECM (Parker and Ingber, 2007) and therefore, one may anticipate a coordinated change in the molecules responsible for this interaction. These changes may not be the same in all heart failure patients supported by a mechanical support device. Some patients' hearts may improve and may be eligible for removal of the support device without a heart transplantation (bridge to recovery and weaning from the device), whereas others do not improve on support or may even deteriorate and these patients remain on the device (destination therapy) or will ultimately receive a heart transplant (bridge to transplantation). To make the proper choice of the type of therapy for each patient a good set of (bio)markers is required (De Weger and De Jonge, 2009).

In this chapter, we describe whether mRNA expression patterns could be indicative for the state of heart functionality supported by a LVAD (Heart-Mate I, Thoratec, Pleasanton, CA, USA). The changes in mRNA profiles that are detectable in myocardial biopsies taken from patients with end-stage heart failure due to dilated cardiomyopathy (DCM) or ischaemic heart disease (IHD) before and after LVAD support were analyzed, and compared with biopsies taken from control hearts as a reference (Table 1). Furthermore, the expression of 109 genes is described, which are involved in the process of mechanotransduction in the heart. Their expression was studied by Quant*i*tative(Q)-PCR. The cohort comprised selected genes coding for ECM filaments (such as collagens), transmembrane proteins (molecules that connect cells and matrix components like integrins and sarcoglycans), intracellular molecules, adhesion molecules related to mechanotransduction and signal transduction, ion-channel molecules, and factors involved in pro- and anti-fibrotic processes. The expression of mRNA is not always directly related to protein production, due to post-transcriptional regulation. Recently, it is has been shown that intracellular gene expression is regulated in part by small RNA molecules: microRNAs (miRs). These miRs are highly expressed in heart tissue (Ji et al., 2007; Cheng et al., 2007) and have also been related to heart diseases (Chen, 2007; Van Rooij et al., 2006). The list of regulatory miRs involved in heart disease is constantly increasing (Coutinho et al., 2007; Markham and Hill, 2010). Each miR can regulate various mRNA expressions and which mRNA is

Nr	*Age*	*Diagnosis*	*Gender*	*Days on LVAD*	*Medication during LVAD-support*
1	56	IHD	Male	138	None
2	57	IHD	Male	225	None
3	45	IHD	Male	259	2,5 mg Ramipril
4	57	IHD	Male	263	None
5	36	IHD	Male	325	2x 4 mg Perindopril
6	26	IHD	Male	357	None
7	39	IHD	Male	548	3x 6,25 mg Capoten
8	34	DCM	Female	55	3x 6,25 mg Capoten
9	17	DCM	Male	111	None
10	47	DCM	Male	190	None
11	35	DCM	Male	196	None
12	32	DCM	Female	219	3 mg Captopril
13	25	DCM	Male	263	1x 25 mg Losartan
14	32	DCM	Male	286	4 mg Perindopril
15	25	DCM	Male	330	2x 10 mg Fosinopril
16	46	DCM	Male	484	3x 50 mg Capoten

DCM: dilated cardiomyopathy, IHD: ischemic heart disease, LVAD: left ventricular assist device.

Table 1. Patient characteristics.

regulated by which miR is not determined with certainty for most genes (see www.targetscan.org; Schuldt, 2010).
An additional goal of this study was therefore, to analyse the changes in expression of 4 miRs that are known to be expressed in the myocardium (Chen, 2007; Ikeda et al., 2007): miR-1, miR-133a, miR-133b and miR-208. These miRs have been related to heart failure. The expression of these miRs was measured in the same group of patients used to analyse the mRNA expression after LVAD support. Our purpose was to find out whether the LVAD-induced remodeling of the heart was accompanied by changes in the expression of miRs that could influence the protein expression of the mRNA studied. This could make expression of some mRNAs less suitable as biomarker for the assessment of the functional quality of the supported heart. If this is the case the expression of miRs may serve as better markers either in the myocardium or the serum.

2. Tissue distribution of mRNA and miR in the myocardium

Tissue samples taken form various locations in cross sections of the heart showed that the expression of both miR in the right and left ventricular wall did not show significant variation. Only in the infarcted area the expression of miR was low to absent. Similar data were obtained for mRNA (Figure 1).

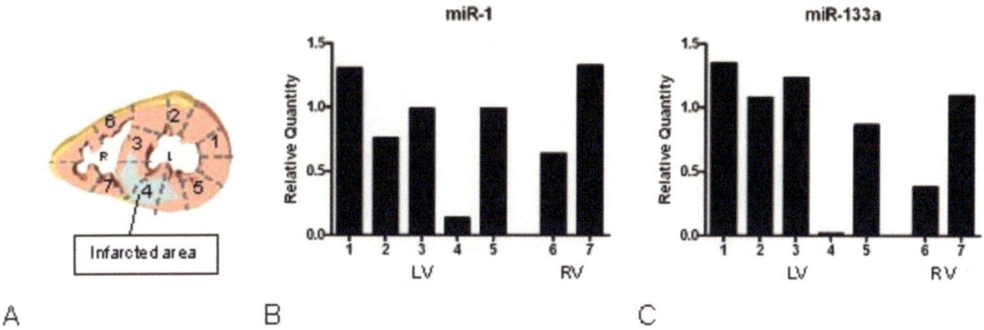

Fig. 1A. Circular cross section of the heart indicating the biopsy areas.
B and C. miRNA expression in and around the infarcted area in the indicated biopsies of a representative case. The miRNA expression in an infarcted area (biopsy 4) is much lower than in the surrounding areas. LV and RV = left and right ventricle.

3. Hierarchical clustering of gene expression in myocardial tissue of IHD and DCM patients

The gene profiles in DCM and IHD heart tissue, detected by Q-PCR, were compared using TIGR software (www.tm4.org). Figure 2 shows the whole data set for all pre-LVAD samples versus the median of control samples. Hierarchical clustering was performed on all 92 detectable genes. The genes that were not detectable (n=14) and house keeping genes (n=3) were excluded (Table 2). The clustering segregated two groups: one group consists of 6 DCM and 1 IHD patients and the other group consists of 5 IHD patients with 2 DCM patients. One DCM and one IHD patient were clustered outside both groups. So, there is a strong tendency of segregation between IHD and DCM. Therefore, the DCM and IHD patient groups were analyzed separately in this study.

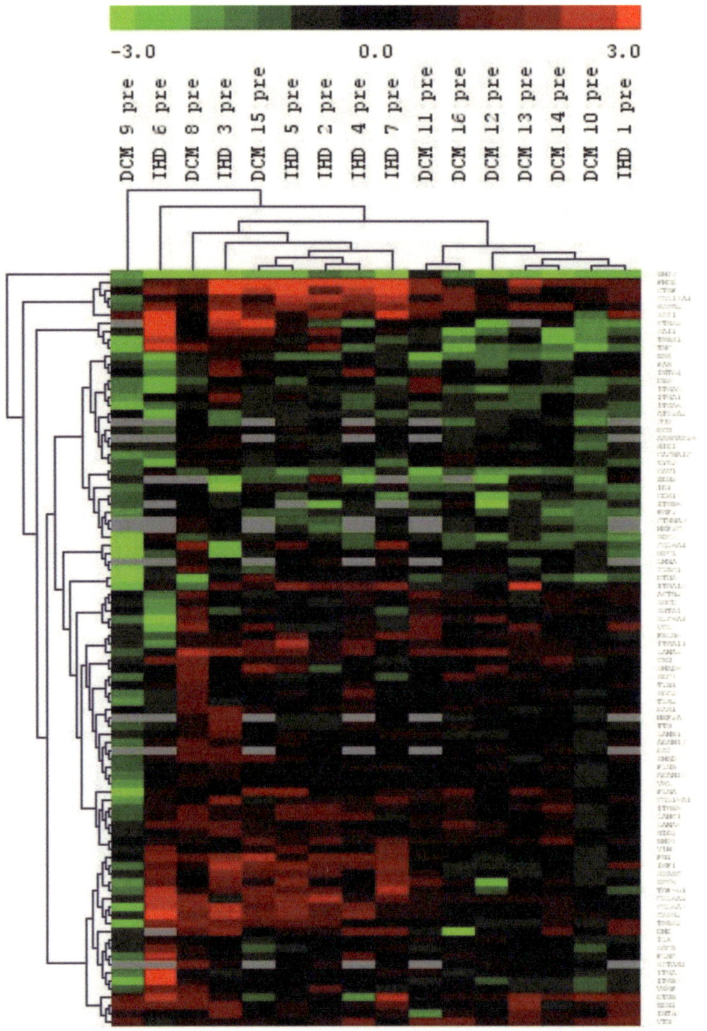

Fig. 2. Unsupervised hierachical clustering of myocardial gene expression profiles pre-LVAD in IHD and DCM patients. Clustering was performed on all 92 detectable genes. Unsupervised hierarchical clustering was performed on normalized data using the multi-experiment viewer (MeV, version 4.3) of the TIGR software (www.tm4.org). The Reletive quantity (RQ) of each sample per gene was normalized:
Normalized signal of sample x = Log2 (RQ sample x / median RQ).
To compare DCM and IHD the median was taken from the RQ (relative quality) of control hearts. To compare pre- and post-LVAD in DCM and IHD samples, the median of all DCM or all IHD samples were taken, respectively. Clustering was performed on the whole dataset, and distance metric selection (Euclidean distance) and linkage metric selection (Complete linkage clustering) were used (www.tm4.org). This segregated two groups; one group consisting of 6 DCM patients with 1 IHD patient, and the other of 5 IHD patients with 2 DCM patients. Two patients (one DCM and one IHD) clustered outside these groups. Red: mRNA expression is higher than the median of control hearts. Green: mRNA expression is lower than the median of control hearts. Grey: not done.

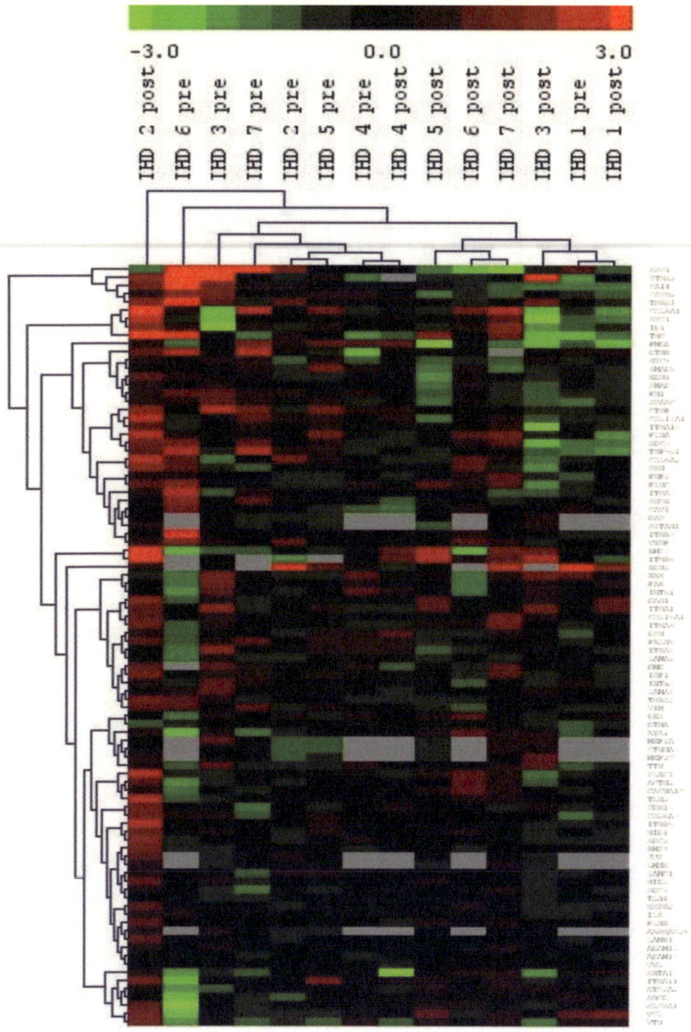

Fig. 3. Unsupervised hierarchical clustering of myocardial gene expression profiles pre- and post-LVAD in IHD patients.
Clustering was performed on all 92 detectable genes and it segregated the patient group into a pre- and post-LVAD group. See for explanation Figure 2. Red: mRNA expression is higher than the median of all IHD samples. Green: mRNA expression is lower than the median of all IHD samples. Grey: not done.

The expression of 14 genes was below level of detection and are therefore not included in this table: ADAM 12 (ADAM metallopeptidase domain 12), ADAM 15 (ADAM metallopeptidase domain 15), AGC1 (aggrecan 1), ANK1 (Ankyrin 1), DSPG3 (dermatan sulfate proteoglycan 3), EDN3 (endothelin 3), LAMC3 (laminin, gamma 3), MMP-7 (matrix metallopeptidase 7), MUC16 (mucin 16), NOS1 (nitric oxide synthase 1), SCN1A (sodium channel, voltage-gated, type I, alpha), SCN2A2 (sodium channel, voltage-gated, type II, alpha 2), SDC1 (syndecan 1), TNXB (tenascin XB).

				DCM						IHD					
Category	Gene name	Gene code AB	assay code AB	p-value pre vs post	fold change pre vs post	p-valua pre vs control		p-value post vs control		p-value pre vs post	fold change pre vs post	p-valua pre vs control		p-value post vs control	
ECM	collagen, type XIV, alpha 1	COL14A1	Hs00385388_m1	0,033	1,75	0,576		0,055	>	0,542		0,014	>	0,197	
	collagen, type XV, alpha 1	COL15A1	Hs00266332_m1	0,003	1,76	0,353		0,131		0,079		0,645		0,161	
	collagen, type VI, alpha 1	COL6A1	Hs00242448_m1	0,104		0,716		0,181		0,374		0,903		0,451	
	collagen, type VI, alpha 2	COL6A2	Hs00242484_m1	0,154		0,129		0,121		0,488		0,061		0,195	
	collagen, type VI, alpha 3	COL6A3	Hs00365098_m1	0,042	1,53	0,842		0,048	>	0,703		0,075		0,081	
	chondroitin sulfate proteoglycan 2 (versican)	CSPG2	Hs00171642_m1	0,990		0,470		0,547		0,078		0,065	>	0,472	
	decorin	DCN	Hs00370385_m1	0,049	0,56	0,051	<	0,903		0,273		0,382		0,964	
	fibulin 5	FBLN5	Hs00197064_m1	0,343		0,490		0,662		0,721		0,481		0,660	
	fibromodulin	FMOD	Hs00157619_m1	0,250		0,097		0,196		0,062	-0,67	0,009	>	0,134	
	fibronectin 1	FN1	Hs00415006_m1	0,445		0,587		0,885		0,024	-0,76	0,023	>	0,589	
	heparan sulfate proteoglycan 2 (perlecan)	HSPG2	Hs00194179_m1	0,024	0,96	0,491		0,067	>	0,805		0,052	>	0,122	
	osteonectin	SPARC	Hs00277762_m1	0,592		0,260		0,236		0,190		0,018	>	0,195	
AFF	bone morphogenetic protein 4	BMP4	Hs00370078_m1	0,029	0,93	0,215		0,023	>	0,120		0,017	>	0,064	>
	bone morphogenetic protein 7	BMP7	Hs00233476_m1	0,034	2,14	0,006	<	0,732		0,072		0,018	<	0,693	
	inhibitor of DNA binding 1	ID1	Hs00357821_g1	0,031	0,87	0,099		0,288		0,323		0,166		0,540	
	prostaglandin-endoperoxide synthase 2/COX2	PTGS2	Hs00153133_m1	0,464		0,911		0,358		0,752		0,445		0,490	
	mothers against DPP homolog 7	SMAD7	Hs00178696_m1	0,300		0,522		0,876		0,295		0,065	>	0,681	
PFF	connective tissue growth factor	CTGF	Hs00170014_m1	0,258		0,318		0,082		0,398		0,048	>	0,112	
	endothelin 1	EDN1	Hs00174961_m1	0,710		0,332		0,442		0,913		0,040	>	0,184	
	endothelin 2	EDN2	Hs00266516_m1	0,431		0,084		0,185		0,419		0,267		0,150	
	fibroblast growth factor 2	FGF2	Hs00266645_m1	0,306		0,022	<	0,369		0,143		0,113		0,849	
	insulin-like growth factor 1	IGF1	Hs00153126_m1	0,084		0,938		0,114		0,903		0,003	>	0,076	
	mothers against DPP homolog 6	SMAD6	Hs00178579_m1	0,089		0,193		0,881		0,125		0,571		0,030	<
	transforming growth factor beta 1	TGF-β1	Hs00171257_m1	0,565		0,728		0,965		0,223		0,318		0,855	
	vascular endothelial growth factor	VEGF	Hs00900054_m1	0,586		0,352		0,134		0,254		0,880		0,538	
BM	glypican 1	GPC1	Hs00157805_m1	0,546		0,738		0,916		0,285		0,330		0,749	
	glypican 6	GPC6	Hs00170677_m1	0,200		1,000		0,373		0,839		0,095		0,104	
	laminin, alpha 2	LAMA2	Hs00166308_m1	0,505		0,072		0,111		0,798		0,078		0,003	>
	laminin, alpha 4	LAMA4	Hs00158588_m1	0,965		0,933		0,949		0,234		0,610		0,935	
	laminin, beta 1	LAMB1	Hs00158620_m1	0,001	0,82	0,338		0,255		0,268		0,696		0,201	
	laminin, gamma 1 (formerly LAMB2)	LAMC1	Hs00267056_m1	0,058	0,91	0,273		0,024	>	0,938		0,026	>	0,019	>
	lamin A/C	LMNA	Hs00153462_m1	0,261		0,287		0,717		0,938		0,055	>	0,112	
	nidogen 1	NID1	Hs00159600_m1	0,264		0,424		0,973		0,763		0,491		0,953	
	nidogen 2 (osteonidogen)	NID2	Hs00201233_m1	0,871		0,950		0,957		0,395		0,718		0,332	
	plasminogen activator inhibitor-2	PAI1	Hs00167155_m1	0,491		0,321		0,476		0,336		0,433		0,657	
	plectin 1	PLEC1	Hs00356977_m1	0,145		0,963		0,138		0,161		0,624		0,294	
	syndecan 4	SDC4	Hs00161617_m1	0,445		0,516		0,903		0,242		0,484		0,905	
	osteopontin	SPP1	Hs00167093_m1	0,001	-1,37	0,805		0,042	<	0,039	-1,82	0,064	>	0,155	
	thrombospondin 1	THBS1	Hs00170236_m1	0,943		0,094		0,118		0,452		0,931		0,322	
	thrombospondin 2	THBS2	Hs00170248_m1	0,656		0,785		0,523		0,764		0,040	>	0,264	
	tenascin C	TNC	Hs00233648_m1	0,654		0,389		0,538		0,890		0,538		0,364	
	vitronectin	VTN	Hs00169863_m1	0,464		0,010	>	0,061	>	0,171		0,366		0,071	
TAM	ADAM metallopeptidase domain 10	ADAM10	Hs00153853_m1	0,960		0,697		0,614		0,378		0,654		0,211	
	ADAM metallopeptidase domain 17	ADAM17	Hs00234224_m1	0,461		0,832		0,294		0,596		0,051	>	0,095	
	ATPase, Ca++ transporting, cardiac muscle	ATP2A2	Hs00155939_m1	0,416		0,096		0,109		0,008	1,02	0,002	<	0,297	
	calcium channel, alpha 1C subunit	CACNA1C	Hs00167681_m1	0,018	0,92	0,296		0,319		0,041		0,125		0,439	
	caveolin 1, caveolae protein, 22kDa	CAV1	Hs00184697_m1	0,267		0,011	<	0,027	<	0,442		0,291		0,126	
	cadherin 13, H-cadherin (heart)	CDH13	Hs00169908_m1	0,002	0,89	0,118		0,356		0,057	0,81	0,168		0,414	
	dystroglycan 1	DAG1	Hs00189308_m1	0,324		0,599		0,126		0,089		0,244		0,054	>
	integrin, alpha 1	ITGA1	Hs00235030_m1	0,014	0,98	0,064		0,500		0,337		0,998		0,511	
	integrin, alpha 10	ITGA10	Hs00174623_m1	0,023	2,47	0,651		0,060	>	0,832		0,017	>	0,072	
	integrin, alpha 11	ITGA11	Hs00201927_m1	0,150		0,264		0,030	>	0,581		0,258		0,049	>
	integrin, alpha 3	ITGA3	Hs00233722_m1	0,309		0,856		0,525		0,364		0,398		0,818	
	integrin, alpha 5	ITGA5	Hs00233732_m1	0,370		0,206		0,945		0,039	-0,41	0,810		0,367	
	integrin, alpha 6	ITGA6	Hs00173952_m1	0,007	1,40	0,035	<	0,457		0,046	1,23	0,249		0,303	
	integrin, alpha 7	ITGA7	Hs00174397_m1	0,062	-0,07	0,102		0,518		0,401		0,237		0,366	
	integrin, beta 1	ITGB1	Hs00559595_m1	0,231		0,313		0,648		0,377		0,747		0,840	
	integrin, beta 3	ITGB3	Hs00173978_m1	0,908		0,643		0,676		0,325		0,406		0,769	
	integrin, beta 5	ITGB5	Hs00609896_m1	0,510		0,252		0,132		0,410		0,012	>	0,288	
	integrin, beta 6	ITGB6	Hs00168458_m1	0,163		0,138		0,602		0,026	9,34	0,070		0,766	
	syndecan 3	SDC3	Hs00206320_m1	0,059	1,03	0,066	<	0,163		0,825		0,345		0,325	
	sarcoglycan, beta	SGCB	Hs00165095_m1	0,107		0,090		0,045	<	0,047	-0,76	0,333		0,083	
	sarcoglycan, delta	SGCD	Hs00165726_m1	0,538		0,152		0,051	>	0,056	1,06	0,589		0,002	>
	solute carrier family 8 ,member 1	SLC8A1	Hs00253432_m1	0,587		0,287		0,285		0,110		0,590		0,188	

				DCM						IHD					
Category	Gene name	Gene code AB	assay code AB	p-value pre vs post	fold change pre vs post	p-valua pre vs control		p-value post vs control		p-value pre vs post	fold change pre vs post	p-valua pre vs control		p-value post vs control	
IF	actinin, alpha 2	ACTN2	Hs00153809_m1	0,685		0,212		0,569		0,171		0,610		0,073	
	Rho GTPase activating protein 26	ARHGAP26	Hs00209395_m1	0,294		0,350		0,876		0,349		0,869		0,445	
	desmin	DES	Hs00157258_m1	0,416		0,617		0,156		0,829		0,109		0,136	
	dystrophin	DMD	Hs00244243_m1	0,196		0,202		0,203		0,882		0,036	>	0,044	>
	desmoplakin	DSP	Hs00189422_m1	0,559		0,869		0,367		0,015	0,59	0,918		0,120	
	dystrobrevin, alpha	DTNA	Hs00263201_m1	0,428		0,375		0,673		0,890		0,981		0,885	
	dystrobrevin, beta	DTNB	Hs00222463_m1	0,458		0,041	>	0,074		0,313		0,143		0,263	
	filamin A, alpha	FLNA	Hs00155065_m1	0,227		0,131		0,095		0,575		0,155		0,214	
	filamin B, beta	FLNB	Hs00181698_m1	0,003	0,92	0,895		0,034	>	0,177		0,161		0,068	
	filamin C, gamma	FLNC	Hs00155124_m1	0,118		0,248		0,564		0,705		0,677		0,804	
	junction plakoglobin	JUP	Hs00158408_m1	0,505		0,050	<	0,076		0,947		0,052	<	0,093	
	paxillin	PXN	Hs00236064_m1	0,077		0,514		0,121		0,393		0,494		0,319	
	syntrophin, alpha 1	SNTA1	Hs00162045_m1	0,312		0,112		0,399		0,454		0,372		0,964	
	spectrin alpha	SPTAN1	Hs00162203_m1	0,948		0,361		0,353		0,065	0,56	0,848		0,232	
	talin 1	TLN1	Hs00196775_m1	0,653		0,210		0,127		0,370		0,113		0,037	>
	talin 2	TLN2	Hs00322257_m1	0,005	1,13	0,936		0,022	>	0,135		0,428		0,286	
	titin	TTN	Hs00399225_m1	0,120		0,803		0,401		0,126		0,951		0,195	
	vinculin	VCL	Hs00247826_m1	0,093		0,154		0,503		0,078		0,934		0,108	
	vimentin	VIM	Hs00185584_m1	0,304		0,833		0,513		0,551		0,160		0,474	
STF	catenin (cadherin-associated protein), alpha 3	CTNNA3	Hs00379052_m1	0,377		0,446		0,900		0,002	1,09	0,163		0,492	
	Integrin-initiated extracellular signal-regulated kinase	ERK	Hs00177066_m1	0,102		0,054	<	0,848		0,433		0,435		0,838	
	Focal adhesion kinase	FAK	Hs00178587_m1	0,016	0,57	0,312		0,496		0,235		0,907		0,471	
	integrin-linked kinase	ILK	Hs00177914_m1	0,526		0,527		0,292		0,947		0,692		0,720	
	myocyte enhancer factor 2A	MEF2A	Hs00271535_m1	0,164		0,239		0,864		0,030	0,94	0,367		0,865	
	myocyte enhancer factor 2C	MEF2C	Hs00231149_m1	0,491		0,564		0,280		0,023	0,69	0,302		0,956	
	ryanodine receptor 2 (cardiac)	RYR2	Hs00181461_m1	0,045	0,70	0,476		0,007	>	0,023	1,73	0,364		0,046	>
	syndecan 1	SDC1	Hs00174579_m1	0,348		0,838		0,495		1,000		0,890		0,920	
	von Hippel-Lindau tumor suppressor	VHL	Hs00184451_m1	0,234		0,762		0,699		0,979		0,762		0,774	

Table 2. Statistical analysis of gene expression profiles in DCM and IHD patients. Significant changes are indicated in yellow. The genes are grouped by function/location. Abbreviations: extracellular matrix proteins (ECM), pro- and anti-fibrotic factors (P/AFF), basal membrane proteins (BM), transmembrane and adhesion molecules (TAM), intracellular filaments (IF), and signal transduction factors (STF). Applied Biosystems (AB). > and < indicate whether gene expression is significantly higher or lower compared to control.

4. Hierarchical clustering of gene expression in myocardial tissue pre- and post-LVAD support

Hierarchical clustering of the IHD samples showed a clear segregation into a pre- and a post-LVAD group (Figure 3). In DCM patients a similar segregation into a pre- and a post-LVAD group was not evident (data not shown).

5. Differential expression of genes in myocardial tissue pre- and post LVAD

Changes in gene expression were tested individually using the paired t-test in DCM and IHD separately. Furthermore, these gene profiles were compared with gene profiles of controls to test whether gene profiles normalized or showed a tendency to deviate from normal after LVAD therapy using the unpaired t-test. Table 2 shows all genes investigated, grouped by function/ location: extracellular matrix proteins (ECM), basal membrane proteins (BM), transmembrane and adhesion molecules (TAM), intracellular filaments (IF), signal transduction factors (STF) and pro- and anti-fibrotic factors (P/AFF) with the p-values and fold changes.

In Table 3 only the genes that show significant changes are indicated for DCM and IHD patients separately. Only a minority of genes showed a significant difference between pre- and post-LVAD: DCM 19/92 genes (21 %) and IHD 12/92 genes (13 %). Most of these genes showed an upregulation post-LVAD (DCM 18/19 genes and IHD 8/12 genes). In DCM pre-LVAD 6 genes and post-LVAD 9 genes were upregulated compared to control. Only one gene, encoding caveolin, showed a decreased expression in both pre- and post-LVAD compared to control. In IHD pre-LVAD 12 genes were upregulated and 2 downregulated compared to control. Post-LVAD 6 were upregulated and 2 downregulated. Among these, two genes (dystrophin and laminin gamma 1) showed an increased expression compared to control in both pre- and post-LVAD samples.

DCM

Gene name	pre vs post	pre vs control	post vs control
osteopontin	▼	=	<
bone morphogenetic protein 4	▲	=	>
collagen, type VI, alpha 3	▲	=	>
filamin B, beta	▲	=	>
laminin, gamma 1	▲	=	>
ryanodine receptor 2 (cardiac)	▲	=	>
talin 2	▲	=	>
cadherin 13, H-cadherin (heart)	▲	=	=
calcium channel, alpha 1C subunit	▲	=	=
collagen, type XIV, alpha 1	▲	=	=
collagen, type XV, alpha 1	▲	=	=
decorin	▲	=	=
focal adhesion kinase	▲	=	=
heparan sulfate proteoglycan 2 (perlecan)	▲	=	=
inhibitor of DNA binding 1	▲	=	=
integrin, alpha 1	▲	=	=
integrin, alpha 10	▲	=	=
laminin, beta 1	▲	=	=
bone morphogenetic protein 7	▲	<	=
integrin, alpha 6	▲	<	=
dystrobrevin beta	=	>	=
vitronectin	=	>	=
integrin, alpha 11	=	=	>
sarcoglycan, beta	=	=	<
fibroblast growth factor 2	=	<	=
junction plakoglobin	=	<	=
caveolin 1	=	<	<

IHD

Gene name	pre vs post	pre vs control	post vs control
fibronectin 1	▼	>	=
integrin, alpha 5	▼	=	=
osteopontin	▼	=	=
sarcoglycan, beta	▼	=	=
ryanodine receptor 2 (cardiac)	▲	=	>
cadherin 13, H-cadherin (heart)	▲	=	=
calcium channel, alpha 1C subunit	▲	=	=
catenin (cadherin-associated protein), alpha 3	▲	=	=
desmoplakin	▲	=	=
integrin, alpha 6	▲	=	=
integrin, beta 6	▲	=	=
myocyte enhancer factor 2A	▲	=	=
myocyte enhancer factor 2C	▲	=	=
spectrin alpha	▲	=	=
ATPase, Ca++ transporting, cardiac muscle	▲	<	=
dystrophin	=	>	>
lamin, gamma 1	=	>	>
bone morphogenetic protein 4	=	>	=
collagen, type XIV, alpha 1	=	>	=
connective tissue growth factor	=	>	=
fibromodulin	=	>	=
insulin-like growth factor 1	=	>	=
integrin, beta 5	=	>	=
integrin, alpha 10	=	>	=
integrin, alpha 6	=	>	=
osteonectin	=	>	=
thrombospondin 2	=	>	=
integrin, alpha 11	=	=	>
laminin, alpha 2	=	=	>
sarcoglycan, delta	=	=	>
talin 1	=	=	>
mothers against DPP homolog 6	=	=	<
bone morphogenetic protein 7	=	<	=

Table 3. Summary of significant alterations in gene expression.
▼: decreased or ▲: increased gene expression after LVAD support, =: no change, >:higher or <:lower expression pre- or post-LVAD compared to control. The shaded (green) genes are significantly altered in both DCM and IHD.

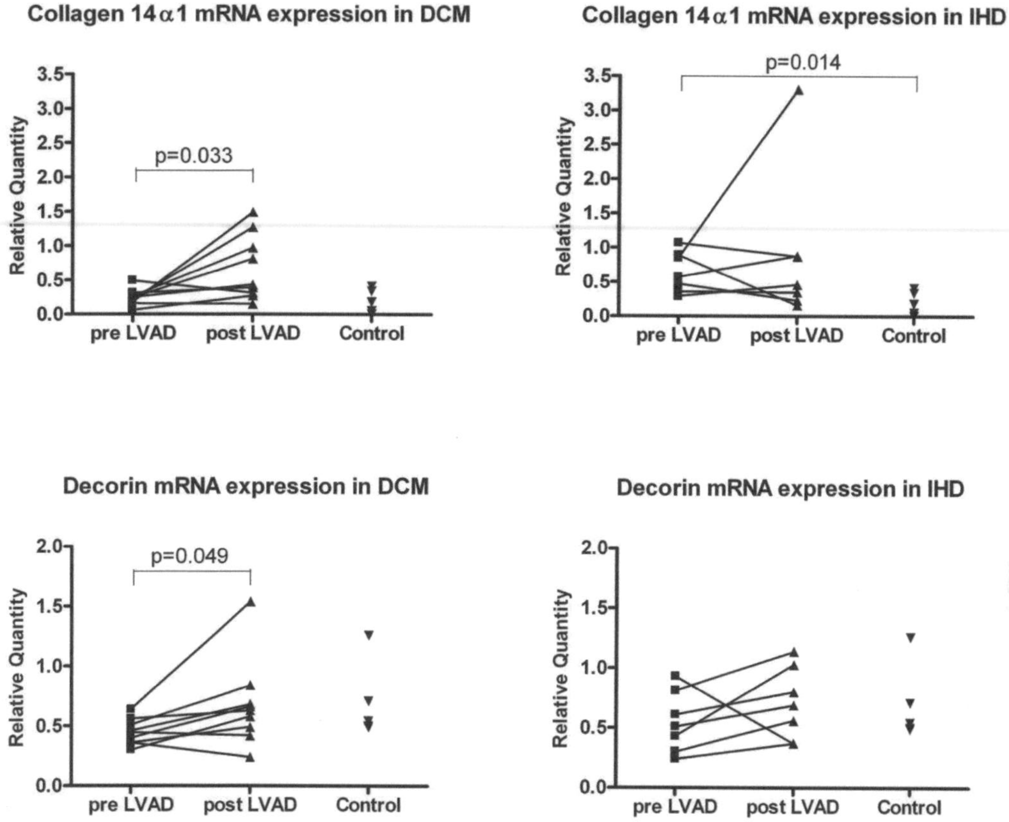

Fig. 4. Relative mRNA expression of genes encoding ECM proteins.

Relative mRNA expression was determined pre- and post-LVAD of DCM and IHD and tested in paired t-test. Increase of collagen 14α1 mRNA expression is significant in DCM but not in IHD. Compared to the control, only the mRNA expression pre-LVAD of IHD patients is significantly higher (unpaired t-test). Decorin is significantly increased post-LVAD in DCM. None of the pre- and post-LVAD samples differed significantly from the control samples.

5.1 Genes encoding extracellular matrix proteins

In DCM, 5 genes encoding ECM proteins were upregulated post-LVAD. However, except for collagen type VI alpha3, these genes did not differ significantly (either pre- or post LVAD) from control. This indicates that the increased expression of these 5 genes induced by the LVAD support is significant but as a group are not different from the control group (Figure 4). In IHD most differences between pre-LVAD and control were observed in genes encoding ECM proteins, but in post-LVAD samples these differences had disappeared, suggesting a high expression of ECM gene activity pre-LVAD (Figure 4).

Relative mRNA expression was determined pre- and post-LVAD of DCM and IHD and tested with the paired t-test. Increase of integrin α6 mRNA expression was significant in both DCM and IHD during LVAD support. Compared to the control, only the mRNA expression pre-LVAD of DCM patients is significantly lower (unpaired t-test). Integrin β6 is only significantly increased post-LVAD in the IHD group. Compared to the control none of the pre- and post-LVAD samples differed significantly.

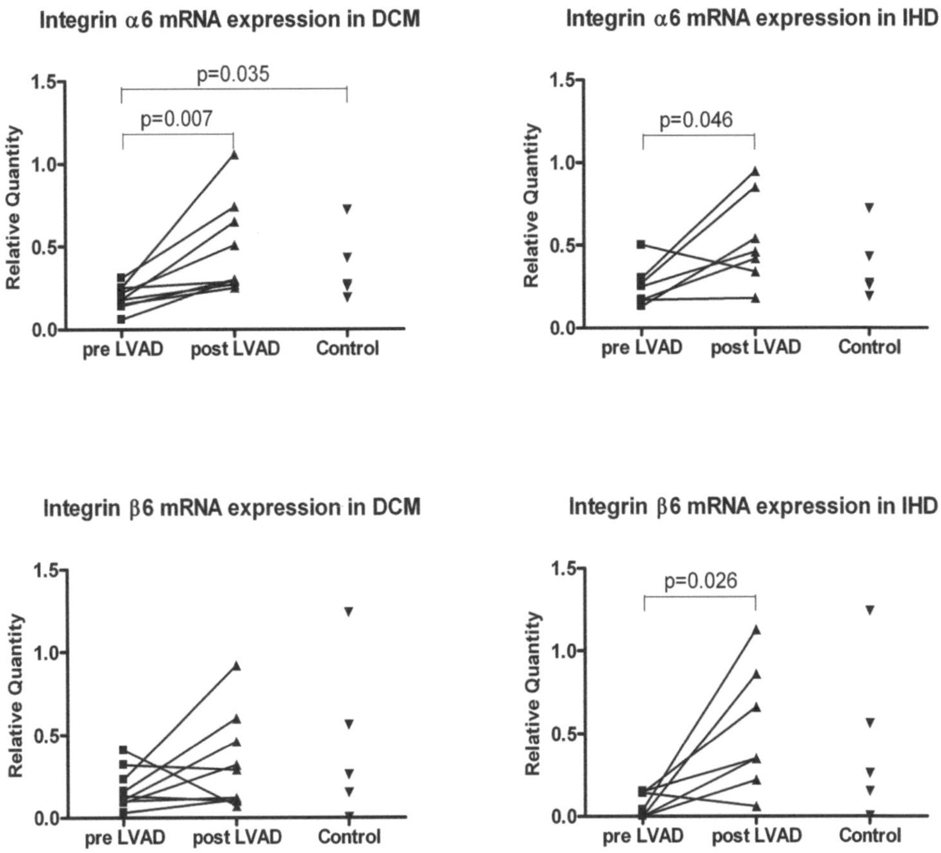

Fig. 5. Relative mRNA expression of genes encoding different integrins.

5.2 Genes involved in the fibrotic pathway

In the fibrotic pathway remarkable differences between DCM and IHD were observed. In DCM patients the expression of genes encoding pro-fibrotic factors (TGFβ1, FGF, IGF, endothelin and CTGF) remained unchanged, whereas the genes encoding anti-fibrotic proteins (BMP-4, BMP-7, decorin and ID1) increased after LVAD support. Pre-LVAD the expression of the pro-fibrotic factor FGF2 and the anti-fibrotic factor BMP-7 was low compared to control. Post-LVAD the expression of the anti-fibrotic factor BMP-4 was increased compared to control. However, in IHD patients these genes showed unchanged expression during LVAD support, but in pre-LVAD samples the pro-fibrotic genes are expressed stronger than in control and the anti-fibrotic gene BMP-7 is expressed less than in control. The post-LVAD expression pattern is comparable to that of control.

5.3 Genes encoding basal membrane proteins

The gene encoding osteopontin is the most remarkable member of the BM group. In both DCM and IHD patients, osteopontin expression is significantly reduced after LVAD

support. Other BM proteins showed hardly any change, apart from laminin, vitronectin and thrombospondin (anchoring proteins).
Several integrins showed differential expression (mostly upregulation) in both DCM and IHD patients. In particular, integrin β6 gene expression showed a strong increase after LVAD in the IHD group (Figure 5). Other membrane molecules, like caveolin, sarcoglycan and ATPase calcium transporting molecule, showed a low expression compared to control either pre- or post-LVAD.

5.4 Genes encoding intracellular proteins

Expression of some intracellular filament genes changed significantly after LVAD support in DCM (2/19: filamin, talin) and in IHD (1/19:desmoplakin), suggesting only a minor intracellular filament involvement. In this group it was remarkable that in IHD the gene encoding dystrophin was upregulated both pre- and post-LVAD.
Relatively many changes in the expression of signal transduction factors were observed after LVAD support both in DCM (2/8: Focal Adhesion Kinase and Ryanodine Receptor 2) and in IHD (4/8: catenin, myocyte enhancer factor 2A and 2C, and Ryanodine Receptor 2).

6. Changes in miR expression during LVAD support

Total RNA was isolated from heart tissue of heart failure patients pre- and post-LVAD. The relative quantities of miRNA1, miRNA133a, miRNA133b and miRNA-208 were established with the Taqman® MicroRNA assay (Applied Biosystems, Foster City, CA, USA). In Figure 6 the expression of miR-1, miR-133a and of miR133b is shown for DCM and IHD patients pre- and post-LVAD. Compared to control levels the miR expression in both heart failure groups was low for all miR tested. These low levels were more significant in IHD than in DCM. After LVAD support the levels did not change significantly, although in IHD there was a tendency that the miR expression levels return to normal. In patients with DCM we observed a tendency of further decrease. The expression of miR-208 showed similar changes (data not shown) as did the other three miRs. However, the expression was too low to make a reliable statistical analysis.

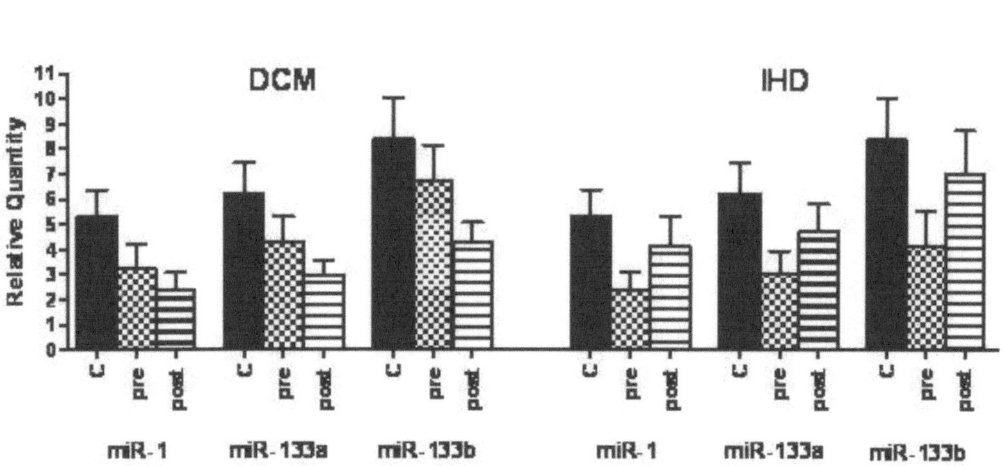

Fig. 6. Changes in miR expression after LVAD support

miR	DCM-patients			IHD-patients		
	1	2	3	1	2	3
miR-1	0.20	0.24	0.06	0.08	**0.05**	0.44
miR-133a	0.73	0.19	**0.04**	0.11	0.07	0.35
miR-133b	**0.02**	0.44	**0.04**	0.11	0.09	0.44

Table 4. Statistical analysis of miR expression changes after LVAD support.
The relative quantities of miR-1, miR-133a and miR-133b measured in heart tissue obtained from patients suffering from IHD (n= 8) or DCM (n=9) or C: controls (n=5; Pre = pre LVAD support ; Post= post LVAD support.
The p-values for the various differences in relative quantitative expression of the miRs in the myocardium obtained from DCM and IHD patients, respectively, before and after LVAD support. $P < 0.05$ is considered significant.
1: pre-LVAD versus post LVAD; 2: pre-LVAD versus control; 3: post LVAD versus control.

The results of the statistical analyses are presented in Table 4. These data confirm that in DCM patients, LVAD support did not increase the low miR-expression. In patients with IHD the values of expression of the miRs after LVAD support were not significantly different from those in the controls, indicating that there was a tendency of the low levels of miRs to increase after LVAD in IHD patients.

7. Discussion

During unloading, the myocardium of the failing heart shows various changes, both macroscopically and microscopically. Major changes include reduction of cardiomyocyte size, and changes in the volumes of ECM and BM components (Goldsmith and Borg, 202; Bruggink et al., 2006; Parker and Ingber, 2007). In many studies analyzing the effect of mechanical support on heart failure, only marginal differences have been observed between IHD and DCM (Bruggink et al., 2006a; De Jonge et al., 2001, 2002; Grady et al., 2003). However, in the present study hierarchical clustering of all expressed genes in end-stage heart failure showed that DCM and IHD segregated and could be identified as separated entities (Figure 2). For this reason both groups were analyzed separately. In the IHD group pre- and post-LVAD samples did segregate by hierarchical clustering (Figure 3). In the DCM group no such separation of pre- and post-LVAD samples was observed. The explanation for this difference between both groups is unknown. DCM may have a genetic background that leads primarily to hypertrophy and fibrosis, leading to gene expression that differs from controls in several aspects, but is not completely reversed by LVAD support. By contrast, in IHD, the gene expression alterations that are induced by infarction are partly normalized by the unloading of the heart. The differences in mRNA expression between IHD and DCM may give an important clue in finding targets that are informative for the state of the (un)supported hearts.
In pre-LVAD samples of DCM patients, the expression of only 7 genes (2 up- and 5 downregulated) differed from control which increased to 10 genes post-LVAD (7 up- and 3 down-regulated). In IHD pre-LVAD samples, the expression of 15 genes (13 up- and 2 down-regulated) differed from control, which decreased to 8 genes post-LVAD (7 up- and only 1 down-regulated). In both groups most genes that were differentially expressed pre-LVAD normalized to control levels after LVAD support. On the other hand, LVAD support can also induce a down- or upregulation of genes of which the pre-LVAD levels did not differ from

control level (Table 2). Eleven genes showed significant changes pre- and post-LVAD in both DCM and IHD. However, only 3 genes showed changes that were the same in DCM and IHD (calcium channel alpha 1C subunit, integrin-α11 and ryanodine receptor 2).

In DCM, the expression of caveolin remained low (both pre- and post-LVAD) compared to control. This is in contrast to the described up-regulation of caveolin protein after LVAD support (Uray et al., 2003). In IHD the expression of dystrophin and laminin (gamma 1) remained high after LVAD support. Changes in expression of both genes after LVAD have been described by others (Vatta et al., 2004; Birks et al., 2005; Refaat et al., 2008).

LVAD-induced changes in ECM and cardiomyocytes have been described by others as well (Milting et al., 2008; Bruggink et al 2006b; Thohan et al., 2005). In this respect, the total number of genes coding for various structural elements, that were differentially expressed pre- and post-LVAD was surprisingly low. Morphological changes during LVAD support were paralleled by changes in collagen turnover and expression of genes encoding for structural collagens (Type I and III; Bruggink et al, 2006b; 2007). So, the minor changes observed in expression of ECM genes in the present study may imply that most ECM changes are induced post-transcriptionally, either by micro-RNA regulation (Schipper et al., 2008) or in the matrix itself (e.g. by MMP). The latter is supported by significant changes in mRNA expression of MMP during LVAD support (Li et al., 2001; Klotz et al., 2005). Interestingly the anchoring and connecting collagens (types VI, XIV and XV) and molecules involved in ECM assembly like fibulin, fibronectin, osteonectin and proteoglycans (fibromodulin, heparan sulfate and decorin; Pollard et al., 2008) changed upon LVAD, although not similar in DCM and IHD patients. The LVAD-induced changes in the expression of these molecules, including collagen, also observed by others (Jahanyar et al., 2007; Gabrielsen et al., 2007), may contribute to the increased rigidity of the heart after LVAD support (Klotz et al., 2005).

Previously, we have shown that unloading of the left ventricle decreased the immunohistochemical expression of collagen IV in the BM (Bruggink et al., 2007). In contrast, immunoreactivity of laminin did not show substantial changes upon LVAD. Of the 17 tested genes that encode BM proteins only few showed expression changes after LVAD, indicating a dysbalance between mRNA expression and protein expression. The few genes that did show changes upon LVAD, either in DCM or IHD, are involved in cell-adhesion (laminin β1 and γ1, osteopontin). Together with the changes observed in the gene expression of the integrin, cadherin and sarcoglycan family members, these results underline the importance of these specific anchoring or connecting proteins in the structural changes observed (Birks et al.,2005; Gabrielsen et al., 2007; Latif et al., 2007; Kim et al.,1999).

Only minor changes were observed in the expression of genes encoding intracellular cytoskeleton proteins. In DCM, alterations after LVAD support in cytoskeletal filaments (dystrobrevin, filamin, junction plakoglobin, and talin) are more pronounced than in IHD (desmoplakin, dystrophin and talin; Gabrielsen et al., 2007). This could indicate that this class of genes is more affected in DCM than in IHD, which may be explained by the different onset of myocardial damage in both diseases.

In the fibrotic pathway a remarkable difference between DCM and IHD is observed. In DCM the expression of pro-fibrotic factors (TGFβ1, FGF, IGF, endothelin and CTGF) did not change upon LVAD support, but the expression of anti-fibrotic genes (BMP-4, BMP-7, decorin, and Id1) increased. This is paralleled by reduced fibrosis in DCM (Bruggink et al., 2006b). In patients with IHD the expression of both anti- and pro-fibrotic factors remain unchanged upon LVAD support. However, in IHD the pre-LVAD expression levels of the pro-fibrotic response genes are stronger than in control whereas the expression of the anti-fibrotic gene BMP-7 is lower than in control. This will favour fibrosis in the hearts of patients with IHD. In these patients, the post-LVAD situation may be associated with a return of gene expression to control values. This may lead to a reduction of fibrosis as is shown in various studies. So, pro- and anti-fibrotic gene expression is in agreement with previously described reduction of fibrosis after LVAD support (Goldsmith and Borg, 2002; Gabrielsen et al., 2007), although the mechanisms responsible differed between the two entities.

In view of the changes in mRNA expression that did not seem to be paralleled by corresponding protein expression, special emphasis was given to miR expression during LVAD support. These miRs are important in the post-transcriptional regulation of mRNAs, also in the heart (Chen, 2007; Couzin, 2008). The miRs tested (miR-1, miR-133a and miR133b) had relatively low expression in the myocardium of heart failure patients compared to controls. In IHD patients the level of miR expression tended to return to control levels upon LVAD support. In DCM, however, the miR expression levels tended to decrease even further, which suggests that genes under the control of these miRs could be expressed even stronger. Chen et al. (2006) have described that miR-1 and miR-133 promote skeletal muscle myogenesis and myoblast proliferation, respectively (Townley-Tilson et al, 2010). Similar data have been produced by Liu et al. (2007) and Ikeda et al. (2008) for the failing myocardium. The relatively low expression of miRs in the failing heart, compared to control, may be related to the presence of myocardial hypertrophy (De Jonge et al., 2002), as overexpression of both miR-1 and miR-133 leads to cardiac hypertrophy (Care et al., 2007).

This difference in miR expression between DCM and IHD patients after LVAD support may be explained by the lack of need for cell proliferation in DCM unlike in IHD where there is a need for cell proliferation. Remodeling of DCM involves mainly a reduction of hypertrophy of cardiomyocytes, whereas IHD involves tissue repair including cell proliferation. This may indicate that the studied miRs are primarily involved in regulation of proliferative processes rather than in reduction of hypertrophy. As already mentioned, the reduction in miRNA expression in IHD patients is not restored completely to control levels during LVAD support, not in patients supported for a short period of time nor in patients supported for more than over one year.

The miR data do show that myocardial expression of miRs changes upon heart failure (Busk and Cirera, 2010) and upon LVAD support. In that respect it is interesting to note that there are initial indications that miR released in the serum (Cheng et al. 2010) may act as biomarkers to screen for cardiac diseases (Adachi et al., 2010) and be targets for therapy (Seok and Wang, 2010).

In conclusion, the set of genes coding for proteins involved in mechanotransduction, selected for the analysis of changes in mRNA expression pre- and post-LVAD, resulted in an identification of IHD and DCM as separate entities. The morphologic and structural changes observed in the failing human heart upon LVAD support are only partly reflected in changes of mRNA expression of genes encoding proteins involved in mechanotransduction. This suggests that most changes in ECM and intracellular filaments are not regulated at the mRNA level. However, expression of genes encoding membrane-bound proteins such as cadherin and integrins, and anchoring proteins such as collagen type VI and proteoglycans, is clearly affected by LVAD support and contributes to adaptation to improved loading conditions. Also the genes involved in fibrosis showed adaptation to LVAD support, and their expression runs parallel to the observed morphological changes. These genes may prove to be important biomarkers in the development of protocols which decide whether LVAD supported patients should undergo heart transplantation, can be weaned from the device, or could rather continue their LVAD therapy for a longer period of time. The role of miR as biomarkers in this decision making, but also as therapeutic targets, is promising but still needs further investigation (Montgomery and van Rooij, 2010).

8. Acknowledgement

MFM van Oosterhout was supported by a grant from the Dutch Heart Foundation; project number 2004T31.

9. References

Adachi , T.; Nakanishi, M.; Otsuka, Y.; Nishimura, K.; Hirokawa, G.; Goto, Y.; Nonogi, H. & Iwai, N. (2010). Plasma microRNA 499 as a biomarker of acute myocardial infarction. *Clin Chem* 56(7), 1183-1185.

Birks, E.J.; Hall, J.L.; Barton, P.J.R.; Grindle, S.; Latif, N.; Hardy, J.P.; Rider, J.E.; Banner, N.R.; Khaghani, A.; Miller, L.W. & Yacoub, M.H. (2005). Gene profiling changes in cytoskeletal proteins during clinical recovery after left ventricular-assist device support. *Circulation* 112(9), 157-164.

Brower, G.L.; Gardner, J.D.; Forman, M.F.; Murray, D.B.; Voloshenyuk, T.; Levick, S.P.;.Janicki, J.S. (2006) The relationship between myocardial extracellular matrix remodeling and ventricular function. *Eur J Cardiothorac Surg* 30(4), 604-610.

Bruggink, A.H.; de Jonge, N.; van Oosterhout, M.F.; Van Wichen, D.F.; de Koning, E.; Lahpor, J.R.; Kemperman, H.; Gmelig-Meyling, F.H.J. & de Weger, R.A. (2006a). Brain natriuretic peptide is produced both by cardiomyocytes and cells infiltrating the heart in patients with severe heart failure supported by a left ventricular assist device. *J Heart Lung Transplant* 25(2), 174-80.

Bruggink, A.H.; van Oosterhout, M.F.; de Jonge, N.; Ivangh, B.; Van Kuik, J.; Voorbij, R.H.A.M.; Cleutjens, J.P.M.; Gmelig-Meyling, F.H.J. & de Weger, R.A. (2006b). Reverse remodeling of the myocardial extracellular matrix after prolonged left ventricular assist device support follows a biphasic pattern. *J Heart Lung Transplant* 25(9), 1091-1098.

Bruggink, A.H.; van Oosterhout, M.F.M.; de Jonge, N.; Cleutjens, J.P.M.; Van Wichen, D.F.; van Kuik, J.; Tilanus, M.G.J.; Gmelig-Meyling, F.H.J.; van den Tweel, J.G.; De Weger, R.A. (2007). Type IV collagen degradation in the myocardial basement membrane after unloading of the failing heart by a left ventricular assist device. *Lab Invest* 87(11), 1125-1137.

Bruggink, A.H.; van Oosterhout, M.F.; De Jonge, N.; Gmelig-Meyling, F.H.; De Weger, R.A. (2008). TNF alpha in patients with end-stage heart failure on medical therapy or supported by a left ventricular assist device. *Transpl Immunol* 19(1), 64-68.

Busk, P.K. & Cirera, S. (2010). MicroRNA profiling in early hypertrophic growth of the left ventricle in rats. *Biochem Biophys Res Commun* 396(4), 989-993.

Carè, A.; Catalucci, D.; Felicetti, F.; Bonci, D.; Addario, A.; Gallo, P.; Bang, M.-L.; Segnalini, P.; Gu Y.S.; Dalton, N.D.; Elia, L.; Latronico, M.V.G.; Hoydal, M.; Autore, C.; Russo, M.A.; Dorn, G.W.; Ellingsen, O.; Ruiz-Lozano, P.; Peterson, K.L.; Croce, C.M.;

Peschle, C. & Condorelli, G. (2007). MicroRNA-133 controls cardiac hypertrophy. *Nat Med* 13(5), 613-618.

Chen, J.F.; Mandel, E.M.; Thomson, J.M.; Wu, Q.L.; Callis, T.E.; Hammond, S.M.; Conlon, F.L. & Wang, D.Z. (2006). The role of microRNA-133 in skeletal muscle proliferation and differentiation. *Nat Genet* 38(2), 228-233.

Chen, K.R. (2007). MicroRNAs and the tell-tale heart. *Nature* 447(7144), 389-922.

Cheng, Y.; Ji, R.; Yue, J.; Yang, J.; Liu, X.; Chen, H.; Dean, D.B. & Zhang, C. (2007). MicroRNAs Are Aberrantly Expressed in Hypertrophic Heart: Do They Play a Role in Cardiac Hypertrophy? *Am J Pathol* 170 (4), 1831-1840.

Cheng, Y.H.; Tan, N.; Yang, J.A.; Liu, X.J.; Cao, X.P.; He, P.C.; Dong, X.L.; Qin, S.S & Zang, C.X. (2010). A translational study of circulating cell-free miRNA-1 in acuite myocardial infarction. *Clin Sc* 119 (1-2), 87-95.

Coutinho, L.L.; Matukumalli, L.K.; Sonstergard, T.S.; Van Tassell, C.P.; Gasbarre, L.C.; Capuco, A.V. & Smith, T.P.L. (2007). Discovery and profiling of bovine microRNAs from immune-related and embryonic tissues. *Physiol Genomics* 29(1), 35-43.

Couzin, J. (2008). MicroRNAs make big impression in disease after disease. *Science* 319(5871), 1782-1784.

De Jonge, N.; Kirkels, H.; Lahpor, J.R.; Klopping, C.; Hulzebos, E.J.; de la Riviere, A.B. & de Medina, E.O.R. (2001). Exercise performance in patients with end stage heart failure after implantation of a left ventricular assist device and after heart transplantation: an outlook for permanent assisting? *J Am Coll Cardiol* 37(7), 1794-1799.

De Jonge, N.; Van Wichen, D.F.; Schipper, M.E.; Lahpor, J.R.; Gmelig-Meyling, F.H.J.; de Medina, E.O. & De Weger, R.A. (2002). Left ventricular assist device in end-stage heart failure: persistence of structural myocyte damage after unloading. An immunohistochemical analysis of the contractile myofilaments. *J Am Coll Cardiol* 39(6),963-969.

De Weger, R. & De Jonge, N. (2009). Editorial comment heart transplantation. *Curr Opin Organ Transplant* 14(5), 552-553.

Estrada-Quintero, T.; Uretsky, B.F.; Murali, S.; Griffith, B.P. & Kormos, R.L. (1995). Neurohormonal activation and exercise function in patients with severe heart failure and patients with left ventricular assist system. A comparative study. *Chest* 107(6), 1499-1503.

Frazier, O.H. & Myers, T.J. (1999). Left ventricular assist system as a bridge to myocardial recovery. *Ann Thorac Surg* 68(2), 734-41.

Gabrielsen, A. ; Lawler, P.R. ; Wang, Y.Z. ; Steinbruchel, D.; Blagoja, D.; Paulsson-Berne, G.; Kastrup, J. & Hansson, G.K. (2007). Gene expression signals involved in ischemic injury, extracellular matrix composition and fibrosis defined by global mRNA profiling of the human left ventricular myocardium. *J Mol Cell Cardiol* 42(4), 870-883.

Goldsmith, E.C. & Borg, T.K. (2002). The dynamic interaction of the extracellular matrix in cardiac remodeling. *J Card Fail* 8(6), S314-S318.

Grady, K.L.; Meyer, P.M.; Mattea, A.; Dressler, D.; Ormaza, S.; White-Williams, C.; Chillcott, S.; Kaan, A.; Loo, A.; Todd, B.; Klemme, A.; Piccione, W. & Costanzo, M.R. (2003). Change in quality of life from before to after discharge following left ventricular assist device implantation. *J Heart Lung Transplant* 22(3) 322-333.

Ikeda, S.; Kong, S.W.; Lu, J.; Bisping, E.; Zhang, H.; Allen, P.D.; Golub, T.R.; Pieske, B. & Pu, W.T. (2007). Altered microRNA expression in human heart disease. *Physiol Genom* 31(3), 367-373.

Jahanyar, J. ; Joyce, D.L. ; Southard, R.E. ; Loebe, M.; Noon, G.P.; Koerner, M.M.; Torre-Amione, G.& Youker, K.A. (2007). Decorin-mediated transforming growth factor-beta inhibition ameliorates adverse cardiac remodeling. *J Heart Lung Transplant* 26(1), 34-40.

Ji, R.R.; Cheng,Y.H.; Yue, J.M.; Yang, J.; Liu, X.; Chen, H.; Dean, D.B. & Zhang, C.X. (2007). croRNA expression signature and antisense-mediated depletion reveal an essential role for microRNA in vascular neointimal lesion formation. *Circ Res* 100(11), 1579-1588.

Kemperman, H.; van den Berg, M.; Kirkels, H. & De Jonge, N. (2004). B-type natriuretic peptide (BNP) and N-terminal proBNP in patients with end-stage heart failure supported by a left ventricular assist device. *Clin Chem* 50(9), 1670-1672.

Kim, H.; Yoon, C.S. & Rah, B. (1999). Expression of extracellular matrix components fibronectin and laminin in the human fetal heart. *Cell Struct Funct* 24(1), 19-26.

Klotz, S.; Foronjy, R.F.; Dickstein, M.L.;Garrelds, I.M.; Danser, A.H.J.; Oz, M.C.; D'Armiento, J. & Burkhoff, D. (2005). Mechanical unloading during left ventricular assist device support increases left ventricular collagen cross-linking and myocardial stiffness. *Circulation* 112(3), 364-374.

Latif, N.; Yacoub, M.H.; George, R.; Barton, P.J. & Birks EJ. (2007). Changes in sarcomeric and non-sarcomeric cytoskeletal proteins and focal adhesion molecules during clinical myocardial recovery after left ventricular assist device support. *J Heart Lung Transplant* 26(3), 230-235.

Li, Y.Y. ; Feng, Y.Q.; McTiernan, C.F. ; Moravec, C.S.; Wang, P.; Rosenblum, W.; Kormos, R.L. & Feldman, A.M. (2001). Downregulation of matrix metalloproteinases and reduction in collagen damage in the failing human heart after support with left ventricular assist devices. *Circulation* 104(10), 1147-1152.

Liu, N.; Williams, A.H.; Kim, Y.; McAnally, J.; Bezprozvannaya, S.; Sutherland, L.B.; Richardson, J.A.; Bassel-Duby, R. & Olson, E.N. (2007). An intragenic MEF-2 dependent enhancer directs muscle-specific expression of microRNAs 1 and 133. *Proc Nat Acad Sci USA* 104(52), 20844-20849.

Markham, D.W. & Hill, J.A. (2010). MicroRNAs and heart failure diagnosis: MiR-acle or MiR-age?. *Circ Res* 106 (4), 1011-1013.

Milting, H.; Ellinghaus, P.; Seewald, M.; Cakar, H.; Bohms, B.; Kassner, A.; Koerfer, R.; Klein, M.; Krahn, T.; Kruska, L.; El Banayosy, A.. & Kramer, F. (2008). Plasma biomarkers of myocardial fibrosis and remodeling in terminal heart failure patients supported by mechanical circulatory support devices. *J Heart Lung Transplant* 27(6), 589-596.

Montgomery, R.L. & Van Rooij, E (2010). MicroRNA regulation as a therapeutic strategy for cardiovascular disease. *Curr Drug Targets* 11 (8), 936-942.

Muller, J.; Wallukat, G.; Weng, Y.G.; Dandel, M.; Spiegelsberger, S.; Semrau, S.; Brandes, K.; Theodoridis, V.; Loebe, M.; Meyer, R. & Hetzer, R. (1997). Weaning from mechanical cardiac support in patients with idiopathic dilated cardiomyopathy. *Circulation* 96(2), 542-549.

Parker, K.K. & Ingber, D.E. (2007). Extracellular matrix, mechanotransduction and structural hierarchies in heart tissue engineering. *Philos Trans R Soc Lond B Biol Sci.* 362(1484), 1267-1279.

Pollard, T.D. & Earnshaw, W.C. (2008). Section VIII Cellular adhesion and the extracellular matrix. In: *Cell Biology*, Philadelphia, Saunders Elsevier, pp 513-598.

Refaat, M.; Chemaly, E.; Lebeche, D.; Gwathmey, J.K. & Hajjar, R.J. (2008). Ventricular arrhythmias after left ventricular assist device implantation. *Pacing Clin Electrophysiol* 31(10), 1246-1252.

Schipper, M.E.; van Kuik, J.; de Jonge, N.; Dullens, H.F. & De Weger, R.A. (2008). Changes in regulatory microRNA expression in myocardium of heart failure patients on left ventricular assist device support. *J Heart Lung Transplant* 27(12), 1282-1285.

Schuldt, A. (2010). Great expectations of small RNAs. Nature Revs Mol Cell Biol 11, 27.

Seok, H.Y. & Wang, D.Z. (2010). The emerging role of microRNAs as a therapeutic target for cardiovascular disease. *Biodrugs* 24(3), 147-155.

Spinale, F.G. (2002). Matrix metalloproteinases: regulation and dysregulation in the failing heart. *Circ Res* 90(4), 520-530.

Stamenkovic, I. (2003). Extracellular matrix remodelling: the role of matrix metalloproteinases. *J Pathol* 200(4), 448-464.

Thohan, V.; Stetson, S.J.; Nagueh, S.F.; Rivas-Gotz, C.; Koerner, M.M.; Lafuente, J.A.; Loebe, M.; Noon, G.P. & Torre-Amione, G. (2005). Cellular and hemodynamics responses of failing myocardium to continuous flow mechanical circulatory support using the DeBakey-Noon left ventricular assist device: A comparative analysis with pulsatile-type devices. *J Heart Lung Transplant* 24(5), 566-575.

Townley-Tilson, W.H.D.; Callis, T.E. & Wang, D.Z. (2010). MicroRNAs 1, 133, and 206: Critical factors of skeletal and cardiac muscle development, function and disease. *Int. J. Biochem. Cell Biol* 42 (8), 1252-1255.

Uray, I.P.; Connelly, J.H. & Frazier, O.H.; Taegtmeyer, H. & Davies, P.J. (2003). Mechanical unloading increases caveolin expression in the failing human heart. *Cardiovasc Res* 59(1), 57-66.

Van Rooij, E.; Sutherland, L.B.; Liu, N.; Williams, A.H.; McAnally, J.; Gerard, R.D.; Richardson, J.A. & Olson, E.N. (2006). A signature pattern of stress responsive microRNAs that can evoke cardiac hypertrophy and heart failure. *Proc Natl Acad Sci USA* 103(48), 18255-60.

Vatta, M,; Stetson, S.J.; Jimenez, S.; Entman, M.L.; Noon, G.P.; Bowles, N.E.; Towbin, J.A. & Torre-Amione, G. (2004). Molecular normalization of dystrophin in the failing left and right ventricle of patients treated with either pulsatile or continuous flow-type ventricular assist devices . *J Am Coll Cardiol* 43(3), 811-817.

Part 4

Types of Ventricular Assist Device

4

Ventricular Assist Device – How to Obtain Optimal Benefits?

Agata Bielecka-Dabrowa[1], Maciej Banach[1], Jacek Rysz[2] and Gerry O'Driscoll[3]
[1]Department of Hypertension, Chair of Nephrology and Hypertension, Medical University of Lodz
[2]Department of Nephrology, Hypertension and Family Medicine, Chair of Nephrology and Hypertension, Medical University of Lodz
[3]Department of Heart Failure and Cardiac Transplant Service, Royal Perth Hospital,
[1,2]Poland
[3]Western Australia

1. Introduction

Heart failure is now acknowledged to be the most common malignant disease in industrialized countries, with advanced heart failure having a worse prognosis than most forms of cancer (Garg, Yusuf 1993). Advances in pharmacological treatment have helped patients in all stages of systolic dysfunction, even those with NYHA IV symptoms (the Captopril-Digoxin Multicenter Research Group 1988, Packer et al. 1996, the RALES Investigators 1996). The Working Group on Heart Failure of the European Society of Cardiology has promoted a number of initiatives aimed at improving the treatment of heart failure (ESC guidelines for the diagnosis and treatment of acute and chronic heart failure 2008).

Despite advances in pharmacological treatments aimed at a neurohormonal blockade for heart failure, there is still a growing number of patients with advanced symptoms who suffer significant morbidity and mortality.

Mechanical stresses on the myocardium (increased preload and afterload) and chronic neurohormonal activation conspire to propagate the maladaptive ventricular remodeling responsible for the insidious nature of heart failure. Recent studies suggest that further pharmacological neurohormonal blockade may be neither safe nor effective (Mann 2004). This finding has led to the concept that the limit to which neurohormonal and cytokine mechanisms can be blocked in heart failure patients has already been reached (Cohn, Tognoni 2001). The problem of how to treat patients worldwide who develop advanced heart failure despite optimal medical therapy has not yet been resolved (Gronda, Vitali 1999).

Transplantation provides the most effective therapy for this condition, but the shortage of donor organs results in <10% of potential recipients actually receiving a transplant (Deng et al. 2001). This situation has forced scientists to search for alternative methods of treatment.

At present end-stage chronic heart failure is a significant clinical problem as well as a subject of scientific interest. Transplant candidates whose disease reaches its final stage before an appropriate donor heart becomes available might be considered eligible for temporary or permanent mechanical circulatory support (MCS). This is why ventricular assist devices (VADs) capable of completely supporting the circulation are taking on an increasingly important role in heart failure therapy. The concept of circulatory assistance is not new. The need for such temporary support for hours or days has been recognized for over 60 years and still exists (Norman 1974). It is recognized that device-based approaches, ranging from the use of devices for monitoring patient status in order to anticipate exacerbation of congestive heart failure and preemptively adjust therapy to the application of devices for supporting pre-terminal patients with end-stage disease, will assume an increasingly important role in treating the growing number of patients with advanced heart failure (Kantrowitz et al. 1968). Mechanical circulatory support was first used clinically in 1953 with the implementation of cardiopulmonary bypass (Gibbon 1954). This breakthrough led to numerous surgical treatments for a variety of cardiac disorders. The success of cardiopulmonary bypass stimulated research into other innovative techniques for supporting the circulation. Counterpulsation with the intra-aortic balloon pump (IABP) was first applied clinically in 1967 to support patients with acute heart failure (Kantrowitz et al. 1968). From 1953 congestive heart failure patients were occasionally supported temporarily by cardiopulmonary bypass (Dennis 1966), an implantable ventricular assist device (VAD) (De Bakey et al. 1966) or a totally artificial heart (TAH) (Cooley et al. 1969). Although the overall success rate was limited, this early experience did prove that mechanical circulatory support could adequately sustain a patient's circulation until cardiac function recovered or a donor heart could be obtained. In the early 1980s the introduction of cyclosporine-based immunosuppression allowed heart transplantation to become a widely accepted therapeutic alternative. During the same decade clinical trials were initiated to evaluate the safety and efficacy of MCS systems in supporting terminally ill transplant candidates until a suitable donor heart could be found. VADs are important bridges to cardiac transplantation. The Randomized Evaluation of Mechanical Assistance for the Treatment of Congestive Heart Failure (REMATCH) trial revealed that they could be used as long-term destination therapy for non-transplant candidates (Rose et al., 1999). The use of a wearable ventricular assist device (VAD) in the treatment of advanced heart failure has steadily increased since 1993, when these devices became generally available. Since this time there has been rapid progress in the development of left ventricular assist device technology and artificial hearts.

2. VADs — indications for support

Patients with end-stage heart failure have a poor quality of life, a very high mortality rate, and are potential candidates for implantation of a ventricular assist device (VAD). Although cardiac transplantation (CTX) is associated with high 1- and 10-year survival rates, organ supply is limited. The technical improvements and proven success of implantable VADs have made it a reasonable treatment option in these patients, either as a bridge to cardiac transplantation or as destination therapy - Table 1 (2010 Focused Update of ESC guidelines on device therapy in heart failure).

Mechanical circulatory support is life saving in patients who fail to improve or stabilize with intravenous inotropes or vasodilators, IABP support and mechanical ventilation.

Hemodynamic criteria for VAD insertion are as follows (Oz et al., 1995):

- cardiac index < 2 L/min/m2;
- systolic blood pressure < 90 mm Hg;
- pulmonary capillary wedge > 20 mm Hg;
- urine output < 20 mL/h;

when these are found despite pharmacological support, optimal fluid loading and use of IABP as appropriate.

Patient selection for VAD is crucial. Most patients are on continuous inotropic support. Patients with severe renal, pulmonary, or hepatic dysfunction as well as patients with active infection, carcinoma with metastases, significant blood dyscrasias, cerebral vascular disease or cardiogenic shock should not be considered as candidates (Lund et al., 2010).

Each case is assessed individually and criteria are used as a guide only. Some patients have the VAD inserted prior to these criteria being met. In planning the application of the assist device we must decide whether one or both ventricles require support. Insertion of an implantable VAD complicated by early right ventricular failure has a poor prognosis and is largely unpredictable. Patients with risk factors for right ventricle dysfunction (the need for circulatory support, female gender, non-ischemic etiology) may best be treated with a biventricular assist device or a TAH. The next questions arising are whether the VAD should be implanted as a bridge to transplantation or as destination therapy and how long mechanical support will be required. Selection of the appropriate device depends on a number of considerations, including the anticipated duration of patient support, the need for right-side support and the patient's size. Excluding the strict contraindications to VAD, insertion is very important.

Recommendations	Patient population	Class of recommendation	Level of evidence
LVAD may be considered as destination treatment to reduce mortality	NYHA functional class IIIB/IV LVEF≤25% Peak VO_2<14 mL/kg/min	IIb	B

LVAD = left ventricular assist device; LVEF = left ventricular ejection fraction; NYHA = New York Heart Association.

Table 1. Recommendation in patients with severe heart failure ineligible for transplant (2010 Focused Update of ESC guidelines on device therapy in heart failure).

One recent study was conducted in 200 patients, who were randomized in a 2:1 ratio to a continuous-flow device (HeartMate I) or a pulsatile device (Slaughter et al., 2009) as destination therapy. Patients were in NYHA function class IIIB/IV with an LVEF of ≤25%. A peak VO_2 of ≤14 mL/kg/min was an inclusion criterion in HEART MATE II but gas-exchange data during exercise are not routinely available in clinical practice and may be inconclusive. The primary composite endpoint was, at 2 years, freedom from disabling stroke or reoperation to repair or replace the device. Secondary endpoints included actuarial survival. The mean age of the patients was 64 years, and the mean left ventricular ejection fraction was 17%. The primary endpoint was achieved in more patients with the continuous-flow device (46 vs. 11%, $P < 0.001$) and actuarial survival at 2 years was higher (58 vs. 24%, $P = 0.008$). Another study examined 281 patients in whom the continuous device was implanted as a bridge to cardiac transplantation (Pagani et al., 2009). After 18 months, 222 patients (79%) underwent cardiac transplantation, left ventricular assist device removal for cardiac recovery, or required ongoing LVAD support (Drews et al., 2010). The INTERMACS registry, an National Institutes of Health (NIH)-supported initiative, demonstrates that in practice ~10% of patients receiving an LVAD are not considered candidates for CTX at the time of implantation (Kirklin et al., 2010).

3. Patient selection and preoperative considerations

The highest risk of death after ventricular assist device implantation is before hospital discharge. Thus, patient selection and the timing of implantation are two of the major determinants of success. Main selection criteria include assessment of the patient's severity of illness and ability to successfully undergo the implant procedure. Preoperative selection criteria which predict successful outcome are difficult to evaluate. The selection of appropriate candidates with a potentially good outcome is of major importance in VAD implantation.

Patients are assessed for appropriateness for LVAD support based on the degree of illness, ability to successfully undergo the operative procedure and ability to be discharged home with adequate family/caregiver support for long-term success. Mortality rates are high after implantation of a ventricular assist device, occurring mainly in the early phase post-implant during the time in the intensive care unit.

4. Patient assessment before LVAD support

The Heart Failure Survival Score (Aaronson et al., 1997) and the Seattle Heart Failure Model (Levy et al., 2006) estimate a heart failure patient's expected survival during the next 1 to 2 years on medical management and identify patients at high risk of death who might benefit from LVAD support.

The Interagency Registry for Mechanically Assisted Circulatory Support (INTERMACS) registry, which follows all long-term mechanical circulatory support systems in the United States, has defined patient profiles that can help identify risks associated with the timing of implantation (Holman et al., 2009; Stevenson et al., 2009) - Table 2. The current 6-month survival data for patients receiving pulsatile LVADs indicate that patients in profile 1, cardiogenic shock, have the lowest survival, and those in profile 3, stable on inotropes, have the best survival (Kirklin et al., 2010).

These data indicate that patients with cardiogenic shock may be too sick for permanent LVAD support. Thus, for these patients, consideration should be given to immediate stabilization with biventricular support, using temporary percutaneous or surgically placed systems or other appropriate treatments, to optimize their condition before implant surgery. This is especially true for the destination therapy indication because most patients can be stabilized and their risks assessed and reduced before implantation. Implantation of a long-term LVAD should not be considered for patients with irreversible major end-organ failure, uncertain neurological status, severe hemodynamic instability, major coagulopathy, prolonged need for mechanical ventilation, sepsis, or right-heart failure (Slaughter et al. 2010).

Profile	Description	Time to MCS
1	"Crashing and burning"—critical cardiogenic shock	Within hours
2	"Progressive decline"—inotrope dependence with continuing deterioration.	Within a few days
3	"Stable but inotrope dependent"—describes clinical stability on mild-to-moderate doses of intravenous inotropes (patients stable on temporary circulatory support without inotropes are within this profile).	Within a few weeks
4	"Recurrent advanced heart failure"—"recurrent" rather than "refractory" decompensation	Within weeks to months
5	"Exertion intolerant"—describes patients who are comfortable at rest but are exercise intolerant.	Variable
6	"Exertion limited"—describes a patient who is able to do some mild activity but fatigue results within a few minutes of any meaningful physical exertion.	Variable
7	"Advanced NYHA III"—describes patients who are clinically stable with a reasonable level of comfortable activity, despite a history of previous decompensation that is not recent.	Not a candidate for MCS
INTERMACS, Interagency Registry for Mechanically Assisted Circulatory Support; MCS, mechanical circulatory support; NYHA, New York Heart Association.		

Table 2. INTERMACS Patient Profiles and Timeframe for Initiating Mechanical Circulatory Support (Holman et al., 2009; Slaughter et al. 2010).

5. Risk factors for operative mortality

Lietz and Miller (Lietz et al., 2007) analyzed preoperative clinical data from 222 patients who received the HeartMate XVE LVAD for destination therapy. They established a risk scoring system to estimate survival after implantation. The multivariate analysis produced 9 risk factors for 90-day mortality, which were assigned a weighted score (Table 3). The cumulative scores for each patient were then used to determine the risk category: 0 to 8, low risk; 9 to 16, medium risk; 17 to 19, high risk; and >19 very high risk. The survival to hospital discharge was 87.5%, 70.5%, 26%, and 13.7% for the low-, medium-, high-, and very high-risk groups, respectively.

Risk factor	Score
Platelet count < 148 x $10^3/\mu L$	7
Serum albumin < 3.3 g/dL	5
International normalization ratio > 1.1	4
Vasodilator therapy	4
Mean pulmonary artery pressures < 25 mm Hg	3
Aspartate aminotransferase > 45 U/mL	2
Hematocrit < 34%	2
Blood urea nitrogen > 51 mg/dL	2
No intravenous inotropes	2

Table 3. Risk Factors for 90-Day Mortality and the Weighted Scores (Lietz et al., 2007)

In 1995, Oz et al. found 7 preoperative factors that predicted poor outcome in a group of 56 patients. These consisted of urine output <30 mL/h, central venous pressure >16 mm Hg, mechanical ventilation, prothrombin time (PT) >16 seconds, re-operation, leukocyte count >15,000/mm^3 and temperature >101.5°F. However, they used only a first-generation device and prediction of urine output <30 mL/h takes at least 1 hour (Oz et al. 1995).

Therefore, this score was revised by Rao et al. based on 130 patients and more easily obtained and quickly accessible parameters (ventilation, post-cardiotomy, pre-VAD, CVP >16 mm Hg, prothrombin time > 16 seconds) (Rao et al. 2003). In 2001, Deng et al. reviewed the Novacor registry data in 464 patients and highlighted 5 parameters - respiratory failure with septicemia, preexisting right heart failure, age >65 years, acute post-cardiotomy, and acute infarction - predicting mortality during VAD support (Deng et al., 2001). In 2004, Chen et al. showed that lactate, and lung and kidney injury are predictive of poor outcome among patients on extracorporeal membrane oxygenation (ECMO) support that was switched to VAD support (Chen et al., 2004). In addition, some studies showed that predictors of poor outcome were similar in total artificial heart or biventricular VAD implantation as compared with VAD implantation. Scientists also tried to use existing intensive care scores, such as the APACHE II score, to predict VAD mortality (Gracin et al., 1998). However, these already existing scores, which attempt to predict mortality after VAD implantation, are based on first-generation pulsatile devices and not on modern second- or third-generation devices, and they assess overall death after VAD as the primary outcome. They do not specifically focus on mortality in the intensive care unit, which is especially dependent on preoperative clinical status. Klotz et al. implemented a pre-operative risk score to predict mortality in the intensive care unit after VAD implantation by using easily obtained and quickly accessible clinical parameters (Klotz et al., 2010).

By focusing on mortality in the intensive care unit, they tried to evaluate preoperative patients who were too sick for mechanical support and may not have survived their stay in the ICU. In 241 VAD patients, 100 preoperative markers were related to mortality in the ICU using univariate analysis and ROC curves, followed by multinomial logistic regression analyses. The mortality rate in the ICU was 32.0%.

The parameters with the highest negative impact on survival in the ICU were: age>50 years, ischemic cardiomyopathy, re-do surgery, on ECMO, on IABP, previous cardiac surgery, ventilation, emergency implant, inotropic support, renal replacement therapy, preoperative resuscitation, transfusion, blood urea nitrogen >40 mg/L, creatinine>1.5 mg/dL, lactate >3 mg/dL, platelets <100 x 1000/μL, whole blood cell count >13,000/μL, C-reactive protein > 8 mg/dL, hemoglobin <12 g/dL, hematocrit <35%, lactate dehydrogenase >500 U/liter, creatinine kinase>200 U/liter, troponin >20 ng/mL.

The risk for mortality in the intensive care unit was as follows: low <15 points, medium 16-30 points, high >30 points.

This score distinguishes clearly between the different urgencies of VAD implantation - Figure 1.

These observations suggest that in-hospital mortality can be predicted preoperatively with easily obtained and quickly accessible parameters. Patients who initially present as high-risk or very high-risk are most likely to benefit from a period of optimization therapy to attempt to lower their risk score (for example: coagulation, nutrition, renal function, right atrial pressure) and then become more suitable candidates for LVAD support. Patients with a low risk should be considered for prompt elective LVAD implantation before their condition worsens.

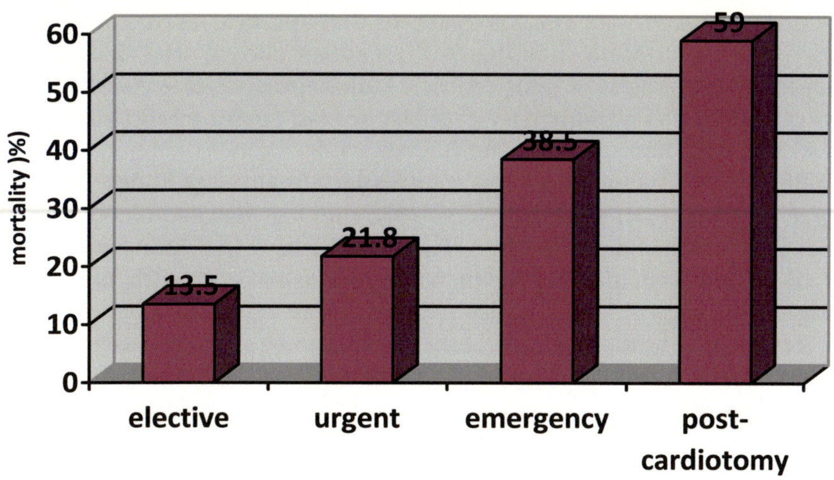

Fig. 1. Mortality in the ICU, depending on VAD implant urgency. Post-cardiotomy is defined as patients with unsuccessful weaning from bypass and on ECMO support.

Pre-implant optimization of comorbid conditions is very important in minimizing the incidence and severity of postoperative adverse events and for enhancing survival. The most influential pre-implant measures are:

- **Improving nutritional status**

Malnutrition is very common in patients with advanced heart failure. If not improved, it increases the risk of infection, decreases the body's ability to recover after surgery, and is generally associated with poor outcomes. Studies have shown that cachexia (BMI <22 kg/m^2) is associated with a high risk for peri-operative death, often due to infection (Manop et al., 2009; Holdy et al., 2005).

Markers of severe malnutrition include a BMI <20 kg/m^2, albumin <3.2 mg/dL, pre-albumin <15 mg/dL, total cholesterol <130 mg/dL, lymphocyte count <100, and purified protein derivative skin test anergy. The nutrition needs to be improved before LVAD implantation (a pre-albumin level >15 mg/dL). For patients with pre-albumin <15 mg/dL, enteral feedings are often helpful preoperatively and should be continued after implantation until the patient is taking adequate nutrition.

It is equally important to maintain adequate nutrition after the implant surgery. Data from Lockard et al. have shown that patients with a pre-albumin level of <15 mg/dL at 2 weeks after LVAD implantation had a significantly greater risk of dying in the hospital (Lockard et al., 2009).

- **Lowering pulmonary vascular resistance to optimize right-heart function and to reduce right atrial pressure and secondary hepatic congestion**

Left ventricular unloading with a LVAD should decrease right ventricular after-load by reducing pulmonary artery pressures (PAPs) (Farrar et al. 1985).

However, mechanical support may increase systemic venous return to a myopathic right heart that is unable to accommodate the additional volume. Furthermore, reduction in left ventricle pressure can cause the interventricular septum to shift leftward, potentially causing disadvantageous geometric changes in the right ventricle that reduce the septal contribution to right ventricle stroke volume and exacerbate tricuspid regurgitation (Farrar et al. 1985). Importantly, right ventricle failure after implantation can be anticipated preoperatively and improved with various therapies that optimize its function. An analysis of 484 patients in the HeartMate II Bridge to Transplant clinical trial demonstrated the following independent predictors of right ventricle failure: preoperative ventilatory support, central venous pressure (CVP)/pulmonary capillary wedge pressure ratio >0.63, and blood urea nitrogen >39 mg/dL (Kormos et al., 2010).

Univariate predictors also included a right ventricular stroke work index (RVSWI) <300 mm Hg × mL/m^2, central venous pressure (CVP) >15 mm Hg, elevated blood urea nitrogen (BUN), and elevated white blood cell count. The HeartMate II trial found no difference in the incidence of right ventricular failure in heart failure patients with non-ischemic vs ischemic etiology.

Other signs of poor right ventricle function can be found with pre-implant echocardiography. Close attention should be paid to RV size, with particular caution extended to patients who have a dilated, poorly contracting right ventricle. Severe tricuspid regurgitation also can be associated with early postoperative RV failure. Some have advocated repair of the tricuspid regurgitation at the time of LVAD implantation if its severity is judged to be more than moderate, either preoperatively or intraoperatively by echocardiogram.

Patients at risk for postoperative right ventricle failure should not necessarily be eliminated from LVAD support. However, the implanting team should promptly treat RV failure using pharmacotherapeutics and mechanical RV support, as appropriate or needed (Slaughter et al. 2010).

- **Aggressively managing volume to minimize right ventricular workload and hepatic congestion**

A pulmonary artery catheter 24 hours before implantation is useful in most patients to assess the cardiac index and volume status as well as to guide diuretic, vasodilator, and inotropic support. One of the main objectives is to reduce the central venous pressure (CVP) to 15 mm Hg or less. This will aid in reducing the right ventricle workload and minimizing hepatic congestion and the possible need for a right ventricular assist device (RVAD). When the CVP exceeds 20 mm Hg, ultrafiltration and inotrope and vasodilator therapy should be used; also consider temporary RVAD support. Increasing the cardiac index with vasodilators, inotropes, and using an IABP will improve conditions for all organ systems. Medications that can lower pulmonary vascular resistance (PVR) and improve the cardiac index before surgery may be beneficial in reducing the incidence of right ventricular failure after implantation (Galie et al., 2005; Klodell et al., 2007).

Medications that have been shown to reduce PVR include angiotensin-converting enzyme (ACE) inhibitors, hydralazine, nitroglycerin, nitroprusside, nitric oxide, sildenafil, prostaglandins, and inotropes (milrinone and dobutamine).

- **Optimizing coagulation**

Preoperative abnormal coagulation is common in heart failure patients due to hepatic dysfunction and the use of anticoagulant or antiplatelet medications. When possible, these medications should be stopped before implantation. Vitamin K may be given to reverse the effects of warfarin. For patients who are at high risk of preoperative thrombosis, a continuous infusion of heparin should be given. Because the continuous-flow left ventricular assist device requires systemic anticoagulation, its use in patients with a history of gastrointestinal (GI) bleeding should be carefully considered. Active GI blood loss should be assessed for 3 to 4 weeks before left ventricular assist device implantation (Slaughter et al. 2010).

- **Optimizing renal, hepatic, pulmonary and neurological function**

Renal dysfunction is a predictor of adverse outcomes in LVAD-supported patients (Sandner et al., 2009; Ma et al., 2008; Butler at al. 2006). Patients in the HeartMate II Bridge to Transplant trial were excluded if their creatinine level was <3.5 mg/dL or if they needed chronic dialysis; 11% of patients had some degree of renal dysfunction after implantation (Miller et al., 2007).

Optimizing renal function preoperatively entails measures to increase renal perfusion and reduce central venous pressure. Renal dysfunction generally improves after LVAD implantation if decreased glomerular filtration rate is due to low cardiac output before implantation.

Liver dysfunction is associated with greater need for intraoperative and perioperative blood transfusion, which can result in worsened right-heart function and the need for RVAD support. Many centers screen patients with clinical evidence of significant right heart failure or serological evidence of hepatic dysfunction using hepatic ultrasound imaging or liver biopsy to rule out cirrhosis.

As with renal function, there is evidence that hepatic function improves after implantation of a continuous-flow LVAD (Radovancevic et al., 2007; Letsou et al., 2003).

Specific management strategies should be initiated to improve hepatic function before an LVAD is implanted in individuals with abnormal values for prothrombin time (PT), partial thromboplastin time (PTT), and international normalized ratio (INR). Right heart pressure and pulmonary vascular resistance should be decreased using combinations of drugs to reduce pre-load and after-load, ultrafiltration, or both.

Patients with severe obstructive or restrictive pulmonary disease are not eligible for LVAD therapy. When pulmonary function testing can be performed reliably, and the forced vital capacity, forced expiratory volume at 1 second, and carbon monoxide diffusing capacity are all less than 50%, exclusion from LVAD implantation should be considered.

Patients with neurological or psychiatric disease that compromises their ability to use and care for external system components, or to ambulate and exercise, are not appropriate candidates for LVAD support (Tylus-Earl et al. 2009).

Psychiatric disorders, drug abuse, and other psychosocial issues must be investigated to assess the patient's ability to understand and comply with care instructions.

All patients with an audible bruit or peripheral arterial disease, diabetes, or age >60 years, should undergo a carotid ultrasound study to rule out significant stenosis or the presence of unstable plaque. Patients with previous stroke also warrant computed tomography (CT) scan or magnetic resonance imaging (MRI) to establish a preoperative baseline study. Patients must have a reliable means of transportation for follow-up visits and a convenient, reliable telephone service to call for medical help in an emergency.

- **Treating any infection or providing prophylactic antibiotic therapy**

Patients with active systemic infection should not be considered for LVAD support because infection is one of

the leading causes of morbidity and death. Implantation should be delayed for patients with localized infections that can be effectively treated, if clinically feasible.

We should try to cope with patients with established or suspected infections, prolonged intubation, cutaneous lesions at surgical sites, or other comorbidities, including multisystem organ dysfunction, immunosuppression, poorly controlled diabetes, renal failure, malnutrition, or debilitation (Slaughter et al. 2010).

6. Device selection

Mechanical support can be applied short-term in an individual patient as a bridge to transplantation or can be applied long-term as in destination therapy. For example, if a patient with myocardial infarction and cardiogenic shock experiences a cardiac arrest that requires prolonged resuscitation, the heart failure specialist would know that percutaneous mechanical support could precede a potential LVAD until the neurological status is determined. If an LVAD is subsequently implanted, the patient's candidacy for transplantation versus discharge and long-term LVAD maintenance therapy (i.e., destination therapy) must be considered.

Numerous devices are now approved by the Food and Drug Administration (FDA) for therapy in acute heart failure and in chronic decompensated congestive heart failure - Table 4.

Company	Device	Position
Abiomed, Inc	Abiocor Total Artificial Heart	Total artificial heart
MicroMed Technology, Inc	MicroMed DeBakey Ventricular Assist Device - Child	Left ventricle
SynCardia Systems, Inc	SynCardia CardioWest	Total artificial heart
Thoratec Corp	HeartMate II Left Ventricular Assist Support HeartMate Implantable Pneumatic HeartMate Vented Electric HeartMate Extended Vented Electric Thoratec Implantable Ventricular Assist Device Thoratec Paracorporeal Ventricular Assist Device	Left ventricle Left ventricle Left ventricle Left ventricle Left or right ventricle Left or right ventricle
WorldHeart, Inc	Novacor PC Novacor PC	Left ventricle Left ventricle

Table 4. Food and Drug Administration-Approved Durable Devices (Potential for Patient Discharge)

These devices can be divided according to site of placement (commonly extra-, para- or intracorporeal) and type of flow generator system (centrifugal, axial or diaphragm).

Intracorporeal ventricular assist device are presented in Figure 2.

Device selection depends not only on specific patient characteristics and the pathology of the patient's heart failure but also on device characteristics, device availability and the experience of the surgical team (D'Alessandro et al. 2002, Goldstein et al. 1998).

Patients in profound cardiogenic shock require support to avoid permanent end-organ dysfunction and increase their chances of survival. The preferred devices are the ABIOMED BVS 5000 or Thoratec device. These devices may provide full biventricular support, re-establishing near normal hemodynamics while myocardial recovery is awaited. If prolonged

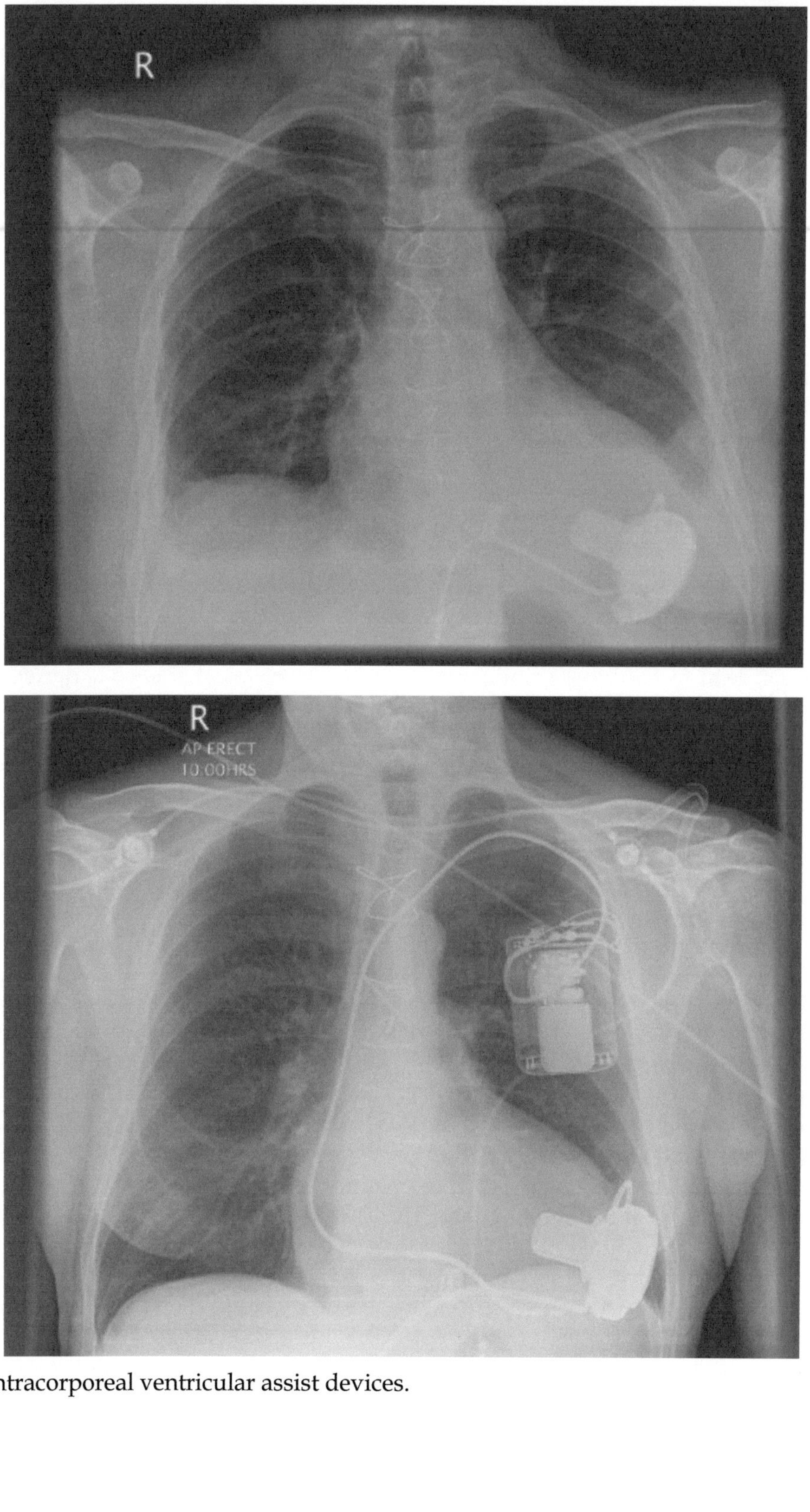

Fig. 2. Intracorporeal ventricular assist devices.

support is expected, conversion to a longer-term device such as an implantable LVAD or TAH should be considered. The Thoratec device has the advantage of providing long-term, extracorporeal support. Device selection for long-term support is much more complicated and is often subjective and based on the surgeon's experience. For smaller patients (body surface area < 1.5 m^2) the Thoratec device and perhaps a continuous-flow pump are the only options (Delgado et al. 2002).

7. Continuous versus pulsatile-flow pumps

Long-term implantable mechanical circulatory assistance as a clinically viable entity started with the approval of the HeartMate XVE as a bridge to transplantation. Results of the REMACH trial led to the device being approved for destination therapy (Lietz et al., 2007).

The other implantable pulsatile devices approved in the United States are the WorldHeart Novacor left ventricular assist device and SynCardia total artificial heart. These first-generation pumps were designed to mimic nature and produce pulsatile blood flow. There has been much debate over the need for pulsatility. Animal data suggest that non-pulsatile flow might not deliver as much perfusion to the distal vasculature and might lead to weakening of the muscle in the walls of major arteries (Yada et al., 1999; Potapov et al., 2000).

The pulsatile devices are bulky as they have to at least be the size of the bladder displacement (usually 60 to 80 cc) and hence have to be placed in the pre- or intraperitoneal space. A diaphragm or sac is required to eject the blood and flexing of this biomaterial interface can lead to failure after millions of cycles. Mechanical energy is derived from a pusher plate-type motor, which has decreased device resistance. These technical limitations mandated by pulsatile devices have led to decreased reliability and durability and a high incidence of infections. Furthermore, the major surgery required for implantation increases the rate of bleeding, perioperative complications, length of hospital stay and need for rehabilitation.

The next generation of devices consists of continuous-flow pumps. The HeartMate II device is approved as a bridge to transplant and destination therapy. The HeartWare HVAD, Jarvik 2000, Trumo DuraHeart and Ventracor VentrAssist devices are in clinical trials. The Cleveland Clinic TAH (Fumoto et al. 2010; Fukamachi et al. 2010) can transition continuous flow principles to a TAH and allow the technology to be used in patients requiring biventricular support. Compared with previous pulsatile devices, continuous-flow pumps cannot completely decompress the left ventricle as the native heart must have some residual volume to prevent suction events. Therefore, the native heart continues to eject and this provides a moderate amount of pulsatility. This low level of pulsatility is apparently enough to increase end-organ perfusion and allow these patients to recover from chronic congestive heart failure. In many patients, this ejection occurs through the left ventricular assist device and the aortic valve can remain closed. They contain only one moving part, the rotor, which is why they tend to be much more reliable. Continuous-flow LVADs are also silent during operation and create minimal motion and vibration. These features make continuous-flow devices more suitable for use in patients with smaller body size. Because they are much smaller and do not have the constant motion caused by blood displacement, the infection rates have dramatically decreased (Miller et al. 2007; Bielecka et al., 2007).

The trend in circulatory assistance is toward continuous-flow devices. They offer many advantages over the pulsatile devices in terms of size, reliability, durability and infection.

However, long-term results will need to be followed closely, specifically with regard to the perioperative period and the incidence of cerebrovascular accident despite appropriate anticoagulation (Jeevanandam 2010; Boyle 2009).
Table 5 provides a general comparison of the 2 types of LVADs in clinical use.

Attribute	Pulsatile-flow VAD	Continuous-flow VAD
Type of pump	Sac or diaphragm	Centrifugal or axial flow by rotating impeller
Main hemodynamic characteristics	Intermittent unloading of ventricle; pulsatile arterial pressure; asynchronous with heart	Continuous unloading of ventricle
Physiological flow variables	Pre-load dependant	Pre-load and after-load dependant
Mechanical flow variables	Automatic or fixed rate and stroke volume capacity	Set speed of the impeller rotation
Size	Large, intracorporeal devices limited to large patients, extracorporeal devices especially suited for smaller patients or for biventricular support	Smaller, accommodates most patients, excluding infants
Blood flow capacity	Up to 10 liters/min	Up to 10 liters/min

Table 5. Comparison of pulsatile and continuous-flow ventricular assist devices (Slaughter et al. 2010).

8. Axial and centrifugal pumps

Continuous-flow ventricular assist devices use axial-flow or centrifugal-flow blood pumps. The most modern axial flow devices offer significant potential advantages over earlier devices, because they are smaller, simpler and less obtrusive to the patient, yielding a better quality of life. The blood flow is essentially non-pulsatile and pump output is dependent mainly on afterload. In addition, because of their smaller size, they can be used in smaller patients, including children (Frazier et al. 2005). The axial flow pumps in current use are: the MicroMed/DeBakey VAD (MM-D VAD) and the Jarvik 2000 Heart, which have certain similarities in design and function. The Jarvik 2000 Heart, in particular, has many advantages. Its implantation can be performed without median sternotomy, which makes the eventual transplantation operation easier. There is no inflow cannula, which rids the patient of the thrombotic and hemolytic problems encountered with inflow cannulae. Circulation to the coronaries, the brachiocephalic, the left carotid and the subclavian arteries is thus provided by retrograde flow. There is no need for an external pocket in the mediastinum or the peri-peritoneum, which decreases the risk of infection (Westaby et al. 2000). The MicroMed/DeBakey VAD consists of a titanium inflow cannula that is inserted into the left ventricular apex and leads to the pump proper, which connects to the ascending aorta via a vascular graft. The pump is implanted through a median sternotomy in a small extracardiac pocket (Noon et al. 2000).

The HeartMate II device is an axial flow pump that has a spinning rotor as its only moving part and the direction of blood is parallel to the rotor. The HeartMate II has a left ventricular apical inflow cannula with a sintered titanium blood-containing surface. No compliance chamber or valves are necessary. The outflow cannula is connected to a Dacron graft, which is then anastomosed to the ascending aorta in a similar fashion to that achieved with the original HeartMate XVE. The pump is designed to deliver as much as 10 L/min of cardiac output and is placed either intraperitoneally or extraperitoneally (Delgado et al. 2005; Noon et al., 1999).
The HeartMate II LVAD is shown in Figure 2.

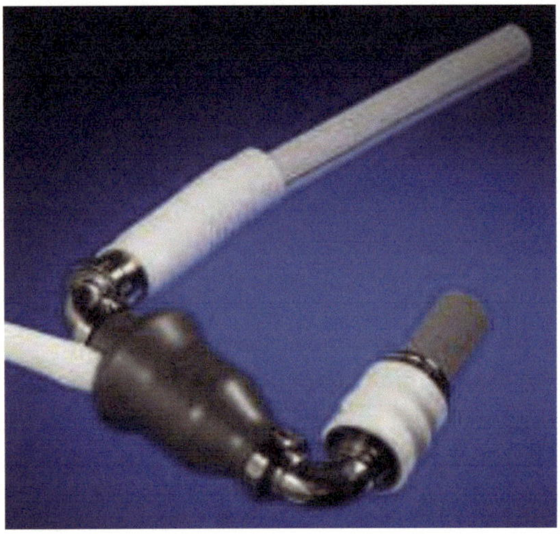

Fig. 3. The HeartMate II LVAD.

HeartMate II has FDA approvals as bridge-to-transplant and destination therapy.
Two other axial-flow pumps are: Incor (left ventricular assist device with magnetic bearing) and Synergy (left ventricular assist device with blood-immersed bearings). Centrifugal pumps use the pump mechanism of a standard heart bypass. In devices such as the HVAD, DuraHeart, Levacor VAD and EVAHEART LVAS the inflow and outflow of blood are in perpendicular directions (Bielecka et al. 2007).
New centrifugal systems include the bearingless system. This drive system is magnetically coupled to an external power source and pump flow is related to rotation speed. The advantages of the centrifugal pump are simplicity of design, versatility and the relatively low costs of manufacture and operation. It can be used as a femoral-femoral bypass or as a left (right) ventricular-to-aortic (pulmonary artery) bypass. Its main disadvantages are the need for heparinization, difficulty in chest closure, the need for intensive monitoring and the inability to generate a pulsatile flow. The pump is used primarily as a bridge to recovery in cardiogenic shock. The total duration of support with a centrifugal pump is usually limited to no more than two to three weeks (Noon et al. 1999).
The Interagency Registry For Mechanical Circulatory Support (INTERMACS) report examined the changing patterns of practice in the application of device type (continuous-flow vs pulsatile) and device strategies during the past 3 years (Kirklin et al., 2010).
The INTERMACS playing field changed dramatically in April 2008 when the HeartMate II axial flow pump (Thoratec) received FDA approval for clinical use as bridge-to-transplant

therapy in the United States. When continuous flow technology is routinely available for long-term destination therapy, and as multiple continuous-flow pumps are approved, INTERMACS offers a unique opportunity to compare and contrast these technologies in the setting of evolving indications, changing patient profiles, and refinement of device strategy in the developing landscape of mechanical circulatory support.

This report focuses on the 1,092 patients who received primary left ventricular assist device implants among the total of 1,420 patients who received primary and secondary devices.

The distribution of pre-implant device strategies continues to focus on bridging patients to cardiac transplantation with the device as a bridge to candidacy or bridge to transplant. The initial strategy was permanent in nearly 10% - Table 6.

Pre-implant device strategy	No. (N=1092)	%
Bridge to transplant	496	45.4
Bridge to candidacy	458	41.9
Planned destination therapy	100	9.2
Bridge to recovery	25	2.3
Rescue therapy	10	0.9
Other	3	0.3
Total	1092	100.0

Table 6. Device strategy at Time of Implant of Primary LVAD (INTERMACS) (Kirklin et al., 2010).

According to INTERMACS data risk factors reflecting older age, greater severity of right ventricular failure and cardiogenic shock at implant predict a higher likelihood of early death among all LVAD patients. The use of a pulsatile pump was a risk factor for death in the constant phase. Because continuous-flow pumps have only accrued a mean follow-up of 4.6 months, adverse events among pulsatile vs continuous-flow pumps during the first 6 months after implantation were assessed. Generally, the events per 100 patient-months are importantly reduced in patients with continuous-flow devices versus pulsatile pumps for device malfunction, infection, hepatic dysfunction, and neurological events - Table 7.

INTERMACS has analyzed the first 1000-plus patients with primary implantation of LVADs during a transitional period from pulsatile technology to continuous-flow pumps. The shift toward implantation of axial flow technology since its approval by the Food and Drug Administration is dramatic. This trend has been accompanied by continued fluctuation in the designation of the primary device strategy as bridge to transplant, bridge to candidacy and destination therapy (Kirklin et al., 2010).

The use of mechanical device support in the congenital heart disease patient requires knowledge of anatomical and physiological factors such as body size, residual intracardiac shunts, the presence of a single ventricle, or venous anomalies and/or arterial anomalies that may impact the success of device implantation, and the effectiveness of the VAD support.

Evidence-based clinical management of LVAD-supported patients is becoming increasingly important for optimizing outcomes. Patient and device selection, preoperative preparation and the timing of LVAD implantation are some of the most important elements critical to successful circulatory support and are principles universal to all devices.

Adverse event	Pulsatile (*n* = 406)		Continuous (*n* = 548)		Pulsatile / continuous	
	Events	Rate	Events	Rate	Ratio	*p*-value
Device malfunction	45	2.95	17	0.82	3.60	<0.0001
Bleeding	369	24.22	360	17.41	1.39	<0.0001
Cardiac/vascular						
Right heart failure	48	3.15	46	2.23	1.41	0.05
Myocardial infarction	2	0.13	2	0.10	1.30	0.37
Cardiac arrhythmia	154	10.11	218	10.54	0.96	0.65
Pericardial drainage	44	2.89	30	1.45	1.99	0.003
Hypertension[1]	75	4.92	17	0.82	6.00	<0.0001
Arterial non-CNS thrombosis	7	0.46	6	0.29	1.59	0.21
Venous thrombotic event	38	2.49	32	1.55	1.61	0.03
Hemolysis	11	0.72	12	0.58	1.24	0.29
Infection	431	28.29	244	11.80	2.40	<0.0001
Neurological dysfunction	66	4.33	40	1.93	2.24	<0.0001
Renal dysfunction	63	4.14	45	2.18	1.90	0.0007
Hepatic dysfunction	24	1.58	14	0.68	2.32	0.009
Respiratory failure	121	7.94	89	4.31	1.84	<0.0001
Wound dehiscence	8	0.53	9	0.44	1.20	0.34
Psychiatric episode	43	2.82	38	1.84	1.53	0.03
Total burden	1549	101.69	1219	58.96	1.72	<0.0001

[1] - with current reporting, identification of hypertension with continuous-flow pumps is unreliable.
CNS - central nervous system

Table 7. Adverse event rates (events/100 patient months) in the first 12 months post-implant for primary LVADs (INTERMACS) (Kirklin et al., 2010).

9. Intraoperative considerations

Moderate to severe aortic insufficiency and mitral stenosis must be corrected during LVAD implantation.

Inflow cannulas must be directed posteriorly toward the mitral valve. Obstruction may result if the cannula is directed or angled toward the septum or free wall or due to changes in position as the left ventricular chamber size is reduced over time.

Proper placement of the percutaneous lead is important for long-term prevention of infection and damage to wires. Tunnel the percutaneous lead to maximize the amount of velour that is inside the body. It may be positioned in a gentle loop or arc, leaving some internal slack for accidental tugs in the perioperative period.

Certain LVAD implant steps can be taken before initiation of cardiopulmonary bypass (CPB) to minimize CPB time: tunnel the percutaneous lead and anastomosis of the outflow graft to the ascending aorta.

Before the patient is taken off CPB, air removal should be conducted at low LVAD speeds. The patient should be weaned off cardiopulmonary bypass or at minimal CPB support (approximately ≤1 liter/min) before increasing revolutions per minute speeds to permit complete filling of the left ventricle (>10 mm Hg) and to prevent aspiration of air around the inflow conduit. The pump should be initiated at low speeds and increases made slowly.

If right ventricle dysfunction occurs, resulting in poor LVAD inflow, temporary right-heart bypass can be used to provide blood flow to the LVAD while transitioning from CPB. For more profound right ventricle failure, a temporary RVAD should be considered and implemented expeditiously. Intraoperative echocardiography is essential for identifying valvular pathology, intracardiac thrombi, and an atrial septal defect or patent foramen ovale (PFO). A PFO should be closed at the time of implantation. Intracardiac thrombus identified in the left atria or ventricle should be removed before LVAD implantation. Echocardiography is critical for assessing left ventricle chamber size, cannula position, septal shifting, and aortic valve opening—factors used to determine optimal pump position and speed setting (Slaughter et al. 2010).

10. Postoperative patient and device management

A patient's right ventricular function can be affected by pump speed. Avoid setting the pump speed so high that it causes a significant leftward septal shift and abnormal right ventricle geometry, which can adversely affect RV function. High pump speeds can also collapse the left ventricle and obstruct flow through the LVAD inlet cannula draining the left ventricle.

Anticoagulation therapy is required during support with continuous-flow LVADs to avoid thrombotic complications. However, results from the HeartMate II Bridge to Transplant trial indicate that anticoagulation requirements for this therapy are less than was initially believed. The results from the clinical trial revealed that the incidence of thrombotic events is very low— much lower than bleeding—which remains one of the most frequent adverse events (Miller et al. 2007; Pagani et al. 2009).

Routine use of heparin is not indicated immediately after the LVAD is implanted. However, there are some clinical conditions of higher thrombotic risk where postoperative heparin may be indicated in the transition to warfarin therapy, such as small patients who have low LVAD flow rates, a small ventricle, previous stroke or transient ischemic attack, chronic atrial fibrillation, or documented left atrial or left ventricle thrombus. Adequate hemostasis should be achieved before anticoagulation is initiated. Patients are usually anticoagulated with warfarin and antiplatelet agents (aspirin) when they are able to take oral medications. Current recommendations are to adjust the warfarin dose to achieve a target INR of 1.5 to 2.5. In addition to warfarin, patients should also be given antiplatelet therapy, such as aspirin (81 to 325 mg daily). If LVAD flow remains low (<3.0 liters/min), consider increasing anticoagulation. If there is a risk of bleeding, decreasing the warfarin dose and increasing or maintaining antiplatelet medications is considered. Anticoagulation and antiplatelet therapy may need to be adjusted for some clinical conditions. Some types of infection, especially bacteremia, are associated with a higher incidence of stroke due to increased endothelial activation and platelet aggregation (Basra et al., 2009).

Therefore, increased antiplatelet therapy may be warranted during systemic bacterial infections.

The major hemodynamic effects of a continuous-flow LVAD are increases in diastolic pressure and flow (Myers et al., 2009).

Because these devices pump continuously throughout the entire cardiac cycle, aortic flow is also present during diastole when normal pulsatile flow is absent. The pulse pressure is influenced by left ventricular contractility, intravascular volume, pre-load and after-load pressure, and by pump speed. Owing to the reduced pulse pressure during continuous-flow LVAD support, it is often difficult to palpate a pulse and measure blood pressure accurately by the usual auscultatory or automated methods. After the arterial catheter is removed, the arterial blood pressure is most reliably assessed using Doppler and a sphygmomanometer. Arterial blood pressure might be controlled with vasoactive and inotropic medications and intravascular fluid volume management. The pump speed should not be adjusted to achieve a desired arterial blood pressure. The goal is to maintain the mean arterial blood pressure in the range of 70 to 80 mm Hg. It should not exceed 90 mm Hg. Unlike a pulsatile LVAD, the amount of cardiac output support by a continuous-flow pump is affected by the after-load, or systemic vascular resistance. Maintaining the mean arterial pressure in the desired range will optimize cardiac support. Hypertension is controlled to avoid decreased LVAD support and cardiac output as well as to avoid cerebrovascular events. Immobilizing the percutaneous lead to prevent exit site trauma reduces infection risk. Care of the percutaneous lead and exit site must be a priority for successful outpatient care (Slaughter et al. 2010).

Multidisciplinary teams are required that allow close collaboration between cardiologists, medical specialists, and cardiac surgeons. The HF specialist must participate in managing these teams. The HF specialist should be familiar with the need to evaluate right ventricular function and associated tricuspid regurgitation prior to placement of an LVAD. Compared with successful cardiac transplantation, exercise capacity is lower following chronic outpatient mechanical support and the patient's daily concerns are typically greater (e.g., battery exchange or recharging, driveline maintenance). A key point in postoperative device management is paying attention that continuous-flow LVADs do not contain valves. If the pump stops, there may be back flow, which can have severe consequences (similar to aortic insufficiency), so we must avoid power interruption or inadvertent power lead disconnection that would lead to loss of support. Pump speed optimization and device monitoring present unique challenges compared with pulsatile devices, because continuous-flow pumps can generate large negative pressures at the pump inlet, which may result in septal shift or ventricular collapse. It is also important to avoid setting the pump speed too high, which can result in ventricular collapse or inlet obstruction and initiate arrhythmias (ACCF/AHA/ACP/HFSA/ISHLT 2010 Clinical Competence Statement on Management of Patients With Advanced Heart Failure and Cardiac Transplant). The system-provided parameters of speed, power, pulsatility index, and estimated flow in conjunction with echocardiography serve as the primary indicators of proper device function. The patient's clinical status should always be assessed when device function is evaluated.

Successful long-term LVAD support depends on comprehensive care from a multidisciplinary team, including the patient and his or her family member(s)/caregiver(s). Training on proper self-care and system operation, with an emphasis on meticulous care of the percutaneous lead and exit site, should begin preoperatively. Training continues throughout hospitalization. Eventually, the patient's demonstration of understanding and competency may be a requirement for discharge.

11. References

Aaronson KD, Schwartz JS, Chen TM, Wong KL, Goin JE, Mancini DM.(1997). Development and prospective validation of a clinical index to predict survival in ambulatory patients referred for cardiac transplant evaluation. Circulation 1997;95:2660-7

Basra SS, Attallab AA, Wagle R, Loyalka R, Kar B (2009). Infections in patients on continuous flow LVAD: epidemiology and role in causation of cerebrovascular accidents. J Heart Lung Transplant 2009;28: S285.

Bielecka A, Wierzbicka M, Goch JH (2007). The ventricular assist device: a bridge to ventricular recovery, a bridge to heart transplantation or destination therapy. Cardiol J. 2007;14(1):14-20.

Boyle A (2009). Current status of cardiac transplantation and mechanical circulatory support. Curr Heart Fail Rep 2009;6:28-33.

Butler J, Geisberg C, Howser R, et al (2006). Relationship between renal function and left ventricular assist device use. Ann Thorac Surg 2006;81:1745-51.

Chen YS, Ko WJ, Chi NH, et al (2004). Risk factor screening scale to optimize treatment for potential heart transplant candidates under extracorporeal membrane oxygenation. Am J Transplant 2004;4:1818-25.

Cohn JM, Tognoni G (2001). A randomized trial of the angiotensin-receptor blocker valsartan in chronic heart failure. N Engl J Med, 2001; 345: 1667–1675.

Cooley DA, Liotta D, Hallman GL, Bloodwell RD, Leachman RD, Milam JD (1969). Orthotopic cardiac prosthesis for two-staged cardiac replacement. Am J Cardiol, 1969; 24: 723–730.

D'Alessandro DA, Rao V, DiGiorgi PL et al (2002). Current options for mechanical heart technology. J Card Surg,2002; 17: 81–88.

De Bakey ME, Liotta D, Hall CW (1966). Left heart bypass using an implantable blood pump. In: Mechanical Devices to Assist the Failing Heart: proceedings of a conference sponsored by the Committee on Trauma, 9–10.09.1964. National Academy of Sciences — National Research Council. Washington, DC 1966: 223.

Delgado DH, Rao V, Ross HJ, Verma S, Smedira NG (2002). Mechanical circulatory assistance. Circulation, 2002;106: 2046–2050.

Delgado R, Bergheim M (2005). HeartMate II left ventricular assist device: a new device for advanced heart failure. Expert Rev Med Devices 2005; 2: 529–532.

Deng MC, Loebe M, El-Banayosy A et al. (2001). Mechanical circulatory support for advanced heart failure. Circulation, 2001; 103: 231–237.

Dennis C (1966). Left heart bypass. In: Mechanical devices to assist the failing heart. National Academy of Sciences — National Research Council. Washington, DC 1966: 1283.

Dickstein K, Vardas PE, Auricchio A et al. (2010). 2010 Focused Update of ESC guidelines on device therapy in heart failure: An update of the 2008 ESC guidelines for the diagnosis and treatment of acute and chronic heart failure and the 2007 ESC guidelines for cardiac and resynchronization therapy Developed with the special contribution of the Heart Failure Association and the European Heart Rhythm Association. Eur Heart J. 2010 Aug 27. [Epub ahead of print]

Drews T, Stepanenko A, Dandel M, Buz S, Lehmkuhl HB, Hetzer R. (2010) Mechanical circulatory support in patients of advanced age. Eur J Heart Fail 2010. May 22 [epub ahead of print]

European Society of Cardiology; Heart Failure Association of the ESC (HFA); European Society of Intensive Care Medicine (ESICM), Dickstein K, Cohen-Solal A, Filippatos G et al. (2008). ESC guidelines for the diagnosis and treatment of acute and chronic heart failure 2008: the Task Force for the diagnosis and treatment of acute and chronic heart failure 2008 of the European Society of Cardiology. Developed in collaboration with the Heart Failure Association of the ESC (HFA) and endorsed by the European Society of Intensive Care Medicine (ESICM). Eur J Heart Fail. 2008;10(10):933-89.

Farrar DJ, Compton PG, Hershon JJ, Fonger JD, Hill, J.D (1985). Right heart interaction with the mechanically assisted left heart. World J Surg 1985;9:89-102.

Frazier OH, Delgado RM, Kar B et al. (2004). First clinical use of the redesigned HeartMate II left ventricular assist system in the United States. Tex Heart Inst J 2004; 31: 157–159.

Frazier OH, Myers TJ, Westaby S, Gregoric ID (2004). Clinical experience with an implantable, intracardiac, continuous flow circulatory support device: physiologic implications and their relationship to patientselection. Ann Thorac Surg 2004; 77: 133–142.

Fukamachi K, Horvath DJ, Massiello AL, et al (2010). An innovative, sensorless, pulsatile, continuous-flow total artificial heart: device design and initial in vitro study. J Heart Lung Transplant 2010;29:13-20.

Fumoto H, Horvath DJ, Rao S, et al (2010). In vivo acute performance of the Cleveland Clinic self-regulating, continuous-flow total artificial heart. J Heart Lung Transplant 2010;29:21-26

Galie N, Ghofrani HA, Torbicki A, et al. (2005). Sildenafil citrate therapy for pulmonary arterial hypertension. N Engl J Med 2005;353:2148-57.

Garg R, Yusuf S (1993). Epidemiology of congestive heart failure. In: Barnett DB, Pouleur H, Francis GS eds. Congestive cardiac failure: pathophysiology and treatment. Marcel Dekker, New York, NY 1993: 9–25.

Gibbon JH (1954). Application of a heart and lung apparatus to cardiac surgery. Minn Med, 1954; 37: 171–180.

Goldstein DJ, Oz MC, Rose EA (1998). Implantable left ventricular assist devices. N Engl J Med, 1998; 339:1522–1533.

Gracin N, Johnson MR, Spokas D, et al (1998). The use of APACHE II scores to select candidates for left ventricular assist device placement. J Heart Lung Transplant 1998;17:1017-23.

Gronda E, Vitali E (1999). Left ventricle assist systems: a possible alternative to heart transplantation for heart failure patients? Patient selection, techniques and benefit. Eur J Heart Fail, 1999; 1: 319–325.

Holdy K, Dembitsky W, Eaton LL, et al (2005). Nutrition assessment and management of left ventricular assist device patients. J Heart Lung Transplant 2005;24:1690-6.

Holman WL, Pae WE, Teutenberg JJ, et al. (2009) INTERMACS: interval analysis of registry data. J Am Coll Surg 2009;208:755-61; discussion 61-2.

Jeevanandam V (2010). The evolution of cardiac assist device technology. The Journal of Heart and Lung Transplantation 2010; 29:20-21.

Kantrowitz A, Tjonneland S, Freed PS, Philips SJ, Butner AN, Sherman JL (1968). Initial clinical experience with the intraaortic balloon pumping in cardiogenic shock. JAMA, 1968; 203: 113–118.

Kirklin JK, Naftel DC, Kormos RL et al. (2010) Second INTERMACS annual report: more than 1,000 primary left ventricular assist device implants. J Heart Lung Transplant 2010;29:1-10.

Klodell CT Jr, Morey TE, Lobato EB, et al (2007). Effect of sildenafil on pulmonary artery pressure, systemic pressure, and nitric oxide utilization in patients with left ventricular assist devices. Ann Thorac Surg 2007;83:68-71.

Klotz S, Vahlhaus Ch, Riehl Ch, Reitz Ch, Sindermann JR, Scheld HH (2010). Pre-operative prediction of post-VAD implant mortality using easily accessible clinical parameters. The Journal of Heart and Lung Transplantation 2010, 29: 45-52.

Kormos RL, Teuteberg JJ, Pagani FD, et al (2010). Right ventricular failure in patients with the HeartMate II continuous flow left ventricular assist device: incidence, risk factors, and impact on outcomes. J Thorac Cardiovasc Surg 2010 [in press].

Letsou GV, Myers TJ, Gregoric ID, et al (2003). Continuous axial-flow left ventricular assist device (Jarvik 2000) maintains kidney and liver perfusion for up to 6 months. Ann Thorac Surg 2003;76:1167-70.

Levy WC, Mozaffarian D, Linker DT, et al.(2006). The Seattle heart failure model: prediction of survival in heart failure. Circulation 2006;113: 1424-33.

Lietz K, Long JW, Kfoury AG, et al (2007). Outcomes of left ventricular assist device implantation as destination therapy in the post-REMATCH era. Circulation 2007;116:497-505.

Lockard KL, Degore L, Schwarm P, et al (2009). Lack of improvement in prealbumin at two weeks predicts a poor outcome after mechanical circulatory support. J Heart Lung Transplant 2009;28:S66.

Lund LH, Matthews J, Aaronson K. (2010) Patient selection for left ventricular assist devices. Eur J Heart Fail 2010;12:434-443.

Ma L, Fujino Y, Matsumiya G, Sawa Y, Mashimo T (2008). Renal function with left ventricular assist devices: the poorer the preoperative renal function, the longer the recovery. Med Sci Monit 2008;14:CR621-7.

Mancini D, Burkhoff D (2005). Mechanical device-based methods of managing and treating heart failure. Circulation, 2005; 112: 438–448.

Mann DL, McMurray JJ, Packer M et al. (2004). Targeted anticytokine therapy in patients with chronic heart failure: results of the Randomized Etanercept Worldwide Evaluation (RENEWAL). Circulation, 2004; 109: 1594–1602.

Mano A, Fujita K, Uenomachi K, et al (2009). Body mass index is a useful predictor of prognosis after left ventricular assist system implantation. J Heart Lung Transplant 2009;28:428-33.

Miller LW, Pagani FD, Russell SD, et al (2007). Use of a continuous-flow device in patients awaiting heart transplantation. N Engl J Med 2007;357:885-96.

Myers TJ, Bolmers M, Gregoric ID, Kar B, Frazier OH (2009). Assessment of arterial blood pressure during support with an axial flow left ventricular assist device. J Heart Lung Transplant 2009;28:423-7

Noon GP, Lafuente JA, Irwin S (1999). Acute and temporary ventricular support with BioMedicus centrifugal pump. Ann Thorac. Surg 1999; 68: 650–654.

Noon GP, Morley D, Irwin S et al (2000). Development and clinical application of the MicroMed DeBakey VAD. Curr Opin Cardiol 2000; 15: 166–171.

Norman JC (1974). An abdominal left ventricular assist device (ALVAD): prospectives and prospects. Cardiovascular Diseases. Bulletin of the Texas Heart Institute, 1974; 1: 251.

Oz MC, Goldstein DJ, Pepino P et al (1995). Screening scale predicts patients successfully receiving long-term implantable left ventricular assist devices. Circulation 1995; 92:II-169-173.

Oz MC, Rose EA, Levin HR.(1995) Selection criteria for placement of left ventricular assist devices. Am Heart J, 1995; 129: 173–177.

Packer M, Bristow MR, Cohn JN et al. (1996). The effect of carvedilol on morbidity and mortality in patients with chronic heart failure. N Engl J Med, 1996; 334: 1349–1355.

Pagani FD, Miller LW, Russell SD et al. (2009) Extended mechanical circulatory support with a continuous-flow rotary left ventricular assist device. J Am Coll Cardiol 2009;54:312-321.

Potapov EV, Loebe M, Nasseri BA, et al (2000). Pulsatile flow in patients with a novel nonpulsatile implantable ventricular assist device. Circulation 2000;102(suppl):III-183-7.

Radovancevic B, Vrtovec B, de Kort E, Radovancevic R, Gregoric ID, Frazier OH (2007). End-organ function in patients on long-term circulatory support with continuous- or pulsatile-flow assist devices. J Heart Lung Transplant 2007;26:815-8.

Rao V, Oz MC, Flannery MA et al (2003). Revised screening scale to predict survival after insertion of a left ventricular assist device. J Thorac Cardiovasc Surg 2003; 125:855-862.

Rose EA, Gelijns AC, Moskowitz AJ et al. (2001). Long-term mechanical left ventricular assistance for endstage heart failure. N Engl J Med, 2001; 345: 1435–1443.

Rose EA, Moskowitz AJ, Packer M et al. (1999). The REMATCH trial: rationale, design, and end points. Randomized Evaluation of Mechanical Assistance for the Treatment of Congestive Heart Failure. Ann Thorac Surg. 1999;67(3):723-30

Sandner SE, Zimpfer D, Zrunek P, et al (2009). Renal function and outcome after continuous flow left ventricular assist device implantation. Ann Thorac Surg 2009;87:1072-8.

Slaughter MS, Pagani FD, Rogers JG et al (2010). for the HeartMate II Clinical Investigators. Clinical management of continuous-flow left ventricular assist devices in advanced heart failure. The Journal of Heart and Lung Transplantation 2010; 29: S4 - S39.

Slaughter MS, Rogers JG, Milano CA et al. (2009) Advanced heart failure treated with continuous-flow left ventricular assist device. N Engl J Med 2009;361:2241-2251.

Stevenson LW, Pagani FD, Young JB, et al. (2009) INTERMACS profiles of advanced heart failure: the current picture. J Heart Lung Transplant 2009;28:535-41.

The Captopril-Digoxin Multicenter Research Group (1988). Comparative effects of therapy with captopril and digoxin in patients with mild to moderate heart failure. JAMA, 1988; 259: 539–544.

The RALES Investigators (1996). Effectiveness of spironolactone added to an angiotensin-converting enzyme inhibitor and a loop diuretic for severe chronic congestive heart failure. Am J Cardiol, 1996; 78: 902–907.

Tylus-Earl N, Chillcott S (2009). Mental health and medical challenges. Management of a depressed patient with a left ventricular assist system in an inpatient psychiatric setting. J Psychosoc Nurs Ment Health Serv 2009;47:43-9; quiz 51.

Westaby S, Banning AP, Jarvik R (2000). First permanent implant of the Jarvik 2000 Heart. Lancet 2000; 356: 900–903.

Writing Committee Members; Francis GS, Greenberg BH, Hsu DT et al. (2010). ACCF/AHA/ACP/HFSA/ISHLT 2010 Clinical Competence Statement on Management of Patients With Advanced Heart Failure and Cardiac Transplant. A Report of the ACCF/AHA/ACP Task Force on Clinical Competence and Training. Circulation. 2010;122:644-672.

Yada I, Mitamura Y (1999). Pulsatile flow versus nonpulsatile flow. J Artif Organs 1999;2:1-2.

5

Cardiac Support and Multiorgan Dysfunction Syndrome

Khurram Shahzad MD MS-candidate, Farhana Latif MD, Hirokazu Akashi MD, Tomoko S. Kato MD PhD, Anshu Sinha PhD, Duygu Onat PhD and Mario C. Deng MD
Columbia University, College of Physicians & Surgeons, New York
United States

1. Introduction

Approximately 5 million Americans suffer from heart failure (HF), the burden of which will grow exponentially over the next 50 years. HF currently results in 3.5 million hospitalizations and 20% of all hospital admissions among individuals >65 years of age. Surgical interventions for HF include cardiac repair (coronary artery bypass grafting, valve repair or replacement), cardiac support (mechanical circulatory support devices) and cardiac replacement (heart transplantation). These modern interventions of cardiac surgery and critical care medicine dramatically improved outcomes. They are offered to patients with increasingly high-risk clinical profiles and a higher likelihood of complications.

The development of vital-organ support therapies (respirator, dialysis, transfusion, etc) in the intensive care units (ICUs) increased the survival of critically ill patients. However, despite these organ-saving therapies, up to 15% of these patients have an unfavourable perioperative course. Frequently, more than one organ system becomes dysfunctional, leading to progressive multiorgan dysfunction (MOD) (**Lietz et al., 2007**). The hallmark of MOD is the development of progressive physiologic dysfunction in two or more organ systems after an acute threat to systemic homeostasis. MOD is the leading cause of morbidity and mortality in the ICUs and after mechanical circulatory support device (MCSD) implantation (**Deng et al., 2005**).

2. Epidemiology

According to a multiyear survey conducted in surgical ICU patients, more than 50% patients develop some degree of MOD during their ICU stay (**Barie et al., 2000**) and currently MOD is the major cause of mortality in surgical ICUs (**Barie et al., 1996**). The recent data from the ICUs around the country show that the severity of MOD correlates significantly with the mortality, the observed incidence of dysfunction of 1, 2, 3, and ≥4 organ systems was 73.6%, 20.7%, 4.7%, and 1% respectively with corresponding mortality rates of 21.2%, 44.3%, 64.5%, and 76.2% (**Angus et al., 2001**).

3. Evolution of mechanical cardiac support

Early descriptions of mechanical support of the human circulation are documented at least back to the early 19th century. The experimental application of mechanical support in animal models was reported in the 1930's. Major interest in mechanical support of the human circulation was generated by the advent of open-heart surgery in the 1950's (**Kirklin et al., 2006**). Basic pump design has remained same over this development period, but power delivery and control has moved from large bedside consoles to wearable components, enabling patient autonomy in an outpatient setting (**Schmid et al., 1999**). This has brought about substantial improvements in patient quality of life (**Dew et al., 1999**) and a reduction in resource use (**Gelijns 1997**). Smaller, inexpensive and less obtrusive blood pumps are undergoing development and some are being tested in clinical trials (**Katsuma 1998, Wieselthaler 2000, Goldstein 2005**). However, while the potential benefits are encouraging, these designs still have to prove their durability, reliability and physiological suitability for chronic applications.

Following the initiative by the US National Heart Lung and Blood Institute in the 1970's to develop long-term artificial heart devices (The Artificial Heart Program 1991), two electrically powered pumps emerged from this initiative and have recently completed trials sponsored by the Food and Drug Administration for evaluating safety and efficacy and have received certification for commercial application in 1998, the HeartMate® 1205 VE (ThermoCardio Systems, Woburn, MA) (**Poirier 1999**), the Novacor® N100 PC (World Heart Corporation, Oakland, CA) (**Portner 1989, Robbins 1999**), and the ABIOCOR total artificial heart (Abiomed, Inc., Danvers, MA), the last under the Humanitarian Device Exemption (HDE) program of the FDA in September 2005. Recently with the introduction of continuous flow devices e.g. HeartMate-II (Thoratec, Inc.) there is increased use of mechanical support in patients with advanced HF.

4. INTERMACS based definition of different forms of organ dysfunction

4.1 Neurological Dysfunction

The INTERMACS database (**Kirklin et al., 2008**) defines neurological dysfunction as any new, temporary or permanent, focal or global neurological deficit ascertained by a standard neurological examination (administered by a neurologist or other qualified physician and documented with appropriate diagnostic tests and consultation note).

4.2 Coagulation dysfunction

According to the INTERMACS database coagulation dysfunction is divided into bleeding and hemolysis. Bleeding as any episode of internal or external bleeding that results in death, the need for re-operation or hospitalization; or necessity of transfusion of red blood cells that is equal or greater than 4 packed units within any 24 hour period during the first 7 days post implant or than 2 packed units within any 24 hour period after 7 days following implant. In patients that are less than 50 kg it is considered 20 cc/kg or 10 cc/kg respectively.

Hemolysis as a plasma free-hemoglobin value that is greater than 40 mg/dl, in association with clinical signs associated with hemolysis (e.g., anaemia, low hematocrit, hyperbilirubinemia) occurring after the first 72 hours post-implant. Hemolysis related to documented non-device-related causes (e.g. transfusion or drug) is excluded from this definition.

4.3 Renal dysfunction

The INTERMACS database distinguishes between two situations of renal dysfunction: Acute renal dysfunction is defined as abnormal kidney function requiring dialysis including hemofiltration) in patients who did not require this procedure prior to implant, or a rise in serum creatinine of greater than 3 times baselines or greater than 5 mg/dl (in children, creatinine greater than 3 times upper limit of normal for age) sustained for over 48 hours. Chronic renal dysfunction is defined as an increase in serum creatinine of 2 mg/dl or greater above baseline, or requirement for hemodialysis sustained for at least 90 days.

4.4 Pulmonary dysfunction

Respiratory dysfunction is defined as impairment of respiratory function requiring reintubation, tracheostomy or (for patients older than age 5 years) the inability to discontinue ventilatory support within 6 days (144hours) post-VAD implant. This excludes intubation for re-operation or temporary intubation for diagnostic or therapeutic procedures.

4.5 Liver dysfunction

The INTERMACS database defines hepatic dysfunction as any increase in any two of the following hepatic laboratory values (total bilirubin, aspartate aminotransferase / AST and alanine aminotransferase/ALT) to a level greater than three times the upper limit of normal for the hospital, beyond 14 days post-implant (or if hepatic dysfunction is the primary cause of death).

5. Clinical scoring systems

Prognostic scoring systems are integral to critical care practice. Composite outcome scales permit the quantification of complex clinical phenomena that cannot be adequately described by a single clinical or biochemical measure. Such scales are used for assessment of clinical status, changes in clinical status, evaluation of therapy, outcome prediction, and resource allocation. Currently, different clinical scoring systems are available to predict outcomes after trauma or injury including the APACHE II, III and IV scores (**Zimmerman et al., 2006**), ISS, MOD-score, EURO-score, and SOFA-score (**Marshall et al., 1995; Vincent et al., 1996; Vincent et al., 1998; Nashef et al., 1999; Minne et al., 2008**). These scoring systems are important in ICU-based research. They allow for MOD-phenotype definition and patient stratification based on objective evaluation of illness severity. While all of these scores have been validated and are in clinical use, they have shortcomings. The EURO-score solely uses pre- and intraoperative risk factors to assess postoperative risk. The APACHE scoring system uses day-1 post-ICU admission data for outcome prediction. In addition, while the APACHE-IV score was developed from APACHE-III to restore discrimination performance, the highest discrimination inaccuracy was seen in the decile of patients at highest risk for death (**Zimmerman et al., 2006**).

The SOFA-score, in contrast to APACHE and other ICU-outcome prediction models based on measurements at one individual time point, has the strength of modelling changes in the patient's status. The SOFA-score is a six-organ dysfunction/failure score measuring MOD daily. Each organ is graded from 0 (normal) to 4 (the most abnormal), providing a daily score between 0 and 24. Shortcomings of the SOFA-score, the best dynamic score currently available, include 1) the treatment-dependent definition of the cardiovascular parameter (positive inotrope medication type and dose) which may reflect variation of practice and not of disease severity, and 2) absence of an immune system parameter.

6. Scoring systems and heart failure

In a pilot study designed to understand the utility of current clinical MOD-scoring systems, we hypothesized that a preoperative diagnosis of HF is associated with an increased risk of postoperative in-hospital mortality independent of the SOFA score. Thus, we analyzed 145 patients requiring a ≥7d postoperative ICU stay and obtained complete maximum postoperative SOFA-score data (5.2% of all 2768 CUMC cardiac surgery cases from January 01 2007 to June 30 2009). Patients were separated into Group-HF (pre-existing HF diagnosis) and Group-NoHF (no known diagnosis of HF). Patients were stratified by a maximum SOFA score of <10, 10-14 and ≥15. In-hospital mortality rates were compared among groups using the Chi-square test. Group-HF (n=66, 46%) had a higher in-hospital mortality rate than Group-NoHF (n=79, 54%) (35% vs. 13 %, p=0.003). Although mortality rates, when the SOFA was <10 and 10-14, were not different in Group-HF and Group-NoHF, patients with SOFA≥15 in Group-HF had a very high mortality rate (71%) (**Figure 1**). Thus, both the SOFA score and pre-existing HF appear to be important risk factors for in-hospital mortality in cardiac surgery patients; in-hospital mortality is exceptionally high in patients with both risk factors. Novel tools are needed to improve our understanding of the interaction between HF and SOFA score, improve outcome prediction and improve management in this emerging cohort.

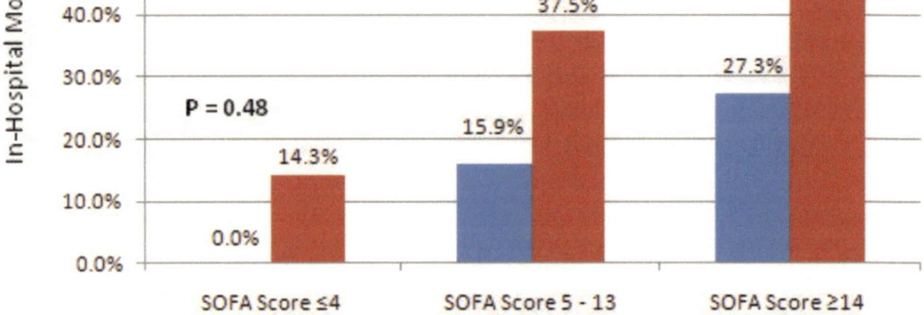

TN	2	7		44	40		11	20	
DN	0	1		7	15		3	15	

Fig. 1.

An ideal descriptor should be simple, routinely and reproducibly measured, and readily evaluable in heterogeneous groups of critically ill patients. It should be derived from independent clinical and/or laboratory data, rather than through subjective clinical evaluation, and should measure physiologic dysfunction directly, rather than the therapeutic intervention employed to support organ function. The descriptor should provide a comprehensive reflection of the physiologic function in the system of interest, and should be specific for the function of that system. Consistent with a definition of MOD as an acute and potentially reversible process, the ideal descriptor should be capable of differentiating the sequelae of an acute homeostatic insult from the chronic effects of primary disease in the organ system of interest. Moreover, the ideal descriptor should be relatively unaffected by transient abnormalities associated with resuscitation or acute reversible complications of therapy, and should be maximally abnormal after resuscitation and well before the time of death. The quantitative value of the descriptor should be minimally affected by therapeutic intervention in the absence of objective functional improvement. Finally, the descriptor should be continuous, rather than dichotomous, and abnormal in one direction only (**Marshall et al., 1995**).

7. Leukocyte gene expression signatures

7.1 Leukocyte gene expression profiling after cardiac surgery

In a pilot project using a transcriptome-wide peripheral blood mononuclear cell (PBMCs) profiling approach we analyzed expression patterns before and after MCSD-implantation in 11 patients with an uncomplicated course (i.e. day -1, day1 and day 7 after surgery). Agilent-44K whole genome microarray analysis was performed on the PBMCs. Data was analyzed using Significance Analysis of Microarrays (SAM) and High-Throughput GoMiner in comparison to baseline. Day 1 profiles included differential expression of 821 genes (SAM, FDR<0.1, fold change >1.5), enriching >60 Gene Ontology (GO) categories. Grouping by component genes revealed GO-clusters including "IL-1 related" (primarily-up-regulated), "T-cell related" (primarily-down-regulated), and "apoptosis related" (up- and down-regulated genes). Day 7 profiles included GO-categories related to repair processes. In conclusion, transcriptome-wide expression profiling of PBMCs suggests a response pattern to MCSD-implantation with pro-inflammatory activation and simultaneous T-cell suppression (**Sinha et al., 2010**).

7.2 Leukocyte gene expression profiling of MOD

As a pilot study on differential leukocyte GEP in MOD, we analyzed the mixed peripheral blood leukocyte GEP in 9 patients after cardiac surgery in comparison to three age-matched healthy control persons. We enrolled 3 healthy controls and 9 consecutive HF patients who underwent MCSD implantation. MOD was defined using sequential organ failure assessment (SOFA) score. Patients were divided into low (≤4), intermediate (5-11), and high (≥12) SOFA-score groups. The blood samples were collected and processed for peripheral blood mononuclear cell separation. Total RNA was purified, amplified and hybridized on Illumina Whole Genome Expression Chips. The expression data was extracted and analyzed using GeneSpring GX 11.0.1. Biological interpretation of the differential signatures was performed using High-Throughput GoMiner. The mean age of the patients was 51±7 years. Using Kruskal-Wallis testing, 1438 unique transcripts were differentially expressed across groups (false discovery rate (FDR) ≤0.02, fold change≥1.5). Based on these genes, hierarchical clustering using Pearson distance metrics separated the high-SOFA groups from all other groups. Gene Ontology analysis (FDR≤0.02) revealed enrichment of 80 categories including "immune response", "defence response", "lymphocyte activation", and "regulation of cell death". AHF patients undergoing MCSD surgery who develop postoperative MOD have unique leukocyte gene expression signatures. Comparing blood samples drawn with CPT and whole blood PAXgene tubes, we found a comparable differentiation using the PAX-samples (**Shahzad et al., 2010**).

7.3 Leukocyte gene network reverse engineering

In a feasibility study for the reverse engineering Aim 2.2, based on 285 microarrays (7370 genes) from 98 heart transplant patients enrolled in the "Cardiac Allograft Rejection Gene Expression" (CARGO) study (**Deng et al., 2006**), we used the information-theoretic, reverse-engineering algorithm called ARACNe (Algorithm for the Reconstruction of Accurate Cellular Networks) and chromatin Immunoprecipitation assay to reconstruct and validate a putative gene PBMC interaction network. We focused our analysis on transcription factor (TF) genes and developed a priority score to incorporate aspects of network dynamics and information from published literature to supervise gene discovery. ARACNe generated a cellular network and predicted interactions for each TF during rejection and quiescence. Genes that were ranked highest by priority score included those related to apoptosis, humoral and cellular immune response such as GABP, NFKB, FADD and CREB. We used the transcription factor CREB to validate our network. ARACNe predicted 29 putative first neighbour genes of CREB. Eleven of these (37%) were previously reported. Out of the 18 unknown predicted interactions, 14 primers were identified and 11 could be immunoprecipitated (78.6%). Overall, 75% (n = 22) inferred CREB targets were validated, a significantly higher fraction than randomly expected ($p<0.001$, Fisher's exact test). We concluded that our results confirm the accuracy of ARACNe to reconstruct the PBMC transcriptional network and show the utility of systems biological approaches to identify possible molecular targets and biomarkers (**Cadeiras et al., 2010**).

8. Future research

Circulating peripheral blood leukocyte populations monitor tissues and blood for agents that pose a danger to the organism (**Matzinger, 2007**). They sense the functional state of all organs in a coordinated way and provide diagnostic information. They constitute a "systemic" organ that can be easily monitored to assess the state of various tissues and the blood. Serial leukocyte GEP can characterize the systemic inflammatory response following intravenous endotoxin administration in healthy individuals (**Calvano et al., 2005**), in heart transplant rejection Deng 2006, and in MOD following trauma (**Laudanski et al., 2006**). Therefore, the information about gene activity in a patient's mixed peripheral leukocyte pool can be used to improve our understanding of organ dysfunction. In particular, knowing the pattern of leukocyte gene expression of a patient at the same time when the patient's organ function status is known can clarify the relationship between these two system levels and may provide a better scoring tool for evaluating MOD.

The integration of a validated leukocyte transcriptome classifier into a clinical MOD scoring system is a novel systems biology strategy that has the potential to improve the prediction, management and outcome of MOD. Developing an immune system GEP parameter needs to proceed in well-defined succinct stages. Establishing a quantitative phenome-transcriptome relationship is an important step in developing a leukocyte GEP-classifier (**Shahzad et al., 2009**). Although this relationship is not necessarily of causal nature, it is critical to identify genes and/or pathways that relate to the biology of the MOD phenotype. The development and independent validation of a GEP-classifier in comparison to a quantifiable clinical phenotype is the critical step in the development of the new GEP parameter. The integration of this GEP-classifier into the clinical MOD-scoring system is an important step towards improving patient outcome and ICU resource use.

The goal is to investigate the interaction between peripheral blood leukocytes and the multi-organ dysfunction syndrome (MOD) in heart failure patients undergoing cardiac support surgery. Specifically, we plan to measure changes in leukocyte gene expression profiles (GEP) in patients developing this postoperative complication in comparison to matched patients who do not develop MOD. From this, we plan to develop and validate a leukocyte GEP test, integrate it into current clinical MOD-scoring systems and demonstrate improved patient outcome prediction. We hope that this will 1) lead to an improved understanding of the mechanisms leading to death in MOD-patients, 2) help identify those patients before cardiac surgery who have a higher probability of MOD, and, after cardiac surgery, to identify 3) those patients who are entering the subclinical phase of MOD, and 4) those patients who are in an advanced state of MOD with very little probability of recovery.

9. Importance & significance

In the United States, MOD develops during 15% of all ICU admissions, causes up to 80% of all ICU deaths, and results in ICU costs of >$100,000 per patient or ~$500,000 per survivor (**ACCP, 1992; Barie et al., 1996; Barie et al., 2000**).

Heart failure related MOD represents a significant healthcare resource challenge (**Ong et al., 2009**). A great amount of resources are spent in the last 6-month period of life of HF patients with a complicated course. The cost of Mechanical Circulatory Support Device therapy with a complicated course, in comparison to an uncomplicated course, is >$100,000 higher (**DiGiorgi 2005**). Overall, HF costs $20-56 billion per year. However, more resource consumption does not necessarily yield better outcomes (**Orszag, 2008**) although higher resource spending increases the likelihood of favourable outcomes (**Ong et al., 2009**). Therefore, the major challenge is to identify 1) before cardiac surgery, those patients who have a higher probability of MOD, 2) after cardiac surgery, those patients who are entering the subclinical phase of MOD, and 3) those patients who are in an advanced state of MOD with very little probability of recovery.

10. Conclusion

With the increased incidence of HF and advances in critical care medicine more patients are undergoing cardiac support surgeries with high-risk clinical profiles. This puts HF patients at increased risk of developing MOD, which is the leading cause of morbidity and mortality in the ICUs. Currently available clinical scoring systems are limited to accurately predict the risk of MOD. The integration of a validated leukocyte transcriptome classifier into a clinical MOD scoring system represents a novel systems biological strategy that has the potential to 1) improve the prediction, management and outcome of MOD and 2) optimize health resource utilization in the ICU.

11. References

American College of Chest Physicians/Society of Critical Care Medicine Consensus Conference: Definitions for sepsis and multiple organ failure and guidelines for the use of innovative therapies in sepsis. Crit Care Med 1992; 20:864-874

Angus DC, Linde-Zwirble WT, Lidicker J, Clermont G, Carcillo J, Pinsky MR. Epidemiology of severe sepsis in the United States: analysis of incidence, outcome, and associated costs of care. Crit Care Med. 2001 Jul;29(7):1303-10

Barie PS, Hydo LJ. Epidemiology of multiple organ dysfunction syndrome in critical surgical illness. Surg Infect (Larchmt). 2000 Fall;1(3):173-85

Barie PS, Hydo LJ. Influence of multiple organ dysfunction syndrome on duration of critical illness and hospitalization. Arch Surg. 1996 Dec;131(12):1318-23

Cadeiras M, von Bayern M, Sinha A, Shahzad K, Lim WK, Grenett H, Tabak E, Klingler T, Califano A, Deng MC. Drawing Networks of Rejection - A Systems Biological Approach to the Identification of Candidate Genes in Heart Transplantation. J Cell Mol Med 2010 (in press)

Calvano SE, Xiao W, Richards DR, Felciano RM, Baker HV, Cho RJ, Chen RO, Brownstein BH, Cobb JP, Tschoeke SK, Miller-Graziano C, Moldawer LL, Mindrinos MN, Davis RW, Tompkins RG, Lowry SF; Inflamm and Host Response to Injury Large Scale Collab. Res. Program. A network-based analysis of systemic inflammation in humans. Nature 2005;437:1032-7

Deng MC, Edwards LB, Taylor DO, et al. Mechanical circulatory support device database of the international society for heart and lung transplantation: third annual report-2005. J Heart Lung Transplant 2005;24:1182-7

Deng MC, Eisen HJ, Mehra RM, Billingham M, Marboe CC, Berry G, Kobashigawa J, Johnson FL, Starling RC, Murali S, Pauly DF, Baron H, Wohlgemuth JG, Woodward RN, Klingler TM, Walther D, Lal PG, Rosenberg S, Hunt SA, for the CARGO Investigators. Non-invasive detection of rejection in cardiac allograft recipients using gene expression profiling. Am J Transplant 2006:6:150-160

Dew MA, Kormos RL, Winowich S et al. Quality of life outcomes in Left Ventricular Assist System inpatients and outpatients. ASAIO J. 1999;45:218-225

Digiorgi PL, Reel MS, Thornton B, Burton E, Naka Y, Oz MC. Heart transplant and left ventricular assist device costs. J Heart Lung Transplant 2005;24:200-4

Gelijns AC, Richards AF, Williams DL et al. Evolving costs of long-term left ventricular assist device implantation. Ann Thorac Surg. 1997;64:1312-9

Goldstein DJ, Zucker M, Arroyo L, Baran D, McCarthy PM, Loebe M, Noon GP.the MicroMed DeBakey VAD. Safety and feasibility trial of the MicroMed DeBakey ventricular assist device as a bridge to transplantation. (MicroMed Technology Inc., Houston, Texas), an axial flow pump (2), has been undergoing clinical evaluation as a bridge to transplantation. J Am Coll Cardiol. 2005;45:962-3

Katsumata T, Westaby S. Implantable axial flow impeller pumps. J Circ Support 1998;1:13-9

Kirklin JK. Developmental History of Mechanical Circulatory Support. In: Frazier OH, Kirklin JK (Eds): Mechanical Circulatory Support (ISHLT Monograph Series Volume 1). Elsevier 2006,Philadelphia, pp 1-8

Kirklin JK, Naftel DC, Stevenson LW, Kormos RL, Pagani FD, Miller MA, Ulisney K, Young JB. INTERMACS database for durable devices for circulatory support: first annual report. J Heart Lung Transplant. 2008 Oct;27(10):1065-72

Lietz K, Long JW, Kfoury AG, Slaughter MS, Silver MA, Milano CA, Rogers JG, Naka Y, Mancini D, Miller LW. Outcomes of left ventricular assist device implantation as destination therapy in the post-REMATCH era: implications for patient selection. Circulation 2007;116:497-505

Laudanski K, Miller-Graziano C, Xiao W, Mindrinos MN, Richards DR, De A, Moldawer LL, Maier RV, Bankey P, Baker HV, Brownstein BH, Cobb JP, Calvano SE, Davis RW, Tompkins RG. Cell-specific expression and pathway analyses reveal alterations in trauma-related human T cell and monocyte pathways. Proc Natl Acad Sci U S A 2006;103:15564-9

Matzinger P. Friendly and dangerous signals: is the tissue in control? Nat Immunol 2007;8:11-3

Marshall JC, Cook DJ, Christou NV, Bernard GR, Sprung CL, Sibbald WJ. Multiple organ dysfunction score: a reliable descriptor of a complex clinical outcome.Crit Care Med 1995 ;23:1638-52

Minne L, Abu-Hanna A, de Jonge E. Evaluation of SOFA-based models for predicting mortality in the ICU: a systematic review. Crit Care 2008;12:R161

Nashef SA, Roques F, Michel P, Gauducheau E, Lemeshow S, Salamon R. European system for cardiac operative risk evaluation (EuroSCORE). Eur J Cardiothorac Surg 1999;16:9-13

Ong MK, Mangione CM, Romano PS, Zhou Q, Auerbach AD, Chun A, Davidson B, Ganiats TG, Greenfield S, Gropper MA, Malik S, Rosenthal JT, Escarce JJ Looking forward, looking back: assessing variations in hospital resource use and outcomes for elderly patients with heart failure. Circ Cardiovasc Qual Outcomes 2009;2:548-57

Orszag PR. Increasing the value of federal spending on health care. Washington, DC: Committee on the Budget, U.S. House of Representatives, July 16, 2008

Poirier V. Worldwide experience with the TCI HeartMate system: issues and future perspective. Thorac Cardiovasc Surg. 1999;47(Suppl. 2):316-20

Portner PM, Oyer PE, Pennington DG et al. Implantable electrical left ventricular assist system: bridge to transplantation and the future. Ann Thorac Surg. 1989;47(1):142-150

Robbins RC, Oyer PE. Bridge to transplant with the Novacor left ventricular assist system. Ann Thorac Surg. 1999;68:695-7

Rose EA, Gelijns AC, Moskowitz AJ, Heitjan DF, Stevenson LW, Dembitsky W, Long JW, Ascheim DD, Tierney AR, Levitan RG, Watson JT, Meier P, Ronan NS, Shapiro PA, Lazar RM, Miller LW, Gupta L, Frazier OH, Desvigne-Nickens P, Oz MC, Poirier VL; Randomized Evaluation of Mechanical Assistance for the Treatment of Congestive Heart Failure (REMATCH) Study Group. Long-term use of a left ventricular assist device for end-stage heart failure. N Engl J Med. 2001 Nov 15;345(20):1435-43

Schmid C, Hammel D, Deng MC et al. Ambulatory care of patients with ventricular assist devices. Circulation. 1999;100[suppl II]:224-228

Shahzad K, Sinha A, Latif F, Deng MC. Standardized operational procedures in clinical gene expression biomarker panel development. In: Scherer A (Ed). Batch effects and experimental noise in Microarray Analysis: sources and solutions. John Wiley & Sons, Chichester 2009

Shahzad K, Sladen RN, Latif F, Akashi H, Onat D, Sinha A, Rodriguez A, Wahlander S, Naka Y, Deng MC. Leukocyte Gene Expression Signatures of MultiOrgan Dysfunction After Mechanical Circulatory Support Device Implantation in Patients with Heart Failure. Circulation (abst), Nov 2010. (in press)

Sinha A, Shahzad K, Latif F, Cadeiras M, von Bayern M, Oz S, Naka Y, Deng MC. Peripheral Blood Mononuclear Cell Transcriptome Profiles Suggest T-cell Immunosuppression after Uncomplicated Mechanical Circulatory Support Device Surgery. Hum Immunol 2010;71:164-9

Vincent JL, Moreno R, Takala J, Willatts S, De Mendonça A, Bruining H, Reinhart CK, Suter PM, Thijs LG. The SOFA (Sepsis-related Organ Failure Assessment) score to describe organ dysfunction/failure. On behalf of the Working Group on Sepsis-Related Problems of the European Society of Intensive Care Medicine. Intensive Care Med 1996;22:707-10

Vincent JL, de Mendonça A, Cantraine F, Moreno R, Takala J, Suter PM, Sprung CL, Colardyn F, Blecher S. Use of the SOFA score to assess the incidence of organ dysfunction/failure in intensive care units: results of a multicenter, prospective study. Working group on "sepsis-related problems" of the European Society of Intensive Care Medicine. Crit Care Med 1998;26:1793-800

Wieselthaler GM, Schima H, Hiesmayr M et al. First clinical experience with the DeBakey VAD continuous-axial-flow pump for bridge to transplantation. Circulation. 2000;101:256-259

Zimmerrman JE, Kramer AA, McNair DS, Malila FM. Acute Physiology and Chronic Health Evaluation (APACHE) IV: Hospital mortality assessment for today's critically ill patients. Crit Care Med 2006;34:1297-1310

6

Future Treatment of Acute Cardiac Collapse - A Role for Percutaneous Circulatory Assist Devices

Vepgard Tuseth MD, PhD and Jan Erik Nordrehaug MD, PhD
Department of Heart Disease, Haukeland University Hospital, N-5021 Bergen, Norway

1. Introduction

1.1 Acute cardiac collapse

Patients with cardiogenic shock and cardiac arrest still have a very poor prognosis despite recent improvements in treatment algorithms. Acute coronary ischemia and myocardial infarction (AMI) is the most frequent cause of cardiogenic shock and cardiac arrest. Improved survival has been shown for patients with AMI treated with urgent coronary revascularization. Also, improved pre-hospital logistics and cooling after successful resuscitation has shown possible benefit for cardiac arrest patients. However, a large proportion of patients with AMI and acute cardiac collapse do not survive until hospital discharge. These represent a group where current treatment options are often unsuccessful.

This far, advances in pharmacological treatment have produced various substances with theoretical and hemodynamic promise but clinical effects have been scarce. The use of vasopressors and inotropes generally has failed to show effect on mortality in cardiogenic shock and cardiac arrest. Recently a large clinical trial showed no effect of intravenous medication on survival for cardiac arrest victims (Figure 1).

Lately, more thought provoking data have emerged indicating a possible negative effect of vasopressor therapy on cardiac and cerebral perfusion during circulatory collapse and resuscitation. Clinical reports have further suggested a possible relationship between the use of adrenaline like drugs and increased mortality in patients with acute myocardial infarction and shock.

Mechanical support with intra-aortic balloon pump (IABP) counter pulsation therapy has been routinely used for several years in cardiogenic shock but the clinical usefulness is currently being strongly questioned. In cardiac arrest, optimally performed chest compressions are critical for successful re-establishment of intrinsic pulse giving rhythm (Figure 2). Mechanical compression-decompression devices have also shown impressive hemodynamic effects experimentally but a benefit compared with conventional chest compressions has not been found in clinical trials.

Both IABP and the compression-decompression devices have been associated with bleeding complications.

The mechanisms behind refractory cardiogenic shock and cardiac arrest may be many and are yet not clearly defined. It seems clear however, that with the pharmacological and

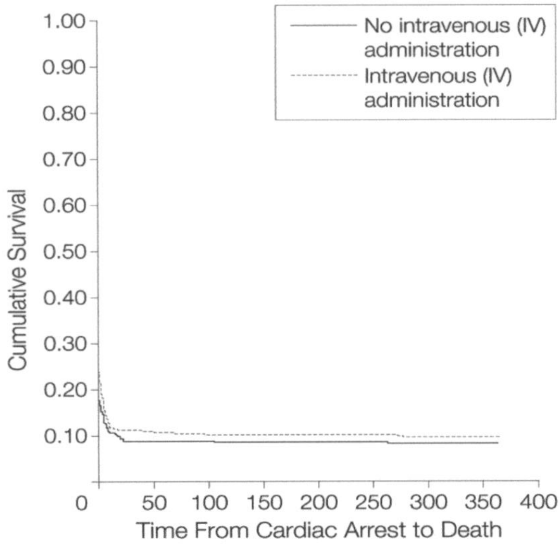

Fig. 1. Survival after witnessed out-of-hospital cardiac arrest with and without any intravenous (IV) drug therapy. Olavsveengen et al. JAMA. 2009 Nov 25;302(20):2222-9

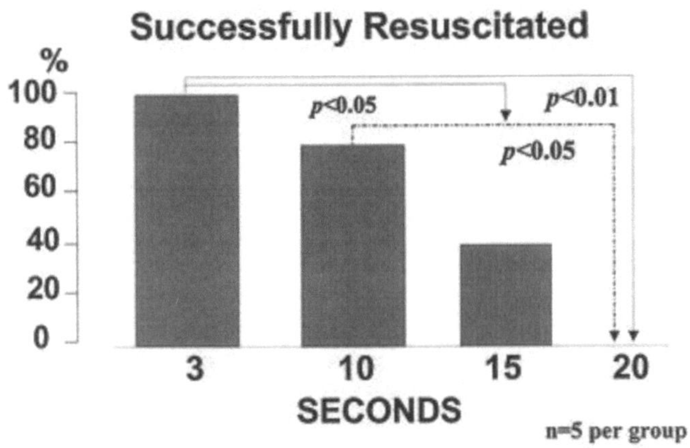

Detrimental effect of interrupted chest compressions

Fig. 2. Interrupted chest compressions (3-10-15 seconds) dramatically reduce the chance of successful defibrillation. Yu et al. Circulation 2002 Jul 16;106(3):368-72

mechanical approaches for hemodynamic support currently in use, vital organ perfusion and cardiac recovery is not reliably obtained sufficiently to have life saving effect.

A major focus for future research in the field of acute cardiac collapse should be on development of approaches for improved circulatory support.

1.2 Cardiac assist therapy in stable patients vs. acute hemodynamic collapse

Left ventricular assist devices (LVADs) can reduce myocardial workload and improve vital organ perfusion in patients with impaired cardiac function. In severe chronic heart failure LVAD therapy has been shown to substantially improve long term survival. Continuous flow devices have shown clinical benefit and are regularly used for long term treatment of terminal heart failure. The theoretical added benefit of additional right ventricular assist device (RVAD) therapy has not been shown to improve results.

Most LVAD systems require surgical implantation and are thus less well suited for acute use in critically ill patients. Patients with acute circulatory collapse require urgent circulatory support in order to prevent irreversible tissue ischemia and vital organ damage. In some cases, the time window for effective treatment may be too short to permit for required logistical and technical procedures related to surgical intervention. Furthermore, the potential to cause further compromise in hemodynamic and metabolic status with complex surgical procedures can be deleterious in these already marginal patients.

Surgical LVADs as well as different types of cardiopulmonary support (CPS) systems, commonly used in routine cardiac surgery have been employed in patients with acute cardiac collapse including cardiogenic shock and cardiac arrest. Results have been encouraging with respect to improving hemodynamics in treated patients. However, clinical results for the most critically ill have not been shown to improve with the devices and technologies tested this far. The lack of a predictable generalised benefit with surgical cardiac assist therapy in acute hemodynamic collapse may be related to complicated implantation procedures and high risk of complications.

1.3 Percutaneous left ventricular assist devices (PVADs)

Recently, cardiac support systems with percutaneous access have been developed. Percutaneous devices could offer rapid placement and reduced risk of complications compared with surgical devices. These obvious advantages compared with surgical assist systems in the critically ill could outweigh limitations in blood delivery related to the smaller size of percutaneous devices.

Two different types of PVAD devices have been approved for clinical use (Impella LP2.5, TandemHeart) (Figure 3). The Impella LP 2.5 is a transfemoraly deployed 12 F impeller pump deployed in the left ventricle on a pigtail shaped catheter. Maximal delivery is 2.5L/min, the pump outlet is situated in the ascending aorta in the level of the coronary artery ostia. The TandemHeart requires 21F venous and 15F arterial groin access as well as trans-septal puncture in order to obtain a left-atrial to femoral-artery blood delivery of maximally 5L/min. Deployment times have been found to be longer with the latter device but the risk of procedure related complications remain low with both systems.

Both devices have been studied in clinical use and have shown potential to improve hemodynamics in cardiogenic shock and acute myocardial infarction. The use of PVAD therapy has also been advocated and tested as backup hemodynamic support in scheduled high risk cardiac intervention including percutaneous coronary intervention (PCI) and trans-catheter aortic valve implantation (TAVI).

In acute hemodynamic collapse and in resuscitated patients requiring immediate circulatory support, the less complicated and more rapidly deployed LP 2.5 may be the technically most attractive of the available devices. The LP 2.5 also offers a more physiological blood delivery and unloading as blood is pumped directly out of the left ventricle into the pre-coronary and pre-cerebral arterial circulation. It is yet unclear however, if the limited delivery of 2.5 liters with the Impella device is sufficient to sustain adequate systemic circulation and cardiac unloading over time in a critical clinical setting. Potentially, improved support can be achieved with the larger (21) Impella LP 5.0 pump for which percutaneous deployment may also be feasible.

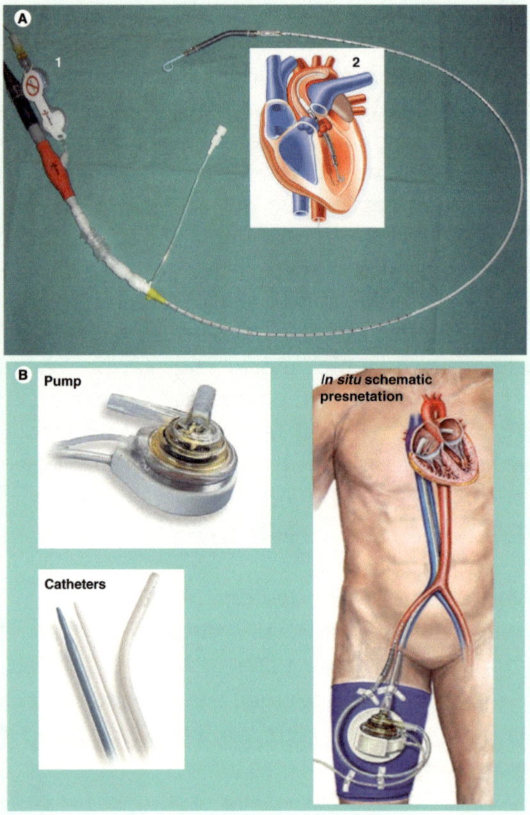

Fig. 3. PVADs in clinical use.
A: 1)Impella LP 2.5, 2) in-situ schematic drawing.
B: TandemHeart-pump, catheters, in-situ schematic drawing

2. Problems to be solved

2.1 Irreversible ischemic injury

Vital organ hypo-perfusion causing ischemic dysfunction and injury is a major challenge. In acute hemodynamic collapse tissue damage due to inadequate blood delivery can be severe. The thresholds for irreversible ischemic injury causing cell death and organ dysfunction are different in different tissues. Vital organs with high metabolic rates as the heart and brain may be particularly prone to injury during short term hypo-perfusion and ischemia. In particular, the risk of acute brain injury is high when cardio-pulmonary resuscitation needs to be performed. Lowering metabolic rates and oxygen consumption with cooling has shown potential to reduce ischemic injury in the heart as well as in the brain after cardiac arrest. Cardiac volume unloading with PVAD therapy can also reduce cardiomyocyte oxygen consumption and may have potential to reduce ischemic injury. Contrarily, vasopressor substances may contribute to increased myocardial injury by increasing metabolic rates in an ischemic heart muscle.

Mechanisms behind cell dysfunction and death during ischemia being investigated and a wide variety of pathways and mediators have been described. Furthermore, Emerging therapeutic targets for pharmacological intervention to prevent ischemic injury have been identified, particularly in the field of reperfusion injury.

Activation of the mithochondrial trans-membrane pore MPTP leads to mithochondrial swelling and subsequent cell death and is by many considered the final common path way for ischemic cell necrosis (Figure 4). A wide range of novel therapies aiming at modulating MPTP and the pathways leading to its activation and inactivation are currently being investigated but a definite clinical breakthrough has not yet been reached.

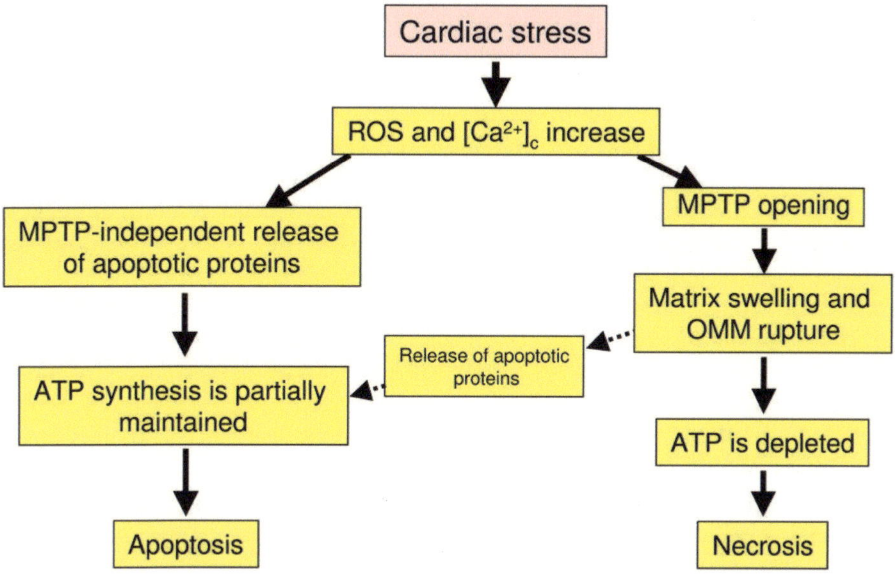

Fig. 4. Mitochondrial permeability transition pore plays a key role in cardiomyocyte necrosis after ischemic stress. Lacerda et al. Cardiovasc Res. 2009;84:201-208

2.2 Persistent cardiac arrest

The most common cause of cardiac arrest is myocardial ischemia.

Cardiac arrest has a high mortality and morbidity despite recent developments in resuscitation methods, educational programs and improved logistics. Clinical results are often poor even after successful re-establishment of intrinsic circulation. Long term neurological sequelae are present in up-to 60% of patients with current advanced therapy including cooling, revascularization and other adjunctive therapy. In patients with persistent cardiac arrest defined as pulseless cardiac rhythm unresponsive to advanced cardiac life support (ACLS) prognosis is even worse.

The setting of persistent cardiac arrest represents the extreme of acute critical cardiac failure where mechanical intervention is absolutely required in order to sustain circulation. Persistent cardiac arrest is present in a substantial portion of cardiac arrest victims; with up to 60%-80% reported in some studies.

Mechanisms behind refractory cardiac arrest remain to be definitely established. There is evidence that sustained coronary ischemia may be an important factor behind shock resistant ventricular fibrillation in ischemic cardiac arrest. Regional ischemic metabolic changes with interstitial hyperkalemia and acidosis contribute to cardiomyocyte electrical instability causing ineffective depolarization patterns which impair re-establishment of spontaneous circulation with defibrillation.

Reports of successful treatment of persistent VF with left ventricular unloading catheters have also been presented indicating that increased left ventricular pressure during cardiac arrest can make the heart refractory to cardioversion. The combined treatment of acute cardiac collapse patients with percutaneous revascularization and a PVAD may in theory be able to improve the return of spontaneous circulation and could also improve cardiac recovery and tissue perfusion after initial stabilisation.

2.3 Life support during revascularization

During ischemic cardiac arrest, chest compressions and coronary revascularisation should be performed optimally in order to maximalise the clinical potential of both treatments. Interruptions of chest compressions and impaired coronary visualisation can reduce the prognostic benefit of acute revascularisation in persistent ischemic cardiac arrest. Chest compressions can cause traumatic injury to the chest and heart which could hamper the effect of otherwise successful treatment. Possibly, the use of percutaneous devices may be more suited for acute treatment in these critically compromised patients.

In the cardiac catheterization laboratory, a percutaneous left ventricular assist device can be deployed within few minutes and may be useful both by improving hemodynamics and by obviating the need for chest compressions during percutaneous coronary intervention during persistent ischemic cardiac arrest.

Of the currently available percutaneous assist devices the Impella 2.5 is likely to be more suited for hyper-acute use during cardiac arrest due to less complicated and faster deployment procedures. This device has been studied in experimental models of persistent ischemic cardiac arrest and results have been promising.

2.4 Previous research

Current resuscitation algorithms are complex and include defibrillation, manual chest compressions and the use of vasopressor drugs. The hemodynamic and clinical effects of conventional resuscitation with external chest compressions and medical therapy are in many cases suboptimal. Results from large clinical trials indicate a substantial potential for improvement of current advanced cardiac life support.

When spontaneous circulation can not be rapidly restored after witnessed resuscitated cardiac arrest (persistent cardiac arrest) reported mortality is close to 100% with conventional treatment.

Sophisticated pharmacological approaches to improve cardiac efficacy and blood pressure have not been able to improve outcomes in this population despite impressive pre-clinical data. Additionally, recent studies indicate vasopressor drugs may have detrimental effects on cardiac and cerebral function. In cardiogenic shock, vasopressor use has been associated with impaired outcomes in the setting of acute myocardial infarction. It may be reasonable to suggest that inotropes and vasopressor substances do not represent the pharmacological agents most likely to make a significant impact on patient survival in this field in the future.

Mechanical assist devices represent an attractive approach in the treatment of cardiac collapse. Intra aortic balloon pump therapy in cardiogenic shock and compression-decompression devices in cardiac arrest are in widespread routine clinical use despite debatable clinical data. Similary as for inotropes and vasopressor therapy, it may be inferred that the encouraging blood pressure augmenting effects of the devices overshadow the lack of survival benefit and the risk of such treatment in clinical practice.

Other treatment modalities such as volume expansion and abdominal compression for increasing venous return have shown hemodynamic benefits comparable to that of vasopressors but clinical use and testing has been limited.

From a hemodynamic standpoint, LVADs as well as CPS represent attractive approaches for improving outcomes in acute cardiac collapse requiring resuscitation. This far, various surgically deployed assist systems and external mechanical compression-decompression devices have been investigated in cardiac arrest. Hemodynamic effects have been promising but clinical results have remained poor.

In the clinical setting, acute myocardial ischemia is a major cause of cardiac arrest. Some studies indicate that urgent PCI may improve outcomes in patients with ST-elevation on the electrocardiogram after return of spontaneous circulation. The subgroup of patients with ROSC and subsequent ST-elevation on ECG constitute only a small part of cardiac arrest patients. Acute coronary revascularisation has not been proven to be beneficial for the large portion of patients without ST elevation or without ROSC.

However, cardiac arrest is commonly caused by acute coronary ischemia in the absence of obvious non-cardiac causes (Figure 5). Furthermore, the presence of coronary ischemia may reduce the success rate of defibrillation causing persistent ventricular fibrillation. On this basis, patients with suspected acute coronary ischemia and persistent cardiac arrest are increasingly being treated with acute revascularization with cardiac catheterization even with ongoing resuscitation.

Table 2. Angiographic Data in the 84 Patients Who Underwent Angiography.*

Variable	Value
Normal coronary arteries — no. (%)	17 (20)
Clinically insignificant coronary artery disease (≤50 percent stenosis) — no. (%)	7 (8)
Clinically significant coronary artery disease — no. (%)	60 (71)
Single-vessel disease	22
Two-vessel disease	13
Three-vessel disease	24
Isolated left main coronary artery disease	1
Left ventricular ejection fraction — %	33.9±10.5
Left ventricular end-diastolic pressure — mm Hg	25.3±9.5

*Plus–minus values are means ±SD. Because of rounding, the percentages do not total 100.

Fig. 5. High incidence of coronary artery disease in cardiac arrest victims. Spaulding et al.N Engl J Med 336:1629-1633 June 5, 1997

3. Our data

3.1 Impella LP 2.5 in cardiac arrest

We performed the first experimental assessment of PVAD therapy during ischemic ventricular fibrillation in 2005. In a randomized porcine model we showed that blood delivery to the systemic circulation could be achieved with a PVAD during cardiac arrest without simultaneous chest compressions and without vasopressor. It was also found that intravenous fluid loading improved pump delivery during cardiac arrest in a randomized comparison with conservative fluid infusion. The complete results have been published previously (Tuseth et al, Crit. Care Med., 2008).

Design and results are outlined below.

16 porcine subjects under general anesthesia were randomized to percutaneous left ventricular assist device support either with conventional or with intensified fluid infusion as only hemodynamic interventions during cardiac arrest. All procedures were performed with percutaneous access.

After randomization for fluid infusion, cardiac arrest was induced by balloon occlusion of the proximal left anterior descending artery. The percutaneous left ventricular assist device and fluid infusions were started after ventricular fibrillation had been induced. Brain, kidney, myocardial tissue perfusion and cardiac index were measured with the microspheres injection technique at baseline, 3 and 15 minutes. Additional hemodynamic monitoring continued until 30 minutes.

At 30 minutes LVAD function was sustained in 11/16 animals (8/8 intensified fluid vs. 3/8 conventional fluid) and was associated with intensified fluid loading ($P<0.001$). Mean cardiac index at 3 minutes of VF was 1.2 L.min/m2 (29% of baseline, $P<0.05$). Mean perfusion at 3 minutes was 65% in the brain and 74% in the myocardium compared to Baseline (P=NS) with no further significant change after 15 minutes.

3.2 Prevention of cerebral ischemia with Impella LP 2.5 during cardiac arrest

In a second study, using a similar protocol, our group investigated the effect of PVAD-assisted circulation during cardiac arrest on cerebral ischemic injury. Using cerebral microdialysis we found that ischemic cerebral metabolism and injury assessed with microdialysis could be avoided during a prolonged period of cardiac arrest. The same study also showed that PVAD function and hemodynamics were maintained for an extended period of 45 minutes of cardiac arrest.

The complete results have been published previously.

Design and results are outlined below. (Tuseth et al, Resuscitation , 2009).

12 anesthetized pigs in narcosis had cerebral microdialysis and pressure catheters implanted via craniotomy; otherwise the principal experimental set-up was comparable to paper 1.

Cerebral microdialysis markers (glucose, pyruvate, lactate, glycerol) were analyzed after 20 and 40 minutes of VF with assisted circulation. Tissue perfusion was measured with microspheres injections.

After 20 minutes of VF, cerebral microdialysis showed no ischemic changes (P=NS to Baseline for glucose, glycerol, lactate, pyruvate and lactate/pyruvate ratio) in subjects with maintained end-tidal CO_2 values above 1.3 kPa (predicted survivors). After 40 minutes only lactate showed a significant change compared to Baseline ($P<0.05$) (Figure 6). Microspheres confirmed blood flow to the brain at 57% and myocardium at 72% of baseline after 15 minutes ($P<0.05$), declining to 22% and 40% after 45 minutes respectively (P=NS). In the predicted non-survivors (end tidal CO_2 below 1.3 kPa after 20 minutes, n=6) microdialysis indicated cerebral ischemia at 20 minutes and tissue perfusion by microspheres was below 1% of Baseline (all P<0.05). End-tidal CO_2 identified subjects with and without successful circulation.

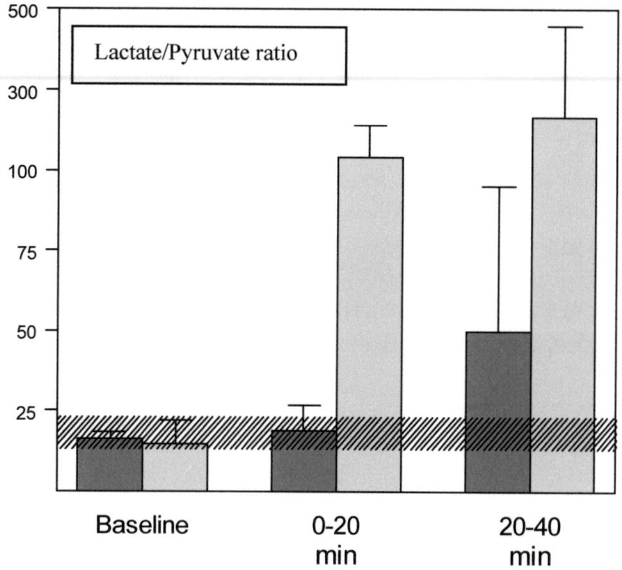

Fig. 6. Lactate/Pyruvate ratio from cerebral microdialysis is a sensitive marker for ischemic cerebral metabolism. Values with PVAD support during ischemic cardiac arrest in dark grey, without in light grey, normal values shaded. Values with PVAD support are normal during the first 20 minutes and moderately pathological between 20 and 40 minutes whereas values without support are immediately critical after onset of ventricular fibrillation. Tuseth et al, Resuscitation.2009 Oct;80(10):1197-203.

3.3 Randomised comparison of PVAD, LVAD and open chest cardiac massage during ischemic ventricular fibrillation

Finally, in a third study, the hemodynamic effects of the PVAD (Impella LP 2.5 (LP2.5)) were compared with optimal manual resuscitation using open chest cardiac massage and with a larger, surgically deployed LVAD (Impella LP 5.0 (LP5.0)) during VF.

This experiment compared clinical outcomes assessed by the rates of successful return of spontaneous circulation (ROSC) with defibrillation after 20 minutes of ischemic cardiac arrest with the three different methods of circulatory support. This study indicated the PVAD outperformed optimal conventional resuscitation with open chest cardiac massage with regards to myocardial perfusion and obtained similar outcomes for ROSC and cerebral perfusion compared to optimal current therapy (OCCM). Compared with a surgical LVAD in this clinical setting the PVAD also showed superior results, likely due to a problem with aortic regurgitation and shunting with the surgical device in the absence of any intrinsic circulation.

The complete results have been published previously (Tuseth et al, Resuscitation, 2010). Design and results are outlined below.

18 pigs were randomized into 3 groups (all n=6). Surgical preparation including thoracotomy was performed in general anesthesia. A Doppler flow probe was placed around the pulmonary artery for direct and continuous cardiac output measurement. A catheter was inserted into the mid-distal LAD for pressure monitoring and the distal LAD was occluded by ligature inducing myocardial ischemia. Microspheres injections were used for measuring of tissue-perfusion. VF was induced with diathermy stimulation of the left ventricle.
After 3 minutes of VF, cardiac output with cardiac massage was 1129 mL.min-1 vs. 1169 mL.min-1 with the percutaneous- and 570 mL.min-1 with the surgical device ($P<0.05$ for surgical vs. others). End-tidal CO_2 was 3.3 kPa with cardiac massage vs. 3.2 kPa with the percutaneous- and 2.3 kPa with the surgical device ($P<0.05$ surgical vs. others). Subepicardial perfusion was 0.33 mL.min-1.g-1 with cardiac massage vs. 0.62 mL.min-1.g-1 with both devices ($P<0.05$ devices vs. massage), cerebral perfusion was not significantly different between groups (all reported values after 3 min cardiac arrest, all $P<0.05$ vs. Baseline, all P= NS for 3 min vs. 15 min). Defibrillation after 20 minutes achieved return of spontaneous circulation in 5/6 subjects with cardiac massage vs. 6/6 with the percutaneous- and 4/6 with the surgical device (P=NS) (Figure 7).

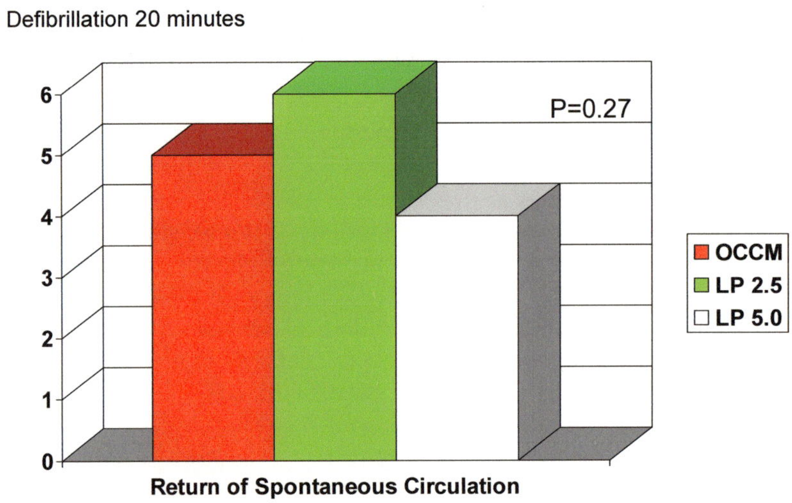

Fig. 7. Rates of successful defibrillation after 20 minutes of persistent ischemic cardiac arrest with open chest cardiac massage (OCCM) or PVAD (Impella LP 2.5) or LVAD (Impella LP 5.0). Tuseth et al. Resuscitation. 2010 Nov;81(11):1566-70.

4. Technical considerations

4.1 Resuscitation

In the routine clinical setting, manual or mechanical chest compressions are the current standard for life support during cardiac arrest. Despite advances in technical performance and monitoring, the hemodynamic effects and clinical outcomes still have potential for improvement. External devices have been employed with promising hemodynamic results, but uncertain clinical benefit. Internal cardiac massage with an open chest has proven superior results compared to external methods both in experimental and clinical studies. However, the method has not been established in the clinical routine as the technique requires surgical access to the heart and may have risk of complications. In experimental cardiac arrest, OCCM may be considered a clinically relevant reference for optimal CPR. A direct comparison of the PVAD to optimal CPR has not been performed previously.

4.2 Hemodynamic considerations

In the absence of myocardial contraction during cardiac arrest, blood flow through the pulmonary circulation depends on thoracic volume compression and decompression in conventional CPR. In addition, sequential variation of thoracic volume and pressure during mechanical ventilation may facilitate blood flow towards the left side circulation. Furthermore, blood flow through the pulmonary vasculature is improved by increasing central venous pressure and TPR. With PVAD support without concomitant chest compressions during VF, LV filling may be limited. However, with optimal filling conditions, the use of the percutaneous impeller device could be feasible during cardiac arrest. Intravenous fluid administration can increase venous return, central venous pressures and left ventricle filling pressures. Consequently, fluid loading may have potential to improve blood delivery to the left ventricle from the right side of the heart in cardiac arrest.

4.3 End-Tidal CO_2

End-tidal CO_2 values can be continuously monitored from the ventilator and may indicate the clinical efficacy of CPR during prolonged cardiac arrest. During resuscitation, end-tidal CO_2 is associated with cerebral perfusion and cardiac output. Cut off values have been identified which can be used to predict survival in cardiac arrest.

4.4 Cerebral injury

Despite novel therapeutic approaches including hypothermia, emergency revascularization, medical intervention and mechanical devices assist devices, ischemic cerebral damage remains a major limitation for outcomes after cardiac arrest. Assessment of cerebral blood flow can be achieved by various techniques. In experimental studies, perfusion measured by microspheres is a reliable approach for assessment of cerebral cortical perfusion and may provide relevant hemodynamic information, but can not detect or quantify ischemic injury.
A recently developed method employs a miniaturized dialysis technique for direct evaluation of biochemical markers related to metabolism and injury in different tissues. In order to assess cerebral injury, cerebral microdialysis can be performed via a miniature dialysis catheter implanted into the cerebral cortex through a small cranial burr hole (Figure 8). This technique can detect and monitor metabolic changes in the brain at an early stage after injury and has been validated in relation to cerebral perfusion and clinical outcomes. Limited data exist from previous experimental studies in circulatory arrest. Normal reference values have been defined. During cardiac arrest, cerebral microdialysis may give highly relevant information for the assessment of the clinical significance of hemodynamic interventions.

4.5 Animal models

Investigation of previously not tested treatment in cardiac arrest has potential to cause harm in a clinical setting. In general, new methodology may have unforeseen complications and may also infer with current optimal standard of care. In cardiac arrest, immediate and aggressive treatment is required for optimal survival which limits assessment of new

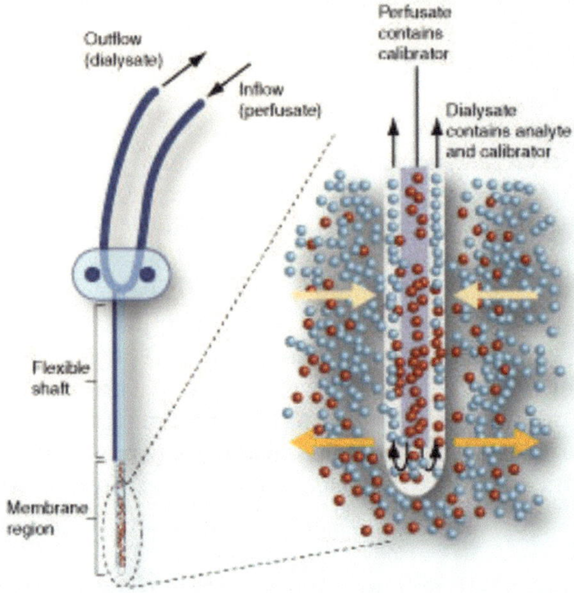

Fig. 8. Principles of cerebral microdialysis catheter. Tuseth et al. Interventional Cardiology.2009 Dec;1(2):197-208

hypotheses in human subjects in this setting. Prognosis is critically poor in this subset of patients and further research aiming on improving the understanding, and possibly the outcomes of cardiac arrest is considered highly relevant. Thus, the use of animal models of human disease may be considered appropriate in order to evaluate novel interventions in cardiac arrest. Research animals have been used in various protocols to study hemodynamics and interventions in cardiac arrest with considerable experimental evidence and validated end-points. In this project, PVAD was used to investigate the use of a miniature blood pump as hemodynamic support during cardiac arrest without concomitant conventional CPR. The device studied is designed for intra-arterial deployment from the femoral artery into the left ventricle and requires anatomy similar to that in humans for optimal assessment. The selected porcine model offers anatomic and hemodynamic conditions close to that in human subjects.

4.6 Animals

All three experimental protocols included Norwegian Land Race swine of either sex and with weight approximately 50 kg. Subjects were fasted overnight with free access to water. The animals were acclimatized for at least 7 days under controlled temperature, lighting and humidity and were fed with a standard diet. The experimental protocols were registered and approved by the Norwegian Animal Research Authority and by the local responsible laboratory animal veterinarian, and was conducted in accordance with national and international laws controlling experiments in live animals. A dose of 330mg acetylsalicylic acid was administered orally the day before the procedure in order to reduce the risk of coronary thrombus formation during intravascular procedures.

4.7 Anesthesia

After intramuscular premedication with ketamine (20 mg/kg) and atropine (1mg) in the neck, ear veins were cannulated. Animals were placed on a warm-water blanket with continuous monitoring of rectal temperature and electrocardiogram. Ventilation (spontaneous on mask) with O2 and 3% (vaporizer setting) isoflurane (Rhodia, Bristol, England) for 2 to 3 min allowed oral intubation. Ventilation was commenced and continued with a mixture of N_2O (56-57%) and oxygen. The mechanical ventilator (Cato M32000, Drägerwerk, Lübeck, Germany) was set to a tidal volume of 10 mL/kg and a frequency of 13 - 15 cycles/min; with small adjustments aiming at an end-tidal CO_2 of 5 %. Anesthesia was induced by intravenous loading doses of fentanyl 0.02 mg/kg, midazolam 0.3 mg/kg and sodium pentobarbital 15 mg/kg and maintained with continuous infusions of fentanyl 0.02 mg/kg per h, midazolam 0.3 mg/kg per h, (pancuronium 0.14 mg/kg per h, paper 1) and pentobarbital 4 mg/kg per h. Thus, the total fluid substitution for anesthesia amounted to 15 mL/kg per h.

4.8 Percutaneous model

After infiltrating the skin with 0.5% xylocaine the femoral arteries and veins were exposed bilaterally and secured by ligatures. Arterial (13F, 6F, 5F) and venous (8F) sheaths were inserted. A bolus of 5000 international units of heparin was administered intra-arterially after placing the sheaths and repeated every 60 minutes for the duration of the study. A 5F-pigtail catheter was placed in the left ventricle for injection of microspheres. A 6F multipurpose hockey stick catheter served as a guide for the left coronary artery. Right side pressures were measured with a Swan Ganz catheter in the pulmonary artery. The Impella LP 2.5 (Abiomed, USA) was implanted with the inlet below and the outlet above the aortic valve. Aortic pressure and pump output in L/min was recorded from the device module. End tidal CO_2 was monitored from the mechanical ventilator system. Samples for arterial acid-base measurements were taken from the arterial sheaths. Additionally, in paper 1, venous blood samples were taken at the same time points as arterial blood.
The Impella Recover LP 2.5 is a true percutaneous LVAD with a diameter of 4 mm (12F). Insertion is by a 13F arterial sheath and deployment into the LV is performed over a 0.14" guide wire under fluoroscopic guidance, usually via the femoral artery. The outlet is in the proximal ascending aorta. Positioning is guided by a pressure sensor.

4.9 Surgical model

Surgical tracheotomy and suprapubic vesical catheterization were performed directly after induction of narcosis. Next, median sternotomy was performed with an oscillating saw. After free-dissection of the aorta, a Doppler-flow probe (Medi-Stim Butterfly Flowmeter Probe, 21mm, MediStim, Oslo, Norway) was placed around the common pulmonary trunk permitting direct measurement of cardiac output. For microspheres administration and pressure monitoring, a soft catheter (Feeding tube CH 6 (2mm, 40cm), UNO Plast A/S, Hundested, Denmark) was deployed in the left atrium using Seldinger-technique and secured by sutures. For pressure monitoring in the LAD, a miniature catheter (ABBOCATH®-T 20 G, Venisystems, Sligo, Ireland) was inserted into the mid-distal portion of the left anterior descending artery (LAD) with Seldinger-technique and fixated with sutures, this also inducing myocardial ischemia distal to the implantation site. Additional fluid supplements were administered to compensate for any fluid- and blood-loss during

the study aiming to maintain a minimum flow in the pulmonary artery of 3 L.min-1 and also optimal filling of the heart visually determined from the surgical field. Trans-esophageal-echocardiography (TEE) with intravenous bubbles contrast was performed to detect potential cardiac defects with shunting of blood at Baseline . Baseline registrations were made during spontaneous circulation after 5 minutes of stabilization post-surgery. VF was induced by stimulation of the LV by surgical diathermy. Open chest cardiac massage was performed using both hands, with the left hand holding the right ventricle and the fingers of the right hand holding the left ventricle, performing anterior-posterior compression at a rate of approximately 80 min−1. Defibrillation with 50 Joules delivered directly to the myocardium was performed after 20 minutes of VF still with mid LAD occlusion.
The Impella Recover LP 5.0 has a diameter of 7mm (21 F) and a maximal output of 5 liters per minute. This device is principally similar to the LP 2.5, but due to its larger diameter, it requires surgical vascular access and hemostasis at the implantation site. The femoral or iliac artery is usually suitable for vascular access in human use. Due to smaller diameter and sharper curves of the vessels in the animals, vascular entry for the LP 5.0 was established through a vascular graft (GORE-TEX®Stretch Vascular Graft, W.L Gore & Associates, Inc., USA) sutured to the distal aorta with retroperitoneal access.

4.10 Sampling techniques

Labelled microspheres (Dye-Trak VII+®, Triton Technology, San Diego, CA) were injected into the left ventricle via a cardiac pigtail catheter with percutaneous technique. In the following two experiments, fluorescent beads were used (Dye-Trak F®, Triton Technology, San Diego, CA). Injections were made percutaneously into the left ventricle in paper 2 and directly into the left atrium in the surgical protocol. In all experiments, microspheres (15μ) dissolved in saline solution were injected. All reference blood samples were drawn from the right femoral artery starting immediately before the start of injections and lasting for 3 minutes. Four different colors were used, in a randomized sequence. Tissue samples were collected from the right and left kidney cortex, the cerebral cortex, right ventricle and from the myocardium. The left ventricular samples were separated between regions and divided into subendocardial and subepicardial halves. Tissue- and reference blood samples were weighed. Next the tissue samples were dissolved in 1M KOH and thereafter the colored or fluorescent markers were separated from the microspheres using a solution of 2-Ethoxyethyl Acetate. Finally, tissue blood flow rates were calculated by spectrophotometry using matched glass cuvettes . In paper 1, readings were made using a color spectrophotometer (Hewlett Packard 8452A). In the two next experiments, readings were made using a fluoro spectrophotometer (Shimadzu RF-5301PC).
Access for cerebral microdialysis and intracranial pressure (ICP) monitoring was established through a 0.5cm burr-hole 1cm lateral to the midline suture and 0.5 cm anterior to the coronal suture. The dura mater was incised with diathermy. The Codman MicroSensor ICP Transducer (Codman, Raynham, MA) was placed 2 cm into brain parenchyma and connected to a Codman ICP Express™ monitor (Codman). A microdialysis catheter with cut off 20 000 Dalton and membrane length 20 mm (CMA 70, Microdialysis AB, Solna, Sweden) was introduced 3 cm into cerebral parenchyma. The microdialysis catheter was perfused with CNS perfusion fluid (CMA Microdialysis AB, Solna, Sweden) at a rate of 0.3 μL/min, using a CMA 107 microdialysis pump (Microdialysis AB, Solna, Sweden). Microdialysis samples were collected in microvials (200μL, Microdialysis AB, Solna, Sweden) that were

changed after 20 minutes and directly analyzed with respect to glucose, glycerol, lactate and pyruvate using photometric assay (CMA 600 Microdialysis Analyzer, Microdialysis AB, Solna , Sweden). A total of 3 vials were analyzed in each experiment, one representing Baseline before VF, the next representing 0-20 minutes of VF and the final representing 20-40 minutes of VF.
Intravascular blood pressures were continuously monitored (HP, M108, Waltham, MA, US). Digital recordings and manual data logs were performed at the pre-specified time points. End-tidal CO2 was directly monitored from the ventilator (Cato M32000, Drägerwerk, Lübeck, Germany) and recordings were made at specified times.
All blood samples were drawn from the intravascular sheaths. Samples were taken immediately before injection of microspheres. Full blood was samples were analyzed directly after sampling. Arterial and venous blood-gas analysis was performed on an automated blood gas/electrolyte analyzer (AVL Opti 3, Critical Care Analyzer, OPTI Medical Systems inc. Roswell, GA, US). Full blood lactate samples were stored on ice and analyzed with amperiometric enzymoassay (ABL 800, Radiometer, Copenhaken, DK). Analysis was performed at the certified laboratory for clinical biochemistry, Haukeland University Hospital.

5. Future perspectives

5.1 Curremt PVAD status

The use of a percutaneous assist device has been shown experimentally to be hemodynamically effective in persistent cardiac arrest. The available data suggest the device may be able to prevent cerebral ischemic injury for a prolonged period of ventricular fibrillation without simultaneous chest compressions and vasopressor. Furthermore, hemodynamic and clinical efficacy was found to be at least as good as optimal conventional therapy with open chest cardiac massage during cardiac arrest in a porcine model.
Data from experimental cardiac arrest have demonstrated a promising area for potential clinical use of percutaneous left ventricular assist devices. The efficacy of the Impella 2.5 during experimental cardiac arrest indicate such a device can be useful as circulatory support for patients with cardiac arrest and extreme heart failure with severe organ hypo-perfusion for a limited period of time. Adjunctive treatment to improve efficacy of such devices, particularly intervention to improve left ventricular filling, may be another focus of further research. The clinical role of percutaneous assist devices in cardiac collapse with absent or severely impaired spontaneous circulation yet remains to be established.

5.2 Practical perspectives with the Impella LP 2.5 in acute hemodynamic collapse

The LP 2.5 may offer rapid and uncomplicated hemodynamic support, can prevent cerebral ischemia and may achieve hemodynamics and outcomes comparable to optimal manual resuscitation during cardiac arrest. These findings indicate the device may find a role in the clinical treatment of cardiac arrest. During acute percutaneous intervention for coronary ischemia in patients with ischemic cardiac arrest, a percutaneous assist device may facilitate coronary revascularization and could improve outcomes in this setting by reducing the need for chest compressions, cardioversion and adrenaline. Further benefit may be achieved by reducing the left ventricular work-load after revascularization.
Potentially, even less complicated deployment algorithms can be developed which may permit use of such devices in a broader clinical setting. Delivery can be performed via the

femoral, axillar, and the subclavian artery (116). Furthermore, trans-apical deployment of the device into the left ventricle through a chest wall puncture could be feasible with a device designed for antegrade delivery. Positioning can be confirmed with echocardiography, and with implantation-techniques independent of fluoroscopy, the device could potentially be useful also without available cardiac catheterization facilities. Accordingly, the clinical potential of the device might theoretically also include out-of hospital use. The future development of percutaneous assist device therapy in cardiac arrest may include percutaneously deployed right heart support systems and possibly the use of adjunctive medical or mechanical intervention for additional hemodynamic benefit. Clinical use for extended time periods during cardiac arrest can not be recommended from the current data. Fluid loading is potentially deleterious over time for patients with compromised left ventricular function due to acute myocardial infarction. As with conventional CPR, the use of LVAD support if spontaneous heart function can not be restored over a longer period of time, have ethical implications that need to be considered.

6. Conclusions

Limited clinical data have demonstrated hemodynamic efficacy and safety of the two PVADs in clinical use. Experimental data with the Impella LP 2.5 have shown this PVAD device is able to sustain perfusion to the brain and myocardium during ischemic cardiac arrest in a porcine model. Fluid loading improved pump efficacy during cardiac arrest. Furthermore, cerebral microdialysis indicated that the percutaneous LVAD can prevent cerebral injury during prolonged cardiac arrest. The hemodynamic effects of the device and its effects on tissue perfusion and cerebral ischemia can be maintained for an extended period of VF and may be continuously assessed with end-tidal CO2 from the ventilator.

The Impella LP 2.5 device maintained hemodynamics and tissue perfusion comparable to open chest cardiac compressions during 15 minutes of VF in a porcine model and obtained similar rates of return of spontaneous circulation after defibrillation compared with open chest cardiac massage. A larger surgically implanted assist device of similar design did not improve results in this experimental model.

Percutaneous left ventricular assist devices may be able to fill a void in the acute treatment of patients with acute hemodynamic collapse. With relative ease of deployment, low risk of procedural complications and beneficial hemodynamic effects, such devices should have potential to improve outcomes in patients with refractory cardiogenic shock and persistent ventricular fibrillation. These patients constitute a significant population in contemporary clinical practice which still have a very high mortality with current treatment. PVAD support can offer myocardial pressure- and ischemia unloading as well as improvement of vital organ perfusion in critically ill patients without the potential hazards of vasopressors and mechanical compression devices. By reducing intra-cardiac pressures, myocardial oxygen consumption and by augmenting myocardial blood delivery, such devices may be able to increase the likelihood for successfully reversing a catastrophic state of refractory hemodynamic collapse as in persistent cardiac arrest and cardiogenic shock. Although limited clinical data are available this far. Experimental studies with the Impella LP 2.5 in ischemic ventricular fibrillation indicate a possible clinical potential. Further clinical studies should be warranted.

7. References

Ewy GA, Zuercher M, Hilwig RW, Sanders AB, Berg RA, Otto CW, Hayes MM, Kern KB. Improved neurological outcome with continuous chest compressions compared with 30:2 compressions-to-ventilations cardiopulmonary resuscitation in a realistic swine model of out-of-hospital cardiac arrest. Circulation. 2007;116: 2525-2530.

Eftestol T, Wik L, Sunde K, Steen PA: Effects of cardiopulmonary resuscitation on predictors of ventricular fibrillation defibrillation success during out-of-hospital cardiac arrest. Circulation. 2004;110:10-15.

Hallstrom AP, Ornato JP, Weisfeldt M, Travers A, Christenson J, McBurnie MA, Zalenski R, Becker LB, Schron EB, Proschan M: Public Access Defibrillation Trial Investigators.Public-access defibrillation and survival after out-of-hospital cardiac arrest. N Engl J Med. 2004;351:637-646.

Hazinski MF, Idris AH, Kerber RE, Epstein A, Atkins D, Tang W, Lurie K: American Heart Association Emergency Cardiovascular Committee; Council on Cardiopulmonary, Perioperative, and Critical Care; Council on Clinical Cardiology. Lay rescuer automated external defibrillator ("public access defibrillation") programs: lessons learned from an international multicenter trial: advisory statement from the American Heart Association Emergency Cardiovascular Committee; the Council on Cardiopulmonary, Perioperative, and Critical Care; and the Council on Clinical Cardiology. Circulation. 2005;111:3336-3340.

Herlitz J, Ekstrom L, Axelsson A, Bang A, Wennerblom B, Waagstein L, Dellborg M, Holmberg S: Continuation of CPR on admission to emergency department after out-of-hospital cardiac arrest. Occurrence, characteristics and outcome. Resuscitation 1997;33:223-231.

Layon AJ, Gabrielli A, Goldfeder BW, Hevia A, Idris AH. Utstein style analysis of rural out-of-hospital cardiac arrest [OOHCA]: total cardiopulmonary resuscitation (CPR) time inversely correlates with hospital discharge rate. Resuscitation 2003;56:59-66.

Ritter G, Wolfe RA, Goldstein S, Landis JR, Vasu CM, Acheson A, Leighton R, Medendrop SV: The effect of bystander CPR on survival of out-of-hospital cardiac arrest victims. Am Heart J. 1985;110:932-937.

Ewy GA, Kern KB. Recent advances in cardiopulmonary resuscitation: cardiocerebral resuscitation.J Am Coll Cardiol. 2009 Jan 13;53(2):149-57.

Zhao D, Abella BS, Beiser DG, Alvarado JP, Wang H, Hamann KJ, Hoek TL, Becker LB. Intra-arrest cooling with delayed reperfusion yields higher survival than earlier normothermic resuscitation in a mouse model of cardiac arrest. Resuscitation. 2008; 77:242-249.

Popp E, Vogel P, Teschendorf P, Böttiger BW. Effects of the application of erythropoietin on cerebral recovery after cardiac arrest in rats. Resuscitation. 2007; 74:344-351.

Spaulding CM, Joly LM, Rosenberg A, Monchi M, Weber SN, Dhainaut JF, Carli P: Immediate coronary angiography in survivors of out-of-hospital cardiac arrest. N Engl J Med 1997;336:1629-1633.

Silfvast T: Cause of death in unsuccessful prehospital resuscitation. J Intern Med 1991; 229:331-335.

Nielsen N, Sandhall L, Schersten F, Friberg H, Olsson SE:Successful resuscitation with mechanical CPR, therapeutic hypothermia and coronary intervention during manual CPR after out-of-hospital cardiac arrest. Resuscitation 2005;65:111-113.

Quintero-Moran B, Moreno R, Villarreal S, Perez-Vizcayno MJ, Hernandez R, Conde C, Vazquez P, Alfonso F, Banuelos C, Escaned J, Fernandez-Ortiz A, Azcona L, Macaya C: Percutaneous coronary intervention for cardiac arrest secondary to ST-elevation acute myocardial infarction. Influence of immediate paramedical/medical assistance on clinical outcome. J Invasive Cardio. 2006;18:269-272.

Müller S, How OJ, Hermansen SE, Stenberg TA, Sager G, Myrmel T.Vasopressin impairs brain, heart and kidney perfusion: an experimental study in pigs after transient myocardial ischemia. Crit Care. 2008;12:R20.

Eftestol T, Sunde K, Steen PA: Effects of interrupting precordial compressions on the calculated probability of defibrillation success during out-of-hospital cardiac arrest. Circulation 2002;105:2270-2273.

Yu T, Weil MH, Tang W, Sun S, Klouche K, Povoas H, Bisera J: Adverse outcomes of interrupted precordial compression during automated defibrillation. Circulation 2002;106:368-372.

Kern KB, Hilwig RW, Berg RA, Sanders AB, Ewy GA: Importance of continuous chest compressions during cardiopulmonary resuscitation: improved outcome during a simulated single lay-rescuer scenario. Circulation 2002;105:645-649.

Henriques JP, Remmelink M, Baan J Jr, van der Schaaf RJ, Vis MM, Koch KT, Scholten EW, de Mol BA, Tijssen JG, Piek JJ, de Winter RJ.Safety and feasibility of elective high-risk percutaneous coronary intervention procedures with left ventricular support of the Impella Recover LP 2.5.Am J Cardiol. 2006; 97: 990-992.

Valgimigli M, Steendijk P, Sianos G, Onderwater E, Serruys PW: Left ventricular unloading and concomitant total cardiac output increase by the use of percutaneous Impella Recover LP 2.5 assist device during high-risk coronary intervention. Catheter Cardiovasc Interv 2005;65: 263-267.

Seyfarth M, Sibbing D, Bauer I, Fröhlich G, Bott-Flügel L, Byrne R, Dirschinger J, Kastrati A, Schömig A. A randomized clinical trial to evaluate the safety and efficacy of a percutaneous left ventricular assist device versus intra-aortic balloon pumping for treatment of cardiogenic shock caused by myocardial infarction. J Am Coll Cardiol. 2008; 52: 1584-1588.

Garatti A, Colombo T, Russo C, Lanfranconi M, Milazzo F, Catena E, Bruschi G, Frigerio M, Vitali E: Different applications for left ventricular mechanical support with the Impella Recover 100 microaxial blood pump. J Heart Lung Transplant 2005;24:481-485.

2005 American Heart Association Guidelines for Cardiopulmonary Resuscitation and Emergency Cardiovascular Care: Circulation. 2005;112:IV1-203.

Boczar ME, Howard MA, Rivers EP, Martin GB, Horst HM, Lewandowski C, Tomlanovich MC, Nowak RMA technique revisited: hemodynamic comparison of closed- and open-chest cardiac massage during human cardiopulmonary resuscitation. Crit. Care Med. 1995; 23: 498–503.

Bircher N. and P. Safar, Comparison of standard and 'new'closed-chest CPR and open-chest CPR in dogs. Crit. Care Med. 1981; 9: 384–385.

Badylak S.F., K.B. Kern, W.A. Tacker, G.A. Ewy, W. Janas and A. Carter, The comparative pathology of open chest vs. mechanical closed chest cardiopulmonary resuscitation in dogs. Resuscitation. 1986; 13: 249–264.

Benson DM, O'Neil B, Kakish E, Erpelding J, Alousi S, Mason R, Piper D, Rafols J. Open-chest CPR improves survival and neurologic outcome following cardiac arrest. Resuscitation. 2005; 64: 209-217.

Bartlett RL, Stewart NJ, Raymond J, et al: Comparative study of three methods of resuscitation: Closed-chest open-chest manual, and direct mechanical ventricular assistance. Ann Emerg Med. 1984; 13: 773-777.

Lindner KH, Pfenninger EG, Lurie KG, Schurmann W, Lindner IM, Ahnefeld FW.Effects of active compression-decompression resuscitation on myocardial and cerebral blood flow in pigs. Circulation.1993; 88:1254-1263.

Halperin HR, Paradis N, Ornato JP, Zviman M, Lacorte J, Lardo A, Kern KB. Cardiopulmonary resuscitation with a novel chest compression device in a porcine model of cardiac arrest: improved hemodynamics and mechanisms. J Am Coll Cardiol. 2004; 44: 2214-2220.

Steen S, Liao Q, Pierre L, Paskevicius A, Sjoberg T: Evaluation of LUCAS, a new device for automatic mechanical compression and active decompression resuscitation. Resuscitation 2002;55: 285-299.

Rubertsson S, Karlsten R: Increased cortical cerebral blood flow with LUCAS; a new device for mechanical chest compressions compared to standard external compressions during experimental cardiopulmonary resuscitation. Resuscitation 2005;65: 357-363.

Lindner KH, Pfenninger EG, Lurie KG, Schurmann W, Lindner IM, Ahnefeld FW:Effects of active compression-decompression resuscitation on myocardial and cerebral blood flow in pigs. Circulation 1993;88:1254-1263.

Swenson RD, Weaver WD, Niskanen RA, Martin J, Dahlberg S: Hemodynamics in humans during conventional and experimental methods of cardiopulmonary resuscitation. Circulation 1988;78: 630-639.

Ma MH, Hwang JJ, Lai LP, Wang SM, Huang GT, Shyu KG, Ko YL, Lin JL, Chen WJ, Hsu KL: Transesophageal echocardiographic assessment of mitral valve position and pulmonary venous flow during cardiopulmonary resuscitation in humans. Circulation 1995;92: 854-861.

Niemann JT, Rosborough J, Hausknecht M, Brown D, Criley JM: Cough-CPR: documentation of systemic perfusion in man and in an experimental model: a "window" to the mechanism of blood flow in external CPR. Crit Care Med 1980;8:141-146.

Niemann JT, Rosborough J, Hausknecht M, Ung S, Criley JM. Blood flow without cardiac compression during closed chest CPR. Crit Care Med 1981;9: 380-381.

Niemann JT, Rosborough JP, Pelikan PC: Hemodynamic determinants of subdiaphragmatic venous return during closed-chest CPR in a canine cardiac arrest model. Ann Emerg Med 1990;19:1232-1237.

Wenzel V, Lindner KH, Prengel AW, Strohmenger HU. Effect of phased chest and abdominal compression-decompression cardiopulmonary resuscitation on myocardial and cerebral blood flow in pigs. Crit Care Med. 2000; 28:1107-1112.

Sanders AB, Kern KB, Fonken S, Otto CW, Ewy GA: The role of bicarbonate and fluid loading in improving resuscitation from prolonged cardiac arrest with rapid manual chest compression CPR. Ann Emerg Med 1990;19: 1-7.

Lewis LM, Stothert J, Standeven J, Chandel B, Kurtz M, Fortney J. Correlation of end-tidal CO2 to cerebral perfusion during CPR. Ann Emerg Med 1992;21:1131-1134.

Sanders AB, Kern KB, Otto CW, Milander MM, Ewy GA: End-tidal carbon dioxide monitoring during cardiopulmonary resuscitation. A prognostic indicator for survival. JAMA 1989;262:347-1351.

Wayne MA, Levine RL. Miller CC. Use of end-tidal carbon dioxide to predict outcome in prehospital cardiac arrest. N Engl J Med 1997; 337:301-306.

Safar P. Cerebral resuscitation after cardiac arrest: research initiatives and future directions Ann Emerg Med 1993; 22:324-349.

Bernard SA, Gray TW, Buist MD, Jones BM, Silvester W, Gutteridge G, Smith K.Treatment of comatose survivors of out-of-hospital cardiac arrest with induced hypothermia. N Engl J Med. 2002; 346:557-563.

Kowallik P, Schulz R, Guth BD, Schade A, Paffhausen W, Gross R, Heusch G. Measurement of regional myocardial blood flow with multiple colored microspheres. Circulation. 1991; 83:974-98258. 47.

Voorhees WD, Babbs CF, Tacker WA. Regional blood flow during cardiopulmonary resuscitation in dogs. Crit Care Med. 1980; 8:134-136.

Johnston AJ, Steiner LA, Coles JP. Effect of cerebral perfusionpressure augmentation on regional oxygenation and metabolismafter head injury. Crit Care Med. 2005; 33: 189–195.

Bahlmann L, Klaus S, Baumeier W, Schmucker P, Raedler C, Schmittinger CA, Wenzel V, Voelckel W, Lindner KH. Brain metabolism during cardiopulmonary resuscitation assessed with microdialysis. Resuscitation 2003; 59:255-260.

Pokela M, Biancari F, Rimpiläinen J, Romsi P, Hirvonen J, Vainionpää V, Kiviluoma K, Anttila V, Juvonen T. The role of cerebral microdialysis in predicting the outcome after experimental hypothermic circulatory arrest. Scand Cardiovasc J 2001;35:395-402.

Reinstrup P, Stahl N, Mellergard P, Uski T, Ungerstedt U,Nordstrom CH. Intracerebral microdialysis in clinical practice:baseline values for chemical markers during wakefulness. Neurosurgery. 2000; 47:701-709.

Massetti M, Tasle M, Le Page O, Deredec R, Babatasi G, Buklas D, Thuaudet S, Charbonneau P, Hamon M, Grollier G, Gerard JL, Khayat A. Back from irreversibility: extracorporeal life support for prolonged cardiac arrest Ann Thorac Surg. 2005;79:178-83.

Martin GB, Rivers EP, Paradis NA, Goetting MG, Morris DC, Nowak RM Emergency department cardiopulmonary bypass in the treatment of human cardiac arrest. Chest. 1998;113: 743-51

Shin JS, Lee SW, Han GS, Jo WM, Choi SH, Hong YS. Successful extracorporeal life support in cardiac arrest with recurrent ventricular fibrillation unresponsive to standard cardiopulmonary resuscitation.Resuscitation. 2007;73:309-13.ECMO

Chen JM, DeRose JJ, Slater JP, Spanier TB, Dewey TM, Catanese KA, Flannery MA, Oz MC: Improved survival rates support left ventricular assist device implantation early after myocardial infarction. J Am Coll Cardiol. 1999;33:1903-1908.

Dang NC, Topkara VK, Leacche M, John R, Byrne JG, Naka Y: Left ventricular assist device implantation after acute anterior wall myocardial infarction and cardiogenic shock: a two-center study. J Thorac Cardiovasc Surg. 2005;130:693-698.

Pagani FD, Lynch W, Swaniker F, Dyke DB, Bartlett R, Koelling T, Moscucci M, Deeb GM, Bolling S, Monaghan H, Aaronson KD:Extracorporeal life support to left ventricular assist device bridge to heart transplant: A strategy to optimize survival and resource utilization. Circulation. 1999;100: II206-II210.

Fannelop T, Dahle GO, Matre K, Segadal L, Grong K. An anesthetic protocol in the young domestic pig allowing neuromuscular blockade for studies of cardiac function following cardioplegic arrest and cardiopulmonary bypass. Acta Anaesthesiol Scand. 2004; 27: 1144-1154.

Segal J, Nassi M, Ford AJ Jr, Schuenemeyer TD Instantaneous and continuous cardiac output in humans obtained with a Doppler pulmonary artery catheter. J Am Coll Cardiol. 1990;16:1398-407.

Kerut EK, Norfleet WT, Plotnick GD, Giles TD Patent foramen ovale: a review of associated conditions and the impact of physiological size. J Am Coll Cardiol. 2001 ; 38: 613-623.

Pinheiro JC, Bates DM: Mixed effects model in S and S-Plus. Springer; 2002

Rubertsson S, Grenvik A, Wiklund L Blood flow and perfusion pressure during open-chest versus closed-chest cardiopulmonary rsuscitation in pigs. Crit Care Med. 1995; 23 :715-725.

DeBehnke DJ, Angelos MG, Leasure JE: Comparison of standard external CPR, open-chest CPR, and cardiopulmonary by-pass in a canine myocardial infarct model. Ann Emerg Med. 1991; 20: 754-760.

Barnett W.M., J.K. Alifimoff and P.M. Paris et al., Comparison of open-chest cardiac massage techniques in dogs. Ann Emerg Med.1986; 15, 408–412.

Wolcke BB, Mauer DK, Schoefmann MF, Teichmann H, Provo TA, Lindner KH, Dick WF, Aeppli D, Lurie KG: Comparison of standard cardiopulmonary resuscitation versus the combination of active compression-decompression cardiopulmonary resuscitation and an inspiratory impedance threshold device for out-of-hospital cardiac arrest. Circulation. 2003;108: 2201-2205.

Casner M, Andersen D, Isaacs SM: The impact of a new CPR assist device on rate of return of spontaneous circulation in out-of-hospital cardiac arrest. Prehosp Emerg Care. 2005;9 :61-67

Steen S, Sjoberg T, Olsson P, Young M. Treatment of out-of-hospital cardiac arrest with LUCAS, a new device for automatic mechanical compression and active decompression resuscitation. Resuscitation. 2005; 67:25-30.

Casner M, Andersen D, Isaacs SM. The impact of a new CPR assist device on rate of return of spontaneous circulation in out-of-hospital cardiac arrest. Prehosp Emerg Care. 2005; 9:61-67.

Lindner KH, Pfenninger EG, Lurie KG, Schurmann W, Lindner IM, Ahnefeld FW.Effects of active compression-decompression resuscitation on myocardial and cerebral blood flow in pigs. Circulation. 1993; 88:1254-1263.

Rittenberger JC, Menegazzi JJ, Callaway CW. Association of delay to first intervention with return of spontaneous circulation in a swine model of cardiac arrest. Resuscitation. 2007; 73: 154-160.

Kitsou V, Xanthos T, Stroumpoulis K, Rokas G, Papadimitriou D, Serpetinis I, Dontas I, Perrea D, Kouskouni E.Nitroglycerin and Epinephrine Improve Coronary Perfusion Pressure in a Porcine Model of Ventricular Fibrillation Arrest: A Pilot Study. J Emerg Med. 2008; Dec19.Epup.

Belli A, Sen J, Petzold A, Russo S, Kitchen N, Smith M. Metabolic failure precedes intracranial pressure rises in traumatic brain injury: a microdialysis study. Acta Neurochir. 2008; 150:461-469.

Vespa PM, McArthur D, O'Phelan K, Glenn T, Etchepare M, Kelly D, Bergsneider M, Martin NA, Hovda DA. Persistently low extracellular glucose correlates with poor outcome 6 months after human traumatic brain injury despite a lack of increased lactate: a microdialysis study. J Cereb Blood Flow Metab. 2003; 23:865-877.

Peerdeman SM, Girbes AR, Polderman KH, Vandertop W.Changes in interstitial glycerol concentration in head-injuredpatients: correlation with clinical events. Intensive Care Med. 2003; 29: 18251828.

Persson L, Valtysson J, Enblad P. Neurochemical monitoringusing intracerebral microdialysis in patients with subarachnoidhemorrhage. J Neurosurg. 1996; 84: 606–616.

Sarrafzadeh AS, Haux D, Lüdemann L, Amthauer H, Plotkin M, Küchler I, Unterberg AW. Cerebral ischaemia in aneurysmal subarachnoid hemorrhage: a correlative microdialysis-PET study. Stroke. 2004 ;35:638-643.

Chaurasia CS, Müller M, Bashaw ED, Benfeldt E, Bolinder J, Bullock R, Bungay PM, DeLange EC, Derendorf H, Elmquist WF, Hammarlund-Udenaes M, Joukhadar C, Kellogg DL Jr, Lunte CE, Nordstrom CH, Rollema H, Sawchuk RJ, Cheung BW, Shah VP, Stahle L, Ungerstedt U, Welty DF, Yeo H. AAPS-FDA workshop white paper: microdialysis principles, application and regulatory perspectives. Pharm Res. 2007; 24:1014-1025.

Ståhl N, Ungerstedt U, Nordström CH. Brain energy metabolism during controlled reduction of cerebral perfusion pressure in severe head injuries. Intensive Care Med .2001; 27:1215-1223.

Frykholm P, Hillered L, Långström B, Persson L, Valtysson J, Watanabe Y, Enblad P. Increase of interstitial glycerol reflects the degree of ischaemic brain damage: a PET and microdialysis study in a middle cerebral artery occlusion-reperfusion primate model. J Neurol Neurosurg Psychiatry. 2001; 71:455-461.

Frykholm P, Hillered L, Långström B, Persson L, Valtysson J, Enblad P. Relationship between cerebral blood flow and oxygen metabolism, and extracellular glucose and lactate concentrations during middle cerebral artery occlusion and reperfusion: a microdialysis and positron emission tomography study in nonhuman primates. J Neurosurg. 2005; 102:1076-1084.

owers WJ. Grubb RL Jr, Darriet D, Raichle ME. Cerebral blood flow and cerebral metabolic rate of oxygen requirements for cerebral function and viability in humans. J Cereb Blood Flow Metab. 1985; 5:600-608.

Baron JC. Perfusion Thresholds in Human Cerebral Ischaemia: Historical Perspective and Therapeutic Implications. Cerebrovasc Dis. 2003; 11: 2-8.

Gedeborg R, Silander HC, Rubertsson S, Wiklund L. Cerebral ischaemia in experimental cardiopulmonary resuscitation--comparison of epinephrine and aortic occlusion. Resuscitation. 2001; 50:319-329.

Newman MF, Croughwell ND, White WD, Lowry E, Baldwin BI, Clements FM, Davis RD Jr, Jones RH, Amory DW, Reves JG. Effect of perfusion pressure on cerebral blood flow during normothermic cardiopulmonary bypass. Circulation 1996; 94:II353-357.

Goodman JC, Valadka AB, Gopinath SP, Uzura M, Robertson CS. Extracellular lactate and glucose alterations in the brain after headinjury measured by microdialysis. Crit Care Med. 1999; 27: 1965–1973.

Haugen O, Farstad M, Lise Kvalheim V, Rynning SE, Hammersborg S, Mongstad A, Husby P. Mean arterial pressure about 40 mmHg during CPB is associated with cerebral ischaemia in piglets. Scand Cardiovasc J. 2006;40:54-61.

Murr R, Stummer W, Schürer L, Polasek J. Cerebral lactate production in relation to intracranial pressure, cranial computed tomography findings, and outcome in patients with severe head injury. Acta Neurochir. 1996;138:928-936.

Nordström CH. Assessment of critical thresholds for cerebral perfusion pressure by performing bedside monitoring of cerebral energy metabolism. Neurosurg Focus. 2003; 15:E5.

Ornato JP: Hemodynamic monitoring during CPR: Ann Emerg Med. 1993;22:289-295.

Falk JL, Rackow EC, Weil MH: End-Tidal Carbon-Dioxide Concentration During Cardiopulmonary Resuscitation. N Engl J Med. 1988;318:607-611.

Gudipati CV, Weil MH, Bisera J, Deshmukh HG, Rackow EC: Expired carbon dioxide: a noninvasive monitor of cardiopulmonary resuscitation. Circulation. 1988;77:234-239.

Weil MH, Bisera J, Trevino RP, Rackow EC: Cardiac output and end-tidal carbon dioxide. Crit Care Med. 1985;13:907-909.

Gazmuri RJ, Kube E: Capnography during cardiac resuscitation: a clue on mechanisms and a guide to interventions. Crit Care Med. 2003;7:411-412.

Weil MH, Bisera J, Trevino RP, Rackow EC. Cardiac output and end-tidal carbon dioxide. Crit Care Med. 1985; 13: 907-909.

Wicker PA, Healy BP. Variability of coronary blood flow measurements with microspheres in the rat: role of injection site and sphere number. Cardiovasc Res. 1989;23:443-52.

Andersen KS, Skjerven R, Lekven J. Stability of 8-, 15-, and 26-micron microspheres entrapped in feline myocardium. Am J Physiol. 1983;244:H121-30.

Domenech RJ, Hoffman JIE, Noble MIM, Saunders KB, Henson JR, Subijanto S: Total and regional coronary blood flow measured by radioactive microspheres in conscious and anesthetized dogs. Circ Res. 1969;25:581-596

Schrock GD, Krahmer RL, Ferguson JL. Coronary flow by left atrial and left ventricular microsphere injection in the rat. Am J Physiol. 1990 Aug;259:H635-8.

Vikenes K, Westby J, Matre K, Farstad M, Nordrehaug JE. Percutaneous assessment of coronary blood flow and cardiac biomarkers. Ultrasound Med Biol. 2002 Jan;28:39-48.

Schosser R, Arfors K-E, Messmer K. MIC-1I -A program for the determination of cardiac output, arterio-venous shunt and regional blood flow using the radioactive microsphere method. Comput Programs Biomed. 1979;9:19-38.

Maslow A, Comunale ME, Haering JM, Watkins J. Pulsed wave Doppler measurement of cardiac output from the right ventricular outflow tract. Anesth Analg. 1996; 83: 466-471.

Ter Minassian A, Dubé L, Guilleux AM, Wehrmann N, Ursino M, Beydon L. Changes in intracranial pressure and cerebral autoregulation in patients with severe traumatic brain injury. Crit Care Med. 2002; 30:1616-1622.

Domanovits H, Schillinger M, Mullner M, Thoennissen J, Sterz F, Zeiner A, Druml W. Acute renal failure after successful cardiopulmonary resuscitation. Intensive Care Med. 2001;2:1194-1199.

Lottes AE, Rundell AE, Geddes LA, Kemeny AE, Otlewski MP, Babbs CF. Sustained abdominal compression during CPR raises coronary perfusion pressures as much as vasopressor drugs. Resuscitation. 2007;75:515-24.

Gueugniaud PY, David JS, Chanzy E, et al. Vasopressin and epinephrine vs. epinephrine alone in cardiopulmonary resuscitation..N Engl J Med. 2008;359:21-30.

Sylvester JT, RD Gilbert, Traystman RJ,Permutt S. Effects of hypoxia on the closing pressure of the canine systemic arterial circulation. Circ. Res.1981;49;980-987.

Nordrehaug JE, Bjørkhaug A, Danielsen R, Vik-Mo H: Arterial and venous measurements in resting forearm of metabolic indicators during rest and leg exercise. Clin Physiol. 1991;11 469-76.

Carden DL, Martin GB, Nowak RM, et al: Lactic acidosis as a predictor of downtime during cardiopulmonary arrest in dogs. Am J Emerg Med. 1985; 3:120-124.

Rivers EP, Martin GB, Smithline H, Rady MY, Schultz CH, Goetting MG, Appleton TJ, Nowak RM: The clinical implications of continuous central venous oxygen saturation during human CPR. Ann Emerg Med. 1992; 21:1094-101.

Karkouti K, Djaiani G, Borger MA, Beattie WS, Fedorko L, Wijeysundera D, Ivanov J, Karski J. Low hematocrit during cardiopulmonary bypass is associated with increased risk of perioperative stroke in cardiac surgery. Ann Thorac Surg. 2005; 80:1381-1387.

Valgimigli M, Steendijk P, Serruys PW, Vranckx P, Boomsma F, Onderwater E, Vaina S, Ligthart J, McFadden E, van der Ent M, de Jaegere P, Sianos G Use of Impella Recover® LP 2.5 left ventricular assist device during high-risk percutaneous coronary interventions; clinical, haemodynamic and biochemical findings. EuroInterv. 2006;2:91-100.

Son HS, Sun K, Fang YH, Park SY, Hwang CM, Park SM, Lee SH, Kim KT, Lee IS.The effects of pulsatile versus non-pulsatile extracorporeal circulation on the pattern of coronary artery blood flow during cardiac arrest. Int J Artif Organs. 2005;28: 609-616.

Feller ED, Sorensen EN, Haddad M, Pierson RN 3rd, Johnson FL, Brown JM, Griffith BP. Clinical outcomes are similar in pulsatile and nonpulsatile left ventricular assist device recipients. Ann Thorac Surg. 2007;83:1082-8.

Niemann JT, Rosborough JP, Youngquist S, Thomas J, Lewis RJ Is all ventricular fibrillation the same? A comparison of ischemically induced with electrically induced ventricular fibrillation in a porcine cardiac arrest and resuscitation model. Crit Care Med. 2007; 35:1356-1361.

Ristagno G, Tang W, Xu TY, Sun S, Weil MH Outcomes of CPR in the presence of partial occlusion of left anterior descending coronary artery. Resuscitation. 2007;75: 357-365.

Lam K, Sjauw KD, van der Meulen J, Symersky P, Biervliet JD, Henriques JP, de Mol BA. A combined surgical and percutaneous approach through the axillary artery to introduce the Impella LP5.0 for short-term circulatory support. Int J Cardiol. 2008;

Initial Experience of Lower Limb Thermal Therapy for Patients with an Extracorporeal Left Ventricular Assist Device Awaiting Heart Transplantation

Kazuo Komamura
Department of Cardiovascular Medicine, National Cardiovascular Center
Japan

1. Introduction

Many researchers have reported that vasodilators, such as angiotensin-converting enzyme inhibitors (The CONSENSUS Trial Study Group, 1987), angiotensin receptor blockers (Cohn et al., 1999), and beta-blockers (CIBIS Investigators et al., 1994), improve prognosis in patients with chronic heart failure (CHF). Furthermore, new technologies to treat CHF, such as cardiac rehabilitation, cardiac resynchronization therapy, left ventricular assist devices, and left ventricular reconstruction surgery, have been developed over the past decade. Despite advances in therapy for heart failure, improving clinical outcomes of patients with acute decompensation of CHF remains a challenge for physicians. Re-hospitalization within 60—90 days occurs in approximately 30% of patients with acute decompensation of CHF (Mann, 2008).

In 1989, Tei et al. developed a form of thermal therapy for heart failure that uses a variation of the traditional dry sauna with temperature maintained at 60°C (Tei et al., 1994; Tei et al., 1995). This new form of thermal treatment is defined as warming the entire body in a uniformly heated chamber for 15 min at a temperature that relaxes both the mind and body. After the core temperature has increased by 1.0–1.2°C, the patient rests outside the sauna for a further 30 min to maintain the soothing effect, and fluids corresponding to perspiration loss are supplied to protect against dehydration at the end of therapy (Tei, 2007).

Tei et al. have previously reported that the repeated use of a dry 60 ◦C sauna by CHF patients improves hemodynamics (Tei et al., 1995), ameliorates symptoms (Tei & Tanaka, 1996), suppresses ventricular arrhythmias (Kihara et al., 2004), and improves vascular function (Kihara et al., 2002). Recently, in a prospective multicenter case-control study, 2 weeks of dry sauna therapy was shown to improve clinical symptoms and cardiac function in CHF patients (Miyata et al., 2008). Repeated sauna therapy also improved survival in TO-2 cardiomyopathic hamsters with heart failure (Ikeda et al., 2002). A recent retrospective follow-up study (Kihara et al., 2009) has shown that sauna therapy decreased cardiac death and re-hospitalization in patients with CHF over a 60-month follow-up period.

A large number of end-stage CHF patients in Japan have been implanted with a left ventricular assist device (LVAD) because of prolonged waiting periods for heart transplants

(Osada et al., 2005). Although we wished to apply sauna thermal therapy to patients with LVAD, we do not have an appropriate sauna facility. Instead, we attempted to apply lower limb thermal therapy to the patients with LVAD awaiting a heart transplant. This paper describes for the first time the safety and effectiveness of this preliminary trial of lower limb thermal therapy for patients with end-stage heart failure.

2. Methods

2.1 Patients and study design

The study subjects included 5 consecutive end-stage CHF patients who were listed on a waiting list for heart transplants in the National Cardiovascular Center, Osaka, Japan. All patients had dilated cardiomyopathy refractory to maximal medical therapy, including angiotensin-converting enzyme inhibitors or angiotensin receptor blockers, beta-blockers, diuretics, and digitalis. Regardless of intensive care with intravenous inotropic agents, heart failure rapidly progressed to cardiogenic shock in the patients. They were fitted with extracorporeal LVAD (VCT-50, Toyobo Ltd., Osaka, Japan) to stabilize their hemodynamics. None of the patients was implanted with a defibrillator device.

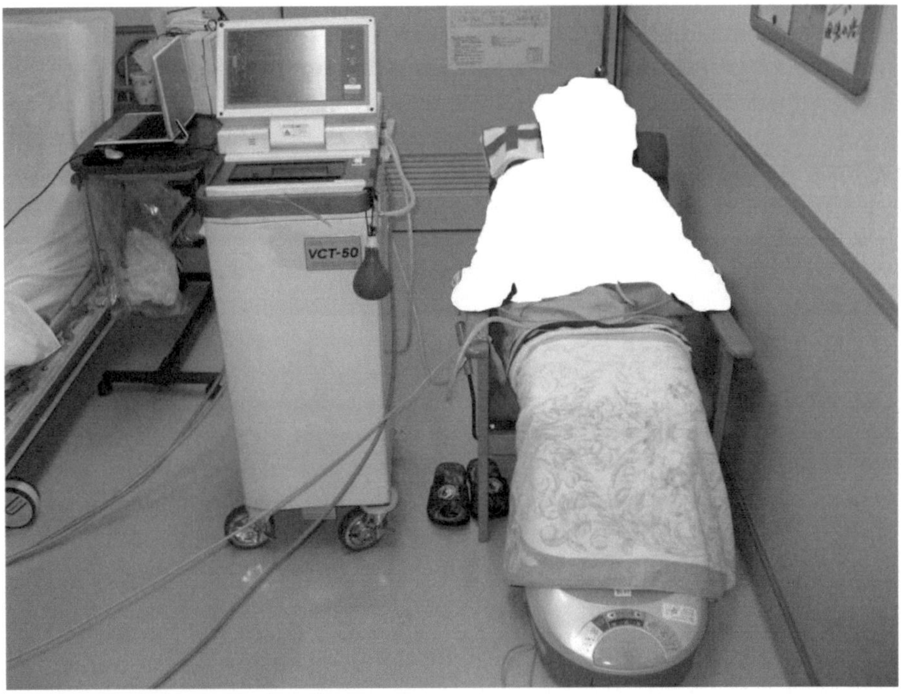

Fig. 1. Typical settings for lower limb thermal therapy for a patient with left ventricular assist device.

The patients' general condition stabilized thereafter and the status of heart failure at the time of study was New York Heart Association (NYHA) class II. Although this status remained stable for at least 6 months, the patients' cardiac function did not sufficiently recover to allow discontinuation of LVAD support. All patients provided written informed consent to enter into the clinical trial for lower limb thermal therapy. The Ethics Committee at the National Cardiovascular Center approved the protocol, and the study was conducted in accordance with the Declaration of Helsinki. The study consisted of clinical examinations before and after a 2-week treatment consisting of daily thermal therapy using a steam bath at 42 ◦C applied to the lower legs and feet (Fig. 1). After 15 min of therapy at 42 ◦C, the patient remained seated in the steam bath with the lower legs and feet wrapped with a blanket for a further 30 min. The procedure was accompanied by electrocardiographic monitoring. The patient remained on the same medications with same dose throughout the study period.

A typical example of lower limb thermal therapy is illustrated in Fig.1. The study protocol for the 2-week treatment was illustrated in Fig.2.

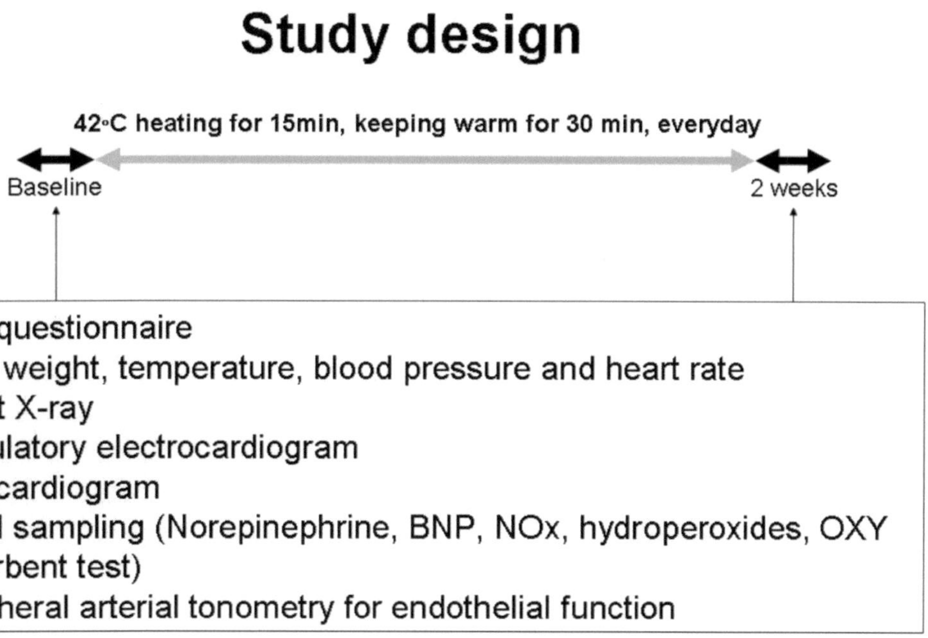

Fig. 2. Illustrative presentation of the study design for lower limb thermal therapy.

2.2 Measurements

Systolic and diastolic blood pressure (BP), heart rate, body weight, and surface and deep body temperature (axillary and sublingual) were measured daily throughout the study. Chest X-ray, ambulatory electrocardiogram, echocardiogram, and peripheral arterial tonometry were recorded and blood was sampled prior to and 2 weeks after the treatment. Blood samples were used for measurement of plasma BNP, serum NT-proBNP, plasma nitrates and nitrites, plasma hydroperoxides and HClO expense test.

Medical interviews were done every morning to evaluate the clinical status of CHF by NYHA functional class, and to estimate the patients' daily life activities using a Specific Activity Scale (SAS). We used the Specific Activity Scale as a measure of QOL, in which self perceived exercise tolerance is expressed by an energy cost spent in the maximal physical activity that the patient can perform (Sasayama et al., 1992). The Specific Activity Scale allows expression of the extent of submaximal physical activity. Sasayama et al. actually measured the metabolic costs of various types of physical activity by hooking subjects up to a mask to measure oxygen consumption and the volume of carbon dioxide exhaled. They then prepared questionnaires about specific physical activities that a patient would perform either customarily or sporadically in daily life and each patient was asked to specify whether he/she could perform each type of activity without symptomatic limitations. Summarizing the questionnaire data, a given number of metabolic costs (Specific Activity Scale) were derived for each patient with regard to their self-perceived exercise tolerance. As a clear linear correlation was observed between Specific Activity Scale and peak oxygen consumption, the Specific Activity Scale was considered to provide a reliable prediction of exercise capacity (Sasayama et al., 1992)

Prior to and 2 weeks after the treatment, the cardiothoracic ratio (CTR) was measured by chest radiography and the count of premature ventricular beats was evaluated daily with an ambulatory electrocardiogram. Prior to and 2 weeks after the treatment, two-dimensional echocardiography were performed to determine left ventricular systolic (LVDs) and diastolic dimension (LVDd), left atrial dimension (LAD), LVEF and degree of mitral regurgitation. The left ventricular (LV) end-diastolic and end-systolic volumes were determined according to a modification of Simpson's method. LVEF was calculated as end-diastolic minus end-systolic volume divided by end-diastolic volume.

Each patient was instructed to lie quietly and undisturbed for at least 30 min, and then a venous blood sample was withdrawn through an indwelling catheter in the forearm. Plasma was immediately separated and stored at 70°C until analysis.

Norepinephrine (NE) concentrations were determined by high performance liquid chromatography and electrochemical detection. Plasma brain natriuretic peptide (BNP) was determined by the chemiluminescent enzyme immunoassay.

For nitric oxide (NO) measurement, the blood specimen was placed immediately in an ice bath and centrifuged within 30 seconds for 5 minutes at 2000*g*. The serum fraction was diluted 1:1 with nitrite- and nitrate-free distilled water, and 400 mL of the diluted sample was centrifuged at 2000*g* in an ultra-free MC microcentrifuge device (Millipore) to remove substances larger than 10 kD. The filtrate was passed through a copper-plated cadmium column to reduce nitrate to nitrite and then reacted with Griess reagents consisting of 0.1% naphthylethylenediamine dihydrochloride in distilled water and 1% sulfanilamide in 5% H_3PO_4, after which absorbance was measured at 540 nm to provide the total amount of plasma NO end products (nitrate plus nitrite). The efficiency of the cadmium column in the conversion of nitrate to nitrite was confirmed to be 100% by measuring both nitrate and nitrite standards before and after sample measurement (Node et al., 1997).

Plasma hydroperoxides, which were determined by the Diacron reactive oxygen metabolites test, were used as a marker of oxidative stress (Cesarone et al., 1999) while the OXY absorbent test was used to measure buffering potential against the oxidant action of hypochlorous acid (HClO), which was quantified by HClO neutralization, and represented a marker of anti-oxidative potency (Trotti et al., 2001).

Endothelial function was quantified by the reactive hyperemic (RH) change in digital blood flow after arm occlusion using a peripheral fingertip arterial tonometry (PAT) device (Endo-PAT 2000 system; Itamar-Medical, Caesarea, Israel)(Bonetti et al., 2004; Hamburg & Benjamin, 2009). After 5 min of baseline recording, a BP cuff was inflated to supra-systolic pressure in the test arm. After 5 min of occlusion, the cuff was rapidly deflated, with PAT tracings recorded. The reactive hyperemic PAT (RH-PAT) response was determined as the ratio of PAT amplitude in the test arm to that in the control arm, averaged over 30-s intervals after cuff deflation, divided by the average PAT ratio measured for the 140-s interval before cuff inflation. RH-PAT ratio was assessed between 60 s and 120 s after occlusion and was the log-transformed value of the post-deflation to baseline pulse amplitude in the hyperemic finger normalized to the contralateral finger.

2.3 Statistical analysis

All data are expressed as means ±S.D. Value of BNP was log-transformed to remove skewness of data distribution. The data prior to and 2 weeks after treatment were compared using a paired *t*-test. A *p*-value of <0.05 was considered statistically significant.

3. Results

3.1 Clinical findings and physical examinations

Table 1 summarizes the results of clinical findings and physical examinations. During the study, none of the patients treated with lower limb thermal therapy showed worsened clinical symptoms. The changes in the clinical findings and variables after 2 weeks are indicated in Table 1. Although the NYHA functional class remained similar, activity of daily life estimated by SAS system tended to decrease (p=0.058). Systolic and diastolic blood pressure and heart rate did not differ between the baseline and 2 weeks after therapy. No significant change was noted in body weight.

	Before	After	p value
Sample size	5	5	
Age (years)	35.4±8.8		
NYHA functional class	2.8±0.4	2.6±0.5	0.374
Activity of Daily Life (METs)	2.66±0.85	3.12±1.11	0.058
Ventricular Premature Beats (per day)	121.8±70.2	71.6±62.2	0.143
Body Weight (kg)	53.0±10.1	52.9±10.1	0.355
Systolic blood pressure (mmHg)	97.4±13.0	99.2±17.0	0.505
Diastolic blood pressure (mmHg)	55.0±10.4	58.2±9.4	0.216
Heart Rate (bpm)	80.0±34.8	79.6±29.7	0.914
Morning Body Temperature (C)	35.9±0.45	36.0±0.39	0.296
Deep Body Temperature (C)	36.0±0.29	36.8±0.23	0.004
Cardiothoracic Ratio (%)	53.7±14.8	52.2±14.7	0.082
Norepinephrine (pg/mL)	974.2±584.8	801.6±482.7	0.041
log BNP (pg/mL)	2.128±0.516	2.080±0.505	0.035
Nitrogen oxide (μmol/L)	25.1±6.7	47.6±19.8	0.028
Hydroperoxides (carr U)	501.4±77.5	430.4±84.2	0.0003
OXY absorbent test (μmol HClO/mL)	397.6±41.9	461.6±56.4	0.096
LAD (mm)	42.8±11.2	42.4±10.0	0.731
LVDd (mm)	54.4±12.0	53.0±13.3	0.184
LVDs (mm)	43.1±15.4	39.7±15.9	0.014
LV Ejection Fraction (%)	43.0±19.3	51.1±18.5	0.0007
Mitral Regurgitation (grade)	2.2±1.1	1.4±0.9	0.016
RH-PAT ratio	1.39±0.24	2.05±0.30	0.02

BNP brain natriuretic peptide, LAD left atrial dimension, LVDd left ventricular diastolic dimension, LVDs left ventricular systolic dimension, NYHA New York Heart Association, RH-PAT reactive hyperemic peripheral arterial tonometry

Table 1. Summary of changes in parameters before and after the thermal therapy

3.2 Chest radiography and echocardiography

Table 1 also presents the results of chest radiography and echocardiography. Chest radiography showed a non-significant decrease of the CTR after 2 weeks of treatment when compared with the baseline.

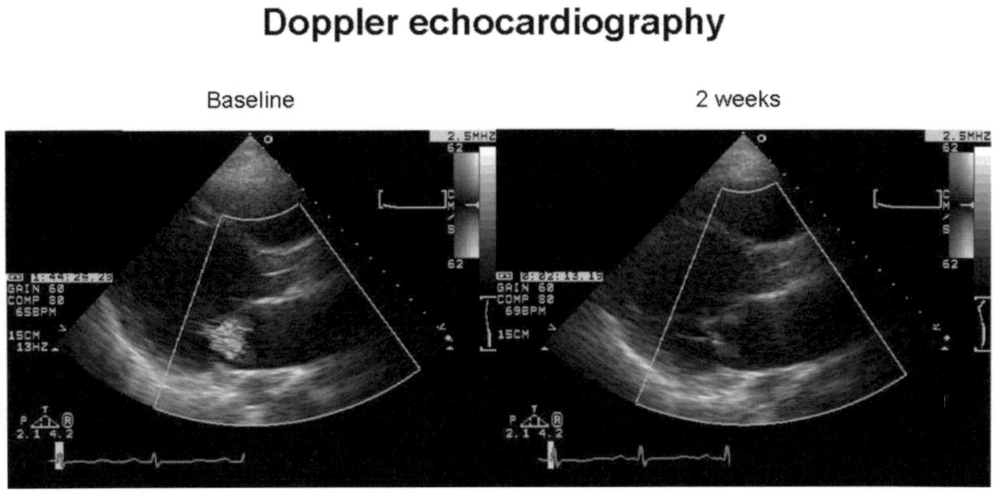

Fig. 3. Representative illustration of the extent of mitral regurgitation prior to and after the therapy

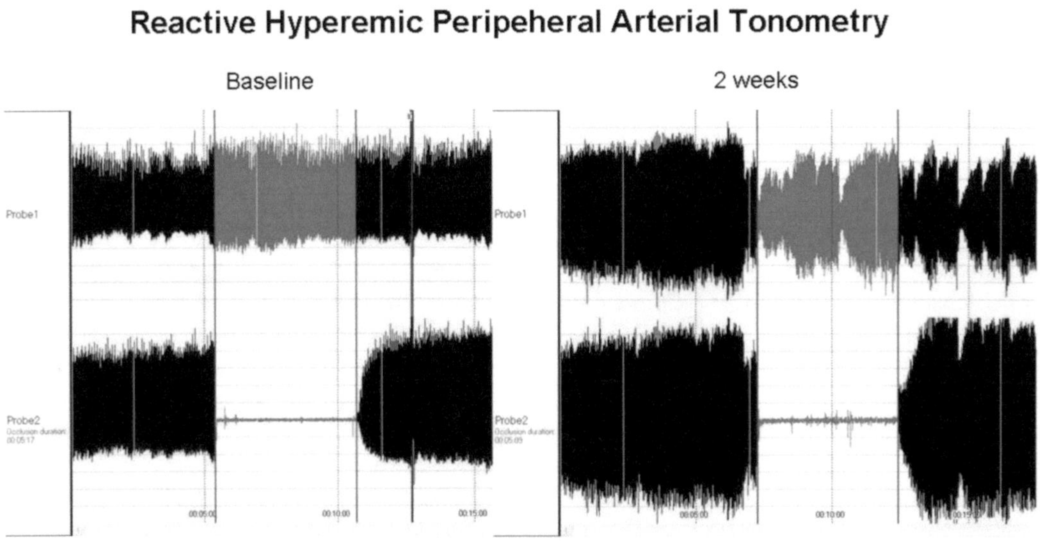

Fig. 4. Representative illustration of the changes in the tracing of peripheral arterial tonometry before and after the therapy

While, echocardiography demonstrated similar dimensions in LAD and LVDd after treatment, LVDs and LVEF significantly decreased after the therapy (Table 1). Doppler echocardiography demonstrated that the extent of mitral regurgitation decreased after treatment (Table 1, Fig. 3).

3.3 Plasma levels of norepinephrine, BNP, nitrogen oxide and hydroperoxides, and result of OXY adsorbent test

Table 1 shows the changes in plasma concentration of norepinephrine, BNP, nitrogen oxide (nitrate plus nitrite) and hydroperoxides. Plasma concentration of norepinephrine significantly decreased after 2 weeks of the therapy. The plasma concentration of BNP significantly decreased after 2 weeks of the therapy. Plasma concentration of nitrogen oxide (nitrate plus nitrite), the stable metabolite of nitric oxide, significantly increased after 2 weeks of the therapy. Plasma concentration of hydroperoxides, a biomarker that reflects oxidative stress, significantly decreased after 2 weeks of the therapy. The OXY absorbent test, a marker of anti-oxidative potency, showed a non-significant increase after 2 weeks of the therapy.

3.4 Endothelial function

The RH-PAT ratio was augmented 2 weeks after the therapy (Table 1, Fig.4).

4. Discussion

This is the first report of lower limb thermal therapy being applied to patients implanted with LVAD and awaiting heart transplantation. Whole body sauna therapy for CHF is widely recognized to result in improved clinical symptoms, cardiac function, quality of life, and ventricular arrhythmia, and in decreased levels of abnormally activated neurohumoral factors (Tei et al., 1995; Tei & Tanaka, 1996; Tei 2007; Kihara et al., 2002; Kihara et al., 2004). However, whole body sauna therapy is impractical for patients with CHF in general hospitals that lack specialized sauna facilities, whereas lower limb thermal therapy using a steam bath can be applied routinely right in the patients' rooms.

Increases in deep body temperature of 1.0−1.2 ◦C during sauna therapy dilate systemic arteries and veins, thereby reducing systemic preload and afterload and resulting in increased cardiac output (Tei et al., 1995; Tei & Tanaka, 1996; Tei 2007; Kihara et al., 2002; Kihara et al., 2004). The sublingual temperature of the patients in the present study was increased by about 0.8 ◦C after the therapy. Nevertheless, the benefits seemed to be similar to those of sauna therapy. Ikeda et al. found that repeated sauna therapy increases endothelial nitric oxide synthase expression and nitric oxide production, and improves cardiac function in animal models of heart failure (Ikeda et al., 2001; Ikeda et al., 2005). Serum nitrate plus nitrite levels doubled in our patients, when compared with the baseline values, as did the index of endothelial function determined by RH-PAT.

Patients implanted with an LVAD for long periods often develop serious hemorrhage in the cerebrum or elsewhere, as well as drive-line infection. We were concerned that the therapy would aggravate hemorrhage or infection in patients through its vasodilatory effects. However, we found that oozing of blood at the insertion site of the LVAD drive-line tended to resolve during therapy. Sauna thermal therapy attenuates psychological stress (Kihara et al., 2004). Because of a donor shortage in Japan, patients must remain attached to an LVAD and stay in hospital for over 2 years while waiting for a heart transplant (Takatani et al., 2005). The decrease in plasma norepinephrine indicated that appendicular thermal therapy also might attenuate psychological, as well as physical stress.

Compared to pharmacological vasodilator therapy and other non-pharmacological therapy, such as cardiac resynchronization therapy and physical therapy, lower limb thermal therapy for CHF has several advantages. First, it is quite safe and has no adverse effects. Second, it is less expensive and more cost-effective. Third, unlike physical therapy,

patients who are elderly or who have severe congestive heart failure, uncontrolled ventricular arrhythmias, and orthopedic limitations are not excluded from undergoing lower limb thermal therapy. Fourth, this treatment promotes mental and physical relaxation. Lower limb thermal therapy may thus be a valuable adjunct to pharmacological or non-pharmacological intervention in the management of CHF.

5. Study limitation

Although the present study is preliminary one, sample size was only five patients. Recruitment of study subjects is still ongoing. In the present protocol, the study subjects were implanted with LVAD for end-stage heart failure, and were therefore unlike typical patients with CHF.

6. Conclusion

Although the study used a very small cohort, I confirmed that lower limb thermal therapy was quite safe and that it improved clinical symptoms and cardiac function in patients with extracorporeal LVAD who were awaiting heart transplantation. The procedure of lower limb thermal therapy might benefit other patients, including those with end-stage heart failure.

7. References

Bonetti PO, Pumper GM, Higano ST, Holmes Jr DR, Kuvin JT, Lerman A. (2004) Noninvasive identification of patients with early coronary atherosclerosis by assessment of digital reactive hyperemia. J Am Coll Cardiol 44:2137–41.

Cesarone MR, Belcaro G, Carratelli M, Cornelli U, De Sanctis MT, Incandela L, Barsotti A, Terranova R, Nicolaides A. (1999) A simple test to monitor oxidative stress. *Int Angiol* 18:127–30.

CIBIS Investigators and Committees. (1994) A randomized trial of beta-blockade in heart failure. *Circulation* 90:1765–73.

Cohn JN, Tognoni G, Glazer RD, Spormann D, Hester A. (1999) Rationale and design of the Valsartan Heart Failure Trial: a large multinational trial to assess the effects of valsartan, an angiotensin-receptor blocker, on morbidity and mortality in chronic congestive heart failure. *J Card Fail* 5:155–60.

Hamburg NM, Benjamin EJ. (2009) Assessment of endothelial function using digital pulse amplitude tonometry. Trends Cardiovasc Med 2009;19:6 -11.

Ikeda Y, Biro S, Kamogawa Y, Yoshifuku S, Eto H, Orihara K, Kihara T, Tei C. (2001) Repeated thermal therapy upregulates arterial endothelial nitric oxide synthase expression in Syrian golden hamsters. *Jpn Circ J* 65:434–8.

Ikeda Y, Biro S, Kamogawa Y, Yoshifuku S, Kihara T, Minagoe S, Tei C. (2002) Effect of repeated sauna therapy on survival in TO-2 cardiomyopathic hamsters with heart failure. *Am J Cardiol* 90:343—5.

Ikeda Y, Biro S, Kamogawa Y, Yoshifuku S, Eto H, Orihara K, Yu B, Kihara T, Miyata M, Hamasaki S, Otsuji Y, Minagoe S, Tei C. (2005) Repeated sauna therapy increases arterial endothelial nitric oxide synthase expression and nitric oxide production in cardiomyopathic hamsters. *Circ J* 69: 722—9.

Kihara T, Biro S, Imamura M, Yoshifuku S, Takasaki K, Ikeda Y, Otuji Y, Minagoe S, Toyama Y, Tei C. (2002) Repeated sauna treatment improves vascular endothelial and cardiac function in patients with chronic heart failure. *J Am Coll Cardiol* 39:754—9.

Kihara T, Biro S, Ikeda Y, Fukudome T, Shinsato T, Masuda A, Miyata M, Hamasaki S, Otsuji Y, Minagoe S, Akiba S, Tei C. (2004) Effects of repeated sauna treatment on ventricular arrhythmias in patients with chronic heart failure. *Circ J* 68:1146—51.

Kihara T, Miyata M, Fukudome T, Ikeda Y, Shinsato T, Kubozono T, Fujita S, Kuwahata S, Hamasaki S, Torii H, Lee S, Toda H, Tei C. (2009) Waon therapy improves the prognosis of patients with chronic heart failure. *J Cardiol.* 53(2):214-8.

Mann DL. (2008) Management of heart failure patients with reduced ejection fraction. In: Libby P, Bonow RO, Mann DL, Zipes DP, editors. *Braunwald's heart disease: a textbook of cardiovascular medicine. 8th ed.* Philadelphia: WB Saunders; 2008. p. 611—40.

Miyata M, Kihara T, Kubozono T, Ikeda Y, Shinsato T, Izumi T, Matsuzaki M, Yamaguchi T, Kasanuki H, Daida H, Nagayama M, Nishigami K, Hirata K, Kihara K, Tei C. (2008) Beneficial effects of Waon therapy on patients with chronic heart failure: results of a prospective multicenter study. *J Cardiol* 52:79—85.

Node K, Kitakaze M, Yoshikawa H, Kosaka H, Hori M. (1997) Reduced plasma concentrations of nitrogen oxide in individuals with essential hypertension. *Hypertension.* 30:405-8.

Osada K, Imaizumi T. (2005) Heart Transplant Candidate Registry Committee of the Japanese Circulation Society. Special report from the heart transplant candidate registry committee in Japan. *J Heart Lung Transplant* 24: 810—4.

Sasayama S, Asanoi H, Ishizaka S, Miyagi K. (1992) Evaluation of functional capacity of patients with congestive heart failure. In: Yasuda H, Kawaguchi H, editors. *New aspects in the treatment of failing heart.* Tokyo: Springer-Verlag; 113 - 117.

Takatani S, Matsuda H, Hanatani A, Nojiri C, Yamazaki K, Motomura T, Ohuchi K, akamoto T, Yamane T. (2005) Mechanical circulatory support devices (MCSD) in Japan: current status and future directions. *JArtif Organs* 8:13—27.

Tei C, Horikiri Y, Park JC, Jeong JW, Chang KS, Tanaka N, Toyama Y. (1994) Effects of hot water bath or sauna on patients with congestive heart failure: acute hemodynamic improvement by thermal vasodilation. *J Cardiol.* 24 (3): 175-183. Japanese.

Tei C, Horikiri Y, Park JC, Jeong JW, Chang KS, Toyama Y, Tanaka N. (1995) Acute hemodynamic improvement by thermal vasodilation in congestive heart failure. *Circulation.* 91(10):2582-2590.

Tei C, Tanaka N. (1996) Thermal vasodilation as a treatment of congestive heart failure: a novel approach. *J Cardiol* 27:29—30.

Tei C. (2007) Waon therapy: soothing warmth therapy. *J Cardiol* 49:301—4.

The CONSENSUS Trial Study Group. Effects of enalapril on mortality in severe heart failure. *N Engl J Med* 1987;316:1429–35.

Trotti R, Carratelli M, Barbieri M, Micieli G, Bosone D, Rondanelli M, Bo P. (2001) Oxidative stress and a thrombophilic condition in alcoholics without severe liver disease. *Haematologica* 86:85–91. 186

Part 5

Complications Following Ventricular Assist Devices

8

Treatment of Ventricular Arrhythmias in Patients Undergoing LVAD Therapy

Mulloy DP, M.D., Mahapatra S, M.D. FHRS and Kern JA, M.D. FACS
University of Virginia
U.S.A.

"When the heart is diseased, its work is imperfectly performed: the vessels proceeding from the heart become inactive, so that you cannot feel them ... if the heart trembles, has little power and sinks, the disease is advanced and death is near."
- Ebers Papyrus of Ancient Egypt: est. 1500 B.C

1. Introduction

Ventricular tachycardia (VT) and ventricular fibrillation (VF) are not uncommon in patients with end-stage heart failure. With the shortage of donor cardiac allografts, most potential heart transplant recipients are now being bridged with continuous-flow left ventricular assist devices (LVADs). In addition, with the recent FDA approval of the HeartMate® II LVAD (Thoratec Corp., Pleasanton, CA) as a destination therapy (DT) device, the potential pool of patients that may benefit from this therapy has expanded almost exponentially. While ventricular arrhythmias are common in patients with all types of cardiomyopathy and heart failure, the effect of LVAD therapy on the incidence of new, or the persistence of old ventricular arrhythmias is unknown. Recent evidence has suggested a possible increase in the rates of VT/VF in patients undergoing LVAD therapy with continuous flow devices as opposed to older pulsatile devices (Ziv et al, 2005);(Andersen et al., 2009). The potential utility of ventricular ablative procedures at the time of continuous flow LVAD placement is unclear. We have implanted 51 continuous flow LVADs over the past 21 months. Because the incidence of clinically significant post-operative VT/VF was initially higher than what he had experienced with earlier generation pulsatile LVADs, we have recently become aggressive at treating VT/VF at the time of LVAD placement. Any patient with a history of previous VT/VF has substrate localization performed via electrophysiologic (EP) mapping or systematic EKG analysis prior to LVAD placement. Intraoperatively, the endocardium is ablated through the LVAD ventriculotomy with cryoablation in addition to epicardial ablation also carried out with cryoablation. Since implementing this algorithm, the incidence of clinically significant post-operative VT/VF requiring additional catheter ablation has fallen to zero. We recommend aggressive localization and subsequent intra-operative ablation for all patients with a history of significant or worsening VT/VF prior to continuous flow LVAD placement to decrease the need for post-operative medical or catheter-based anti-arrhythmic therapy and to improve outcomes.

2. Background

2.1 Heart failure

Cardiovascular disease remains the leading cause of death in the United States and other industrialized nations (Kokolis, 2006). Heart failure represents the end stage of cardiovascular disease and continues to have a high prevalence in the U.S. despite advances in medical therapy. In developing countries, around 2% of adults suffer from heart failure, but in those over the age of 65, this increases to 6–10% (McMurray & Pfeffer 2005). Approximately 5 million Americans suffer from heart failure with over 550,000 new cases diagnosed each year (AHA, 2006). Community-based surveys show that 30–40% of patients die within a year of diagnosis and 60–70% die within 5 years, most from worsening heart failure or suddenly (probably because of a ventricular arrhythmia) (McMurray & Pfeffer, 2005). It is estimated that heart failure causes about 287, 0000 deaths in the US each year (AHA, 2006). In addition to the loss of life, heart failure poses a significant financial burden with estimated annual direct costs in the U.S. of $35 billion dollars (AHA, 2006). Hospitalizations due to heart failure are increasing and this is expected to continue with the progressively aging population (Roger, 2004).

Despite the advances in the management of heart failure, there may be as many as 100,000 persons who have been treated with guidelines-based therapy but have remained relatively unresponsive in New York Heart Association (NYHA) Class IIIb or IV heart failure (O'Connell, 2009). Optimal therapy with angiotensin-converting enzymes inhibitors, angiotensin receptor blockers, beta blockers, aldosterone antagonists, nitric oxide enhancers, implantable cardioverter-defibrillators (ICD) and cardiac resynchronization therapy have reduced hospitalizations and prolonged survival. However, the response is not uniform and at least a quarter of those who receive all therapies fail to respond (Hawkins, 2009). In these end-stage heart failure patients with recurrent hospitalizations, few options exist. Aggressive surgical approaches including cardiac restraint devices, mitral valve repair, and surgical ventricular reconstruction are under evaluation but have yet to demonstrate definitive benefit (Mann et al., 2007);(Jones et al. 2009). Only cardiac transplantation has been shown to definitively improve outcomes with median survival of 13 years, but this is restricted to a select relatively young population (Taylor et al., 2009). The number of heart transplants in the U.S. has remained stable at about 2,000 per year, only 2% to 4% of patients who need definitive therapy. With a growing population of end-stage heart failure patients and a static donor pool, it has become clear that heart transplantation will never meet the demands. Although there is great enthusiasm for innovative approaches, stem cell therapy is only entering preliminary clinical trials, gene therapy of calcium transport proteins is only completing the first step in the cascade of clinical trials, and xenografting research has been stalled (O'Connell 2009). To date, the most promising area of development has been mechanical circulatory support with LVADs, most recently with the Thoratec HeartMate II.

2.2 Left ventricular assist devices

Implantable left ventricular assist devices have become accepted as an important therapeutic modality for patients with end-stage heart failure. The most common uses for LVADs include bridge to heart transplantation (BTT) and long-term destination therapy (DT) for those patients not eligible for transplantation.

The development of ventricular assist devices began in earnest in 1964 with the National Institutes of Health establishment of the Artificial Heart Program, whose stated goal was putting a man-made heart into a human being by the end of the decade (Sahuar 2004). Unlike the moon-landing, this lofty goal was not met. Nevertheless, progress proceeded slowly and clinical use of ventricular assist devices on a more routine basis began in the mid 1980s. Since then, the research and development of ventricular assist device technology, along with clinical progress, has accelerated. Several LVADs have now been designed and developed and are in various phases of clinical and preclinical evaluation. Currently, implantable LVADs can be classified into two main categories: volume-displacement (pulsatile) and continuous-flow (nonpulsatile) pumps. All LVADs are composed of an inflow cannula, the actual pump with its associated mechanical and electrical components, an outflow conduit, a percutaneous lead, and the external system components with varying degrees of portability. LVADs can also be grouped based on the engineering design of the pump with classification broadly as first-, second-, and third-generation devices (Nguyen & Thourani, 2010). First-generation devices are the pulsatile pumps. They include the HeartMate XVE and its predecessors including the HeartMate IP1000 and HeartMate VE (Thoratec Corp., Pleasanton, CA), the Thoratec PVAD and IVAD (Thoratec Corp.), and the Novacor LVAS (World Heart Corp., Oakland, CA). In contrast to the first-generation devices, both second- and third-generation LVADs are continuous flow, rotary pumps. Second-generation pumps, which include the HeartMate II (Thoratec Corp.), Jarvik 2000 FlowMaker (Jarvik Heart, Inc., New York, NY), and MicroMed-DeBakey (MicroMed Cardiovascular, Inc., Houston, TX), have an internal rotor within the blood flow path that is suspended by contact, blood-immersed bearings. Third-generation devices are similar, but lack contact bearings in an effort to prevent wear and prolong device life without failure. Third-generation devices are in varying stages of clinical development, but are not available for commercial use in the U.S.

First-generation LVADs came to clinical use in the mid 1980s and all of the first-generation devices listed above are approved for BTT. Despite this, only the HeartMate XVE is approved by the Food and Drug Administration for DT in the United States. As volume displacement pumps, first-generation LVADs have an internal reservoir chamber with inflow and outflow valves. The pumps function by cyclic filling and emptying of the reservoir chamber either by pneumatic or electrical drive systems. More than 5000 pulsatile HeartMate devices have been implanted worldwide and have been shown to provide excellent hemodynamic support (Frazier et al., 2001). In several studies, mechanical circulatory support with these devices is reported to bridge patients successfully to transplant with a perioperative mortality of 15% to 20% and an overall survival until transplantation of 60% to 70% (El-Banayosy et al., 2000). Unfortunately, first-generation devices have inherent limitations in their design, particularly when used for the purpose of prolonged support or DT. The pump size is quite large, thus requiring extensive surgical dissection with subsequent risk of hematoma formation and infection. The large size also limits implantation to patients with a large body habitus. In addition, a large-diameter percutaneous lead is needed for venting of air, which can lead to an increased risk of driveline infections. Finally, a critical drawback in first-generation devices is the high frequency of eventual device failure, requiring device exchange or causing possible death. In the landmark REMATCH trial, which was used as the basis for LVAD approval for DT, the failure rate of the HeartMate XVE after 2 years was 35%, with a mortality of more than 10% attributed directly to device failure (Rose et al., 2001).

The second-generation have now essentially replaced the first-generation devices for clinical use. The most extensive clinical experience is with the HeartMate II. Currently, this is the only second-generation device approved for both BTT and DT in the United States (Miller et al., 2007); (Slaughter et al., 2009). These continuous flow, rotary pumps were introduced to overcome many of the shortcomings of the first-generation devices. They are simpler in design with only a single moving part: the internal rotor. Advantages over first-generation devices include smaller size requiring less extensive surgical dissection for implantation, the absence of valves that are a primary site of wear, higher efficiency with less energy requirement, and a smaller percutaneous lead (Nguyen & Thourani, 2010). With these improvements, the second-generation devices have shown to be much more reliable with device support of more than 6 years reported (Westaby et al., 2006). While the necessity for device replacement does still occur with the HeartMate II, the underlying causes have been related to thrombosis, infection, or damage to the percutaneous leads and not to mechanical failures of the pumping mechanism (Slaughter et al., 2009). In a recently-published randomized clinical trial for DT comparing the HeartMate II versus the first-generation HeartMate XVE, the HeartMate II was shown to be significantly better than the HeartMate XVE in achieving the primary end point of survival free from device failure or disabling stroke at 2 years (Slaughter et al., 2009). Moreover, patients with HeartMate II support also had significantly superior actuarial survival rates at 2 years (58% vs. 24%). In addition, device failure and other complications including infections were less frequent in patients supported with the HeartMate II.

3. Ventricular arrhythmias

Mortality in patients with heart failure is mostly due to progressive heart failure or sudden death related to ventricular tachyarrhythmias (VAs) (Jessup, 2003). The most important risk factor for VA is a reduced ejection fraction (EF) (Myerburg et al., 1997; Singh et al., 2002). Although medications such as beta-blockers, ACE inhibitors, and ARBs, and devices such as implantable cardiac defibrillators (ICDs) have been shown to decrease morbidity and mortality, the risk of sudden cardiac death (SCD) remains high. In fact, approximately 50% of patients with heart failure die from SCD (Guido et al., 1997).

While the precise mechanism of ventricular tachyarrhythmias is not entirely understood, VAs are generally thought to originate from cardiac scar tissue and from the border between normal myocardium and scar tissue. Ventricular scars are composed of variable regions of dense fibrosis that create conduction block and surviving myocyte bundles with interstitial fibrosis and diminished coupling, which produce the circuitous slow-conduction paths (Stevenson & Soejima, 2007). The effective refractory period in the action potential of this borderline ischemic, viable myocardium is altered and bears the risk of generating the re-entry circuits responsible for ventricular tachyarrhythmias (Doenst et al., 2007).

In all patients with heart failure, the elevation of plasma catecholamines that cause increases in sympathetic outflow along with decrease in parasympathetic activity correlate well with poor prognosis. Also significant in many patients are anatomic and mechanical factors such as wall stretch, abnormal wall motion, left ventricular stress, and increased myocardial length. These factors acting directly, or through alterations in hemodynamic factors, may lead to the genesis of cardiac arrhythmias in the setting of heart failure (Damiano et al., 1985). All of these causative arrhythmogenic factors merge in the dilated and failing ventricle, creating a perfect storm for arrhythmogenesis. The immediate trigger for the development of VT or VF in an individual patient with heart failure is often unclear but a composite of the major interacting factors will reveal those patients at highest risk for sudden death.

To properly understand ventricular tachyarrhythmias, it is necessary to distinguish monomorphic ventricular tachycardia (MMVT) on one hand, and polymorphic ventricular tachycardia (PMVT) and ventricular fibrillation (VF) on the other. Monomorphic VT is generally caused by fixed anatomic abnormalities such as scar from previous MI where border zone areas generate re-entrant circuits causing VT (Stevenson & Soejima, 2007). This ventricular scar can be caused by ischemia or other forms of injury including scar tissue resultant from LVAD cannula placement. In this case, 12-lead electrocardiogram and EP mapping can be used to localize specific areas of the ventricle where scar is present and re-entrant VT is initiated. On the other hand, PVT and VF are generally caused by a functionally deteriorating ventricle and result from repolarization abnormalities of the unhealthy myocardium (Aliot et al., 2009). Congestive heart failure caused by the failing ventricle creates ventricular dilation, increase wall tension, and with that, conditions ripe for subendocardial ischemia. These conditions alter the electric behaviour of the ventricle and can result in the disorganized contractions seen in PVT and VF. As a result of the often direct anatomic correlation between MMVT and myocardial scar, MMVT is usually more receptive to targeted ablation therapies (Aliot et al., 2009). Eliminating PMVT and VF is more difficult and often requires therapy guided toward functional improvement of the failing ventricle rather than ablation alone.

4. Arrhythmias in patients with VADs

4.1 Background

The prevalence of ventricular arrhythmias is highest in those patients with severe end-stage heart failure: the same cohort of patients who stand to benefit most from LVAD therapy. Therefore, it should come as no surprise that ventricular arrhythmias are relatively common in patients supported with LVADs. Despite this, the interaction between LVAD placement and ventricular arrhythmias is not well understood. On one hand, LVAD placement does ease the burden on a diseased left ventricle by decompressing the ventricle. This decompression in turn decreases the neurohormonal, hemodynamic, mechanical, and electrolyte abnormalities which predispose toward arrhythmia development; thereby reducing the frequency of post-op VTE, especially PMVT and VF. In contrast, LVAD placement does not treat areas of existing ventricular scar, and indeed the apical cannula placement necessarily requires creation of new myocardial scar tissue. This new scar tissue created by LVAD implantation places patients at risk for new monomorphic ventricular arrhythmias and does not impact existing MMVT resulting from other areas of scar. Indeed, many reports suggest a higher incidence of ventricular arrhythmias in patients after LVAD placement (Ziv et al., 2005);(Andersen et al., 2009). Postoperative ventricular tachyarrhythmia events (VTE) have been documented to occur in up to 35% of patients within 30 days of LVAD placement (Ziv et al., 2005);(Refaat et al., 2008).

The pathogenesis of increased arrhythmias post-LVAD is likely to be caused by direct mechanical irritation from the inflow cannula of the LVAD as well as scar tissue from the cannula placement. With the LVAD in place the ventricle is decompressed and the aortic root pressure improved, resulting in improved blood flow to scarred regions of the heart and actually allowing for the tissue to conduct and support VT. Post-VAD arrhythmias have also been attributed in the literature to a host of other mechanisms including acute left ventricular unloading with pulsatile VADs, altered ventricular repolarization (Grzywacz et al., 2006), mechano-electrical feedback from the VAD motor (Harding et al., 2001), and alterations in calcium handling gene expression (Rodriguez-Way et al., 2005). In addition, continuous flow devices are theorized to predispose to arrhythmias by causing so-called "suction events" when the ventricle is completely decompressed and the endocardium is sucked against the inflow cannula (Vollkron et al., 2007). This suction phenomenon is thought to account for the apparent increased arrhythmia incidence with continuous flow LVADs as opposed to pulsatile LVADs. While all of these theories are interesting and may contribute to the existing understanding of the interaction between LVADs and ventricular arrhythmias, the reality is that the current paucity of published literature and surplus of theories reflect an inadequate understanding of the relationship. Most of the available data concerning arrhythmias in patients with LVADs constitute results from relatively small case series. In addition, most of these case series review data from patients with pulsatile LVADs, while newer continuous flow devices such as the HeartMate II now dominate the national clinical practice.

While the presence of an LVAD mitigates the profound hemodynamic collapse often seen in unsupported patients with VT or VF, studies have demonstrated a decrease in LVAD flow output with ventricular tachyarrhythmias (Bedi et al., 2007). Additionally, crude mortality as high as 52% has been reported for patients with VT/VF within 1 week postoperatively (Bedi et al., 2007). Ventricular tachyarrhythmias can reduce right ventricle output, thereby reducing left ventricular venous return. Therefore, even though the left ventricle is supported by the LVAD, the arrhythmia prevents adequate preload on left ventricle and can become hemodynamically unstable. Thus, elimination of ventricular tachyarrhythmias in LVAD patients is essential to maximizing outcomes.

4.2 Literature review

In order to begin understanding the relationship between ventricular arrhythmias and LVADs it is necessary to review of the existing literature. In 1991, the first known report of ventricular arrhythmias in patients with LVADs was published (Arai et al., 1991). In 1994, Oz et al. reported that ventricular arrhythmias are well tolerated in the immediate setting in patients LVAD support. Pulmonary perfusion was maintained even during rapid ventricular arrhythmias and cardiac arrest was well tolerated without syncope. Thus, delayed termination of ventricular fibrillation or flutter was reported to be safe and feasible in this setting (Oz et al., 1994). In 1997, the first case report documenting benefit from an implantable cardioverter-defibrillator (ICD) in a patient on LVAD support was published in a 51 year-old male who underwent LVAD implantation for refractory heart failure after having received an ICD five years earlier (Skinner et al., 1997).

Following these reports, it took until 2005 for a relatively large retrospective observational study to be performed (Ziv et al., 2005). This study remains of the best available, and reported a 32% incidence of VT/VF following pulsatile LVAD implantation for advanced heart failure, with particularly high rates during the early post-operative period (Ziv et al., 2005). Notable in this study was the comparison of pre-operative arrhythmias to post-operative arrhythmias. One hundred and eighteen episodes of documented sustained ventricular arrhythmia occurred in 30 (of 100) patients pre-operatively, one hundred and seventy nine episodes occurred in 32 patients post-operatively. Of those 9 patients with pre-operative MVT, 4 patients no longer had MVT and 5 continued to have MVT after LVAD. New-onset MVT was documented in 18 patients who had no pre-LVAD MVT, 12 of whom had no pre-LVAD arrhythmia of any type. With regards to PVT and VF, 23 patients had PVT/VF documented pre-operatively and 17 patients had PVT/VF post-operatively. PVT/VF was no longer observed in 16 patients who had this arrhythmia before LVAD placement, whereas PVT/VF was a new finding in 10 patients who had not had this arrhythmia documented pre-operatively.

Summarizing these results, in 100 patients undergoing pulsatile LVAD implantation, there was a slight decrease in post-operative PVT/VF and a significant increase in post-operative MVT. This is exactly as one might expect given the LVADs role in decompression of the ventricle helping with PVT/VF, but creating a new site of scar and mechanical irritation in the ventricle and causing a new focus for MVT. In addition, the majority of the 32 patients who had post-LVAD ventricular arrhythmias had experienced the first episode by the end of the first postoperative week. Post-LVAD ventricular tachyarrhythmia was nearly incessant in 9 patients and highly frequent (>5 episodes/day) in 7 patients. Whereas the total number of patients with ventricular tachyarrhythmias of any kind before and after LVAD was similar, post-LVAD arrhythmias were more frequent and resistant to drug treatments. Trends were observed in all-cause mortality and stroke, but no statistically significant relationship between arrhythmia and these outcomes was demonstrated (Ziv et al., 2005).

The above retrospective review was followed by another retrospective review of 111 consecutive patients undergoing pulsatile LVAD placement for BTT between 1987 and 2001 (Bedi et al., 2007). In this study, clinically significant ventricular arrhythmias occurred in 24 patients (22%) during device support. 54% of these occurred during the first week post-implantation. The mortality was significantly higher ($p<0.001$) during LVAD support in the group with ventricular arrhythmias (33%) vs. the group without ventricular arrhythmias (18%).

In 2008 a smaller retrospective review of 42 patients (Refaat et al., 2008) documented post-operative ventricular arrhythmias in 15 patients (36%). Analysis of multiple pre- and post-operative factors revealed that non-usage of post-operative beta-blockade was strongly associated with arrhythmia development (odds ratio 7.04, $p=0.001$). Unfortunately, this association has not been borne out in subsequent studies.

A 2009 retrospective review represents the first published description of ventricular arrhythmias in continuous flow LVADs. This study reviewed records of 23 consecutive HeartMate II recipients and documented a 52% incidence (12 of 23) of sustained VT or VF (Anderson et al. 2009). 75% of the patients experienced the arrhythmia within 4 weeks, and in all of these patients the arrhythmia predicted recurrent arrhythmic events. None of these patients died of the arrhythmia but most were symptomatic during the event. 32% of the patients required cardioversion or defibrillation. Based on the high incidence of post-operative arrhythmias, along with the fact that 3 patients experienced hemodynamic instability associated with the event, the authors recommended consideration for prophylactic ICD implantation for all patients expected to be supported by the LVAD for a longer period of time (Anderson et al 2009).

Other more recent reviews have concurred with Anderson et al.'s assertion that ICD implantation should be considered for primary prevention of VT/VF in all patients undergoing LVAD implantation. A Cleveland clinic review looked at all 478 patients undergoing VAD placement between 2001 and 2008; the majority (74%) of these being pulsatile LVADs, 8.2% continuous-flow, and 10.5% with extracorporeal systems (Cantillon et al, 2010). 90 of these patients (18%) had an ICD at the time of VAD implantation. Crude mortality was lower among patients with an ICD (24.4%) when compared to those without an ICD (36.9%; $P=0.026$), Kaplan-Meier curve for survival shows divergence between patients with and without ICD beginning at 20 days and extending throughout the support period. 32% of the patients experienced a sustained ventricular tachyarrhythmia event in the post-operative period with the mean time to first event being 32.4 +/- 47.1 days. While the retrospective nature and large cohort of patients with pulsatile LVADs limit the review, the survival difference in a large number of patients is intriguing.

The only prospective study looking at ventricular arrhythmias in LVAD patients is a recently published study from Hanover Germany. 61 consecutive patients underwent LVAD implantation between 2005 and 2008, 44 of these patients with the HeartMate II and 15 with the Heartware LVAD, a third-generation continuous-flow device (Oswald et al., 2010). After the acute perioperative period, all patients without a pre-existing ICD (40 patients) underwent ICD implantation (17 +/- 15 days after VAD placement). Ventricular arrhythmias leading to ICD interventions were frequent in the study population with 34% of patients receiving appropriate ICD interventions for ventricular arrhythmias during the study follow-up (median 12 months; range 13-1167 days). Even excluding the first 7 days when patients were most prone to arrhythmias, there was a still a 25% rate of appropriate ICD interventions. Observed arrhythmias were 52% monomorphic VT, 35% VF, and 13% polymorphic VT. Of the 21 patients with appropriate ICD interventions, there were a total of 144 episodes of spontaneous ventricular arrhythmias (average 6.8 per patient). Patients with no previous arrhythmia history had an estimated 1-year risk of 24% for appropriate ICD treatment, those with a secondary prevention indication had an even higher 1-year risk of 50%. In these secondary prevention patients, the calculated VTE rate per month was the same both before and after VAD placement. Interestingly, ventricular arrhythmia rate was higher in nonischemic heart failure (50%) than ischemic heart failure (22%) patients.

The observations from all of the above studies yield more questions than answers; however, several basic conclusions can be drawn from them. First, sustained ventricular arrhythmias are common in patients after LVAD implantation with a range of 22% to 52% of patients experiencing sustained VT/VF in the post-operative period. Second, most patients who experience post-operative VT/VF do so within the first few weeks after surgery. Third, patients who experience one episode of sustained VTE are more likely to experience future events. Fourth, while ventricular arrhythmias seem to better tolerated in the LVAD population as compared to patients without assist devices, most ventricular arrhythmias do have associated symptoms, some cause hemodynamic instability, and all may impact long term survival and survival to transplantation. Fifth, prophylactic ICD placement may be indicated and a prospective randomized trial is needed to answer this question. Finally, as is always the case with any emerging medical technology, further prospective analysis is needed.

5. Arrhythmia treatment

5.1 Arrhythmia surgery

Cardiac surgery for arrhythmias was initiated in 1968 by Dr. Will Sealy with the first successful division of an accessory AV connection for the Wolff-Parkinson-White (WPW) syndrome. During the 1980s hundreds of cardiac surgeons learned the technique of open-chest surgical division of accessory AV pathways for the cure of WPW syndrome. However, as the 1980s ended, catheter-based radiofrequency ablation (RFA) emerged as a less invasive method of cure and Dr. Sealy's surgery was relegated to a historical footnote (Cox J, 2004). Subsequently, Cox and colleagues attained the first clinical cure of an AV nodal reentrant tachycardia in 1982 via a discrete cryosurgical procedure (Cox et al., 1987). Again, catheter-based RFA rapidly replaced the use of cryosurgery specifically for the treatment of AV nodal reentrant tachycardias. Nevertheless, this initially use of cryothermal energy in cardiac surgery opened the door for other uses of cryosurgery throughout the 1980s and 1990s for treatment of other supraventricular tachyarrhythmias, atrial tachyarrhythmias via the Cox-Maze procedure, and ventricular arrhythmias via destruction of ectopic foci of excitation (Cox J, 2004).

Experiments in the 1960s had documented the heterogeneity of tissue injury in acute MI and the reentrant basis of ischemic ventricular arrhythmias was defined (Han et al., 1970);(Boineau & Cox, 1973). During the 1970s, it became apparent that simple revascularization with CABG failed to cure ischemic ventricular tachyarrhythmias and that revascularization alone had prohibitively high morbidity and mortality. In 1969, Kaiser and colleagues reported on intraoperative mapping in patients with heart disease to localize the area of ischemia injury (Kaiser et al., 1969). A decade later, Harken and associates described the endocardial resection procedure based on intraoperative mapping (Josephson et al., 1979). In the late 1980s, Dor and colleagues described the technique of both surgical resection and repair of LV aneurysms (Dor et al., 1989). Part of Dor's described procedure included cryoablation of the junction of scar and normal myocardium if spontaneous or inducible tachycardia was present preoperatively. When reporting on results of this procedure, the unexpected effect was that arrhythmias were essentially cured without need for intraoperative mapping (Dor et al., 1994). While ischemic VT remains the most common surgically treated ventricular arrhythmia to this day, these surgical procedures are only rarely performed primarily to treat arrhythmia. Most often, there is another primary indication, such as the improvement of left ventricular function (via the Dor procedure), the removal of apical thrombus, or the alleviation of heart failure symptoms (Doenst et al., 2007). Subsequent advances in the field of electrophysiology have replaced many open surgical techniques for the treatment of arrhythmias, however the use of open cryosurgery for treatment of ventricular arrhythmias in the Dor procedure, and for treatment of atrial fibrillation via the Cox-Maze procedure has persisted (Cox J, 2004).

5.2 Mechanism of cryoablation

Cryothermal energy is the preferred energy source for arrhythmia ablation in open cardiac surgery. Cryothermal energy destroys tissue through the formation of intracellular and extracellular ice crystals. These crystals disrupt the cell membrane and the cytoplasmic organelles. Following cryoablation, there is development of hemorrhage, edema, and inflammation over the first 48 hours. Healing is characterized by extensive fibrosis, which begins approximately 1 week after lesion formation. Cryoablation is the only available energy source that does not disrupt tissue collagen, thus preserving normal tissue architecture (Lall & Damiano, 2007). This makes it an excellent energy source for ablation close to valvular tissue or the fibrous skeleton of the heart. Histologically, cryoablation creates a dense homogenous scar which has been shown to have a low arrhythmogenic potential (Wetstein et al., 1985).

With conventional nitrous oxide cryoablation probes, 2 to 3 minute ablations have been shown to reliably create transmural atrial lesions and penetrate ventricular muscle to adequate depths for effective and reliable ablation. Nitrous oxide cryoablation has a history of extensive clinical use and an excellent safety profile. Thus the benefits of cryoablation include the ability to preserve tissue architecture and collagen structure, as well as a well-defined dose curve and safety profile. The potential disadvantage is the relatively long time necessary to create an ablation (2 to 3 minutes).

Two commercially available sources of cryothermal energy are available for use in cardiac surgery. The older, and more proven, technology utilizes nitrous oxide and is manufactured by Cooper Surgical, now recently purchased by AtriCure® (Cincinnati, OH). A variety of rigid and malleable probes are available for use. More recently, CryoCath Technologies (Montreal, Canada) developed a device using argon gas. This technology uses either a malleable probe or a two-in-one convertible device that incorporates a clamp and surgical probe. At one atmosphere of pressure, nitrous oxide is capable of cooling to -89.5°C, whereas argon has a minimum temperature of -185.7°C. Both types of probes consist of a hollow shaft, an electrode tip, and an integrated thermocouple for distal temperature recording. The liquid is pumped under high pressure to the electrode through an inner lumen. Once the fluid reaches the electrode, it converts to a gas phase, absorbing energy and resulting in rapid cooling of the tissue. The gas is then aspirated by vacuum through a separate return lumen to the console (Lall & Damiano, 2007). In our protocol, the AtriCure device was used with the malleable Cryo1™ probe. The probe is applied to the relevant areas selected for ablation and either a 2 or 2.5 minute cycle is used.

6. Our treatment protocol

6.1 The problem

Over the last 21 months, we have implanted 51 continuous flow HeartMate II LVADs at the University of Virginia. Following the first dozen HeartMate II implantations, we anecdotally noted that the rate of post-operative ventricular arrhythmias seemed higher than with the previously used HeartMate XVE, a pulsatile LVAD. Therefore, after the first 23 implantations of the HeartMate II, we analyzed our single-institution data and noted that the rate of post-operative VT and VF was higher in the HeartMate II population as compared to the 14 previously placed HeartMate XVE LVADs. 34.7% (n=8) of the HeartMate II patients had recurrent post-operative VT/VF, while 21.4% (n=3) of the HeartMate XVE patients had recurrent post-operative VT/VF. Importantly, pre-operative rates of VT/VF were the same in both groups (35%). While this difference did not demonstrate statistical significance, we decided that in conjunction with published data confirming a high rate of VT/VF in post-operative patients with continuous flow LVAD and the potential association of these events with poor outcomes, we needed to become more aggressive in treating for ventricular arrhythmias at the time of LVAD placement. Our group sought to devise with a method to reliably decrease, or completely prevent, the incidence of post-operative ventricular tachyarrhythmias. Through a combination of catheter-based EP approaches along with open surgical ablation techniques, we began instituting a protocol for open cryoablation of mapped arrhythmia loci at the time of LVAD implantation.

6.2 Catheter mapping and ablation

There are several methods for ablating a focus of ventricular tachycardia as mentioned previously. The most common method of ventricular arrhythmia treatment in all patients is via EP catheter-directed mapping and RFA of identified areas of endocardial border zone ischemic tissue (scar mapping) or RFA of other identified foci of arrhythmogenic substrate (activation mapping). While this represents the least invasive of potential methods for ablation of VT/VF, it suffers from several shortcomings, especially in the LVAD population.

First, with a continuous flow LVAD in place, such as the HeartMate II, the left ventricle is decompressed. In this decompressed left ventricle with the LVAD inflow cannula in the apex of the ventricle, there is very little room to maneuver the ablation catheter (see Figure 1), thus making the procedure exceedingly difficult despite the fact that reducing the LVAD flow can mitigate this issue. Second, traditional catheter-based RFA offers access only to endocardial sources of arrthymogenic tissue. Evidence shows that up to 70% of patients with ventricular tachycardia have epicardial substrate as the source of their arrhythmia, especially those patients with non-ischemic cardiomyopathies (Sacher et al., 2009). While trans-cutaneous catheter-based epicardial ablation of ventricular tachycardia via a sub-xiphoid approach is becoming a more frequently used technique at our institution and others, it is associated with several complications including post-procedure atrial fibrillation and pericarditis, right ventricle puncture during access, and others (Aliot et al., 2009; Mahapatra et al., 2009). Third, it is difficult to reliably create transmural ventricular lesions using a catheter-based RFA approach. Therefore, post-operative catheter-based RFA for LVAD-associated ventricular arrhythmias suffers from too many shortcomings to be the primary method of ventricular tachyarrhythmia treatment in LVAD patients.

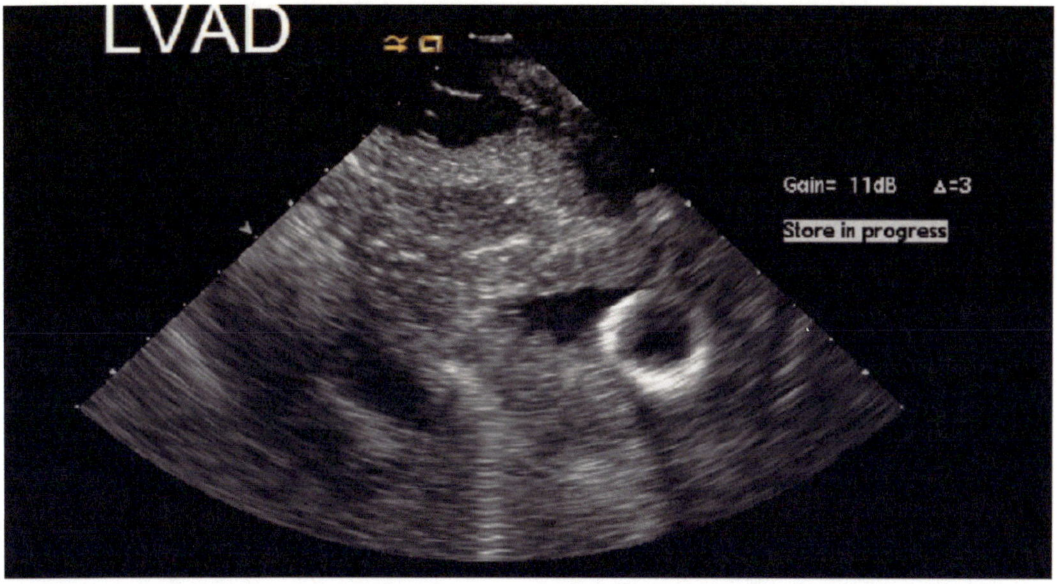

Fig. 1. Echocardiography demonstrating EP catheter in decompressed ventricle

6.3 Other options

Alternatively, given the difficulties and shortcomings associated with catheter-directed RFA, intra-operative ablation of arrhythmogenic substrate can be performed. Ideally this would be performed using simultaneous intra-operative EP scar mapping to identify areas of substrate to maximize the efficacy of cryoablation; however, this technique would require a hybrid EP suite and surgical operating room which is not available at our institution. A second option is mapping prior to planned LVAD implantation to define targeted areas for intra-operative cryoablation. Following localization of arrhythmogenic substrate via EP mapping or EKG analysis, patients can then undergo intra-operative cryoablation of the arrhythmia focus at the time of LVAD implantation.

As mentioned previously, arrythmia surgery has in large part been replaced by catheter-directed EP therapies. However, in a case where another primary indication exists that requires sternotomy or thoracotomy with open access to the heart with or without cardiopulmonary bypass, arrhythmia surgery has remained as a mainstay of treatment. Examples of this include cryoablation at the time of surgical ventricular reconstruction, as seen in the Dor procedure, and the Cox-Maze procedure for atrial fibrillation performed in conjunction with mitral valve repair or replacement. We argue that LVAD implantation offers and equally opportune occasion for arrhythmia treatment via an open surgical approach.

6.4 Substrate mapping technique

Prior to any planned arrhythmia intervention, one must identify the target area for treatment. In our experience, this is done with either targeted EP mapping and/or systematic EKG interpretation. Using an established technique of electrophysiologic substrate mapping, a detailed schematic map of the heart is generated (Figures 3 and 4). This map is generated by measuring endocardial voltage potentials at a variety of locations. In the generated map, voltages greater than 1.5mV represent normal cardiac tissue and appear purple; voltages less than 0.5mV represent dead cardiac muscle and appear red; and voltages in between represent the borderline ischemic areas and are represented by a range of colors (Aliot et al., 2009). After substrate mapping is completed, the electrophysiologist and surgeon are able to carefully review the generated projection and can specifically target the border zone areas of potentially arrhythmogenic substrate for open intra-operative cryoablation at the time of LVAD placement. Note in figure 2 the visualized EP mapping catheter. In a hybrid EP suite/Operating room, the surgeon would be able to visualize and palpate the intra-cardiac catheter at the time of mapping in order to very specifically target the mapped arrhythmogenic substrate in real time.

Unfortunately, a hybrid suite is not available at this time and not all patients are stable enough to tolerate transport to, and mapping in, the EP suite. Given this logistic issue, we have devised a compromise technique for targeting the locus of arrhythmia-generating

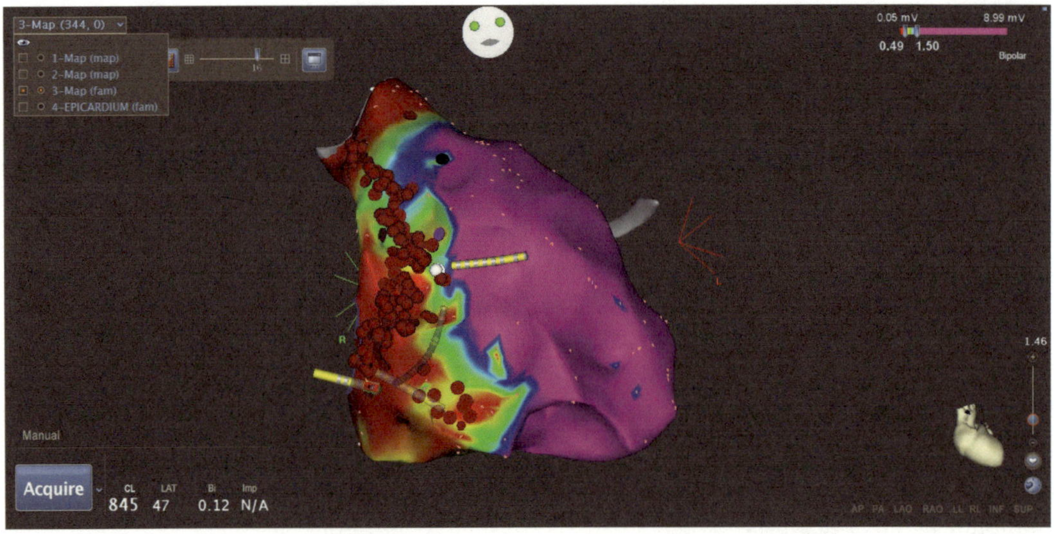

Fig. 2. Electrophysiologic Substrate Map

substrate. In patients with hemodynamic instability who would not tolerate substrate mapping in the EP suite, a systematic interpretation of 12-lead EKG results capturing episodes of ventricular arrhythmia is performed. Systematic EKG analysis of captured ventricular arrhythmia events is then used to localize the arrhythmia origin to an anatomic area of the heart (i.e. LV lateral wall).

Using Figure 3 as a guide, and Figure 4 as an example of sustained monomorphic VT, one first looks at lead V1. If a left bundle branch block (LBBB) is visible, the arrhythmia source comes from the RV or septum; if a right bundle branch block (RBBB) is visible, the arrhythmia is generated in the LV. One can then look at the direction of deflection of the QRS complex to more specifically localize the arrhythmia focus. First, looking at the inferior leads, II, III, and avF, a positive wave localizes the focus to the anterior aspect of the LV. Alternatively, a negative wave indicates posterior LV. Similarly, the precordial leads are analyzed and a positive deflection in avR and V4 indicates an apex source, a negative deflection points to the base of the ventricle. Finally, lead I and avL are analyzed, with a positive deflection indicating a septal source, a negative deflection pointing to a lateral wall source. In this manner, the focus of arrhythmogenic substrate can be localized to a specific area of the heart that allows the surgeon to target this area intra-operatively with cryoablation. For example, using Figure 4 below, the 12-lead EKG of captured ventricular tachycardia can be used to localize the arrhythmia source to the apical LV antero-lateral wall. RBBB points to the LV, then inferior leads point to the anterior surface, then precordial leads indicate an apical source, then I and avL point to the septum. Therefore, the LV antero-lateral wall close to the apex is the likely source.

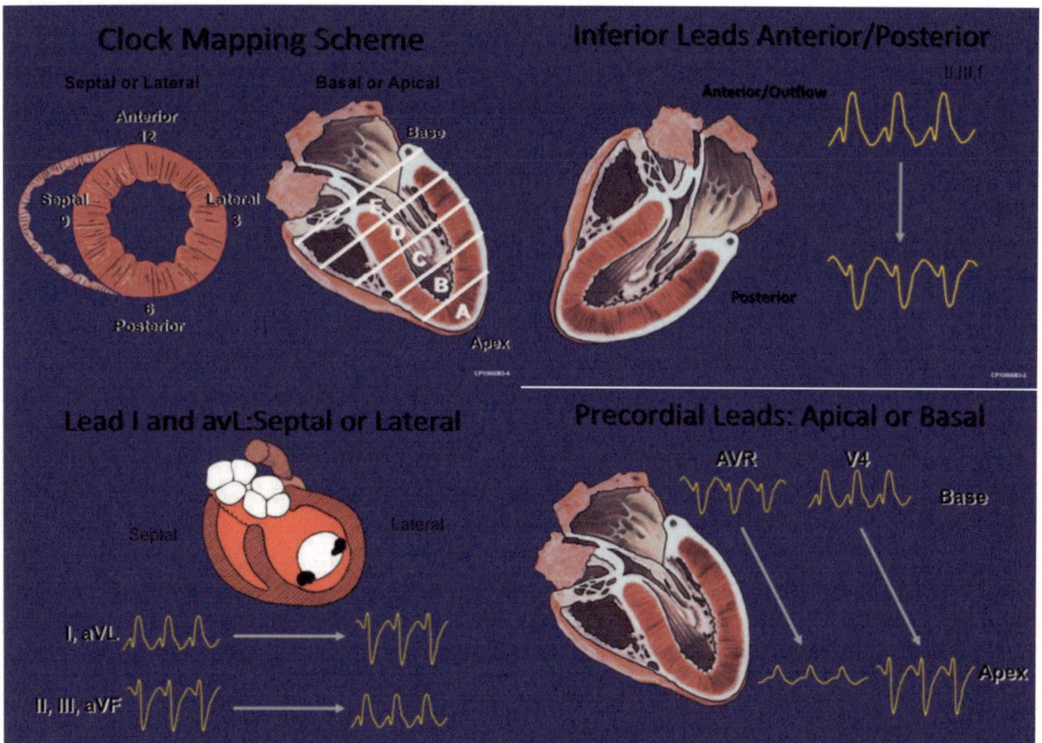

Fig. 3. Schematic for 12-lead EKG analysis of captured VT.

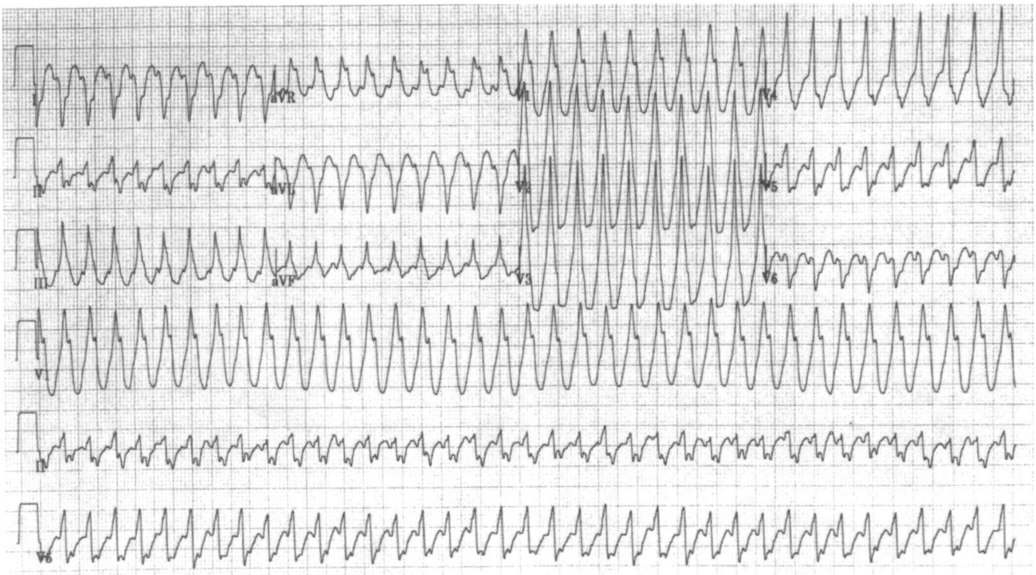

Fig. 4. Monomorphic Ventricular Tachycardia localizing to LV antero-lateral wall.

6.4 Intra-operative cryoablation

LVAD implantation surgery offers a unique opportunity for arrhythmia treatment because of the open access the surgeon is granted to the entire epicardial surface of the heart and the endocardium of the entire left ventricle. In addition, one can proceed with cryoablation with relative impunity on the left ventricle because the LVAD will be in place post-operatively. Given the role of the LVAD in supporting the already failed left ventricle, the preservation and optimization of post-operative left ventricular function does not carry the same supreme importance associated with virtually every other cardiac surgery performed. A common cause of morbidity and mortality in patients with LVADs is RV failure, so care must be exercised to avoid unnecessary ablation on the septum and free wall of the RV, but otherwise one may proceed without excessive concern of damaging healthy myocardium.

The procedure is performed in the same manner as any other LVAD implantation. A median sternotomy is performed followed by pericardiotomy and the preperitoneal pocket is made to accommodate the LVAD pump. Following this, cannulation sutures for cardiopulmonary bypass are inserted, anticoagulation is dosed, cardiopulmonary bypass cannulae are placed, and partial bypass is initiated. Once partial bypass is initiated, epicardial cryoablation is performed using the AtriCure device with the Cryo1 probe. Each pre-identified site of arrhythmogenic substrate is ablated at -70°C for two and a half minutes. If necessary, the malleable Cryo1 probe can be shaped to match the contour of the epicardial surface to facilitate uniform application of the cryothermal energy (see Figure 5).

Following epicardial ablation, full bypass is initiated, the aorta is cross-clamped, and cardioplegia is administered. We prefer to perform the endocardial ablation and LVAD placement on the arrested heart, although these procedures can also be done on the empty beating heart. At this point, the left ventricle apex is identified and the coring device is used to create a ventriculotomy for placement of the LVAD inflow cannula. Subsequently, the AtriCure device is again used with the Cryo1 probe for endocardial ablation via the

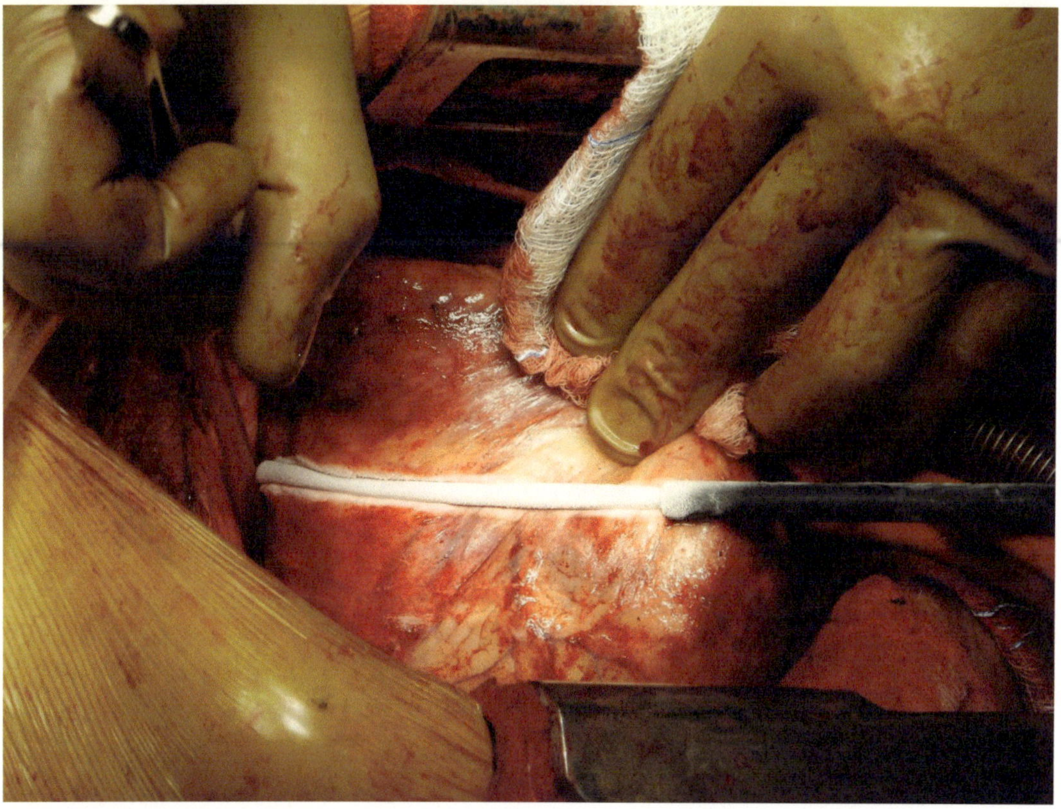

Fig. 5. Epicardial Cryoablation

previously-performed ventriculotomy (see Figure 6). For endocardial ablation in the arrested and non-perfused heart, we opt to reduce cryo time to two minutes, again at -70°C. For effective arrhythmia ablation, care must be taken to ablate the previously identified arrhythmogenic site in addition to creating a surrounding cryoablation tract extending to fixed anatomic sites such as the mitral valve and/or apical LVAD inflow cannula site. Ablation at an arrhythmogenic scar site only, without this extension, could leave the patient prone to recurrent arrhythmias via reentrant conduction around the ablated scar site. Following completion of the endocardial ablation, circumferential stitches are placed at the ventriculotomy, the LVAD inflow cannula is seated, and the remainder of the surgery for standard LVAD placement proceeds as per usual.

7. Results

Since instituting the above protocol for the prevention of post-operative ventricular arrhythmias, we have performed 28 additional HeartMate II LVAD implantations. Of these 28 patients, 9 patients had a history of previous VT/VF and thus underwent pre-operative mapping and intra-operative endocardial and epicardial cryoablation. None of these 9 patients who underwent intra-operative cryoablation have suffered from sustained post-operative ventricular arrhythmias. Of the 21 patients who had no history of pre-operative VT/VF, 3 patients experienced post-operative sustained VT or VF. In all 3 of these cases, the

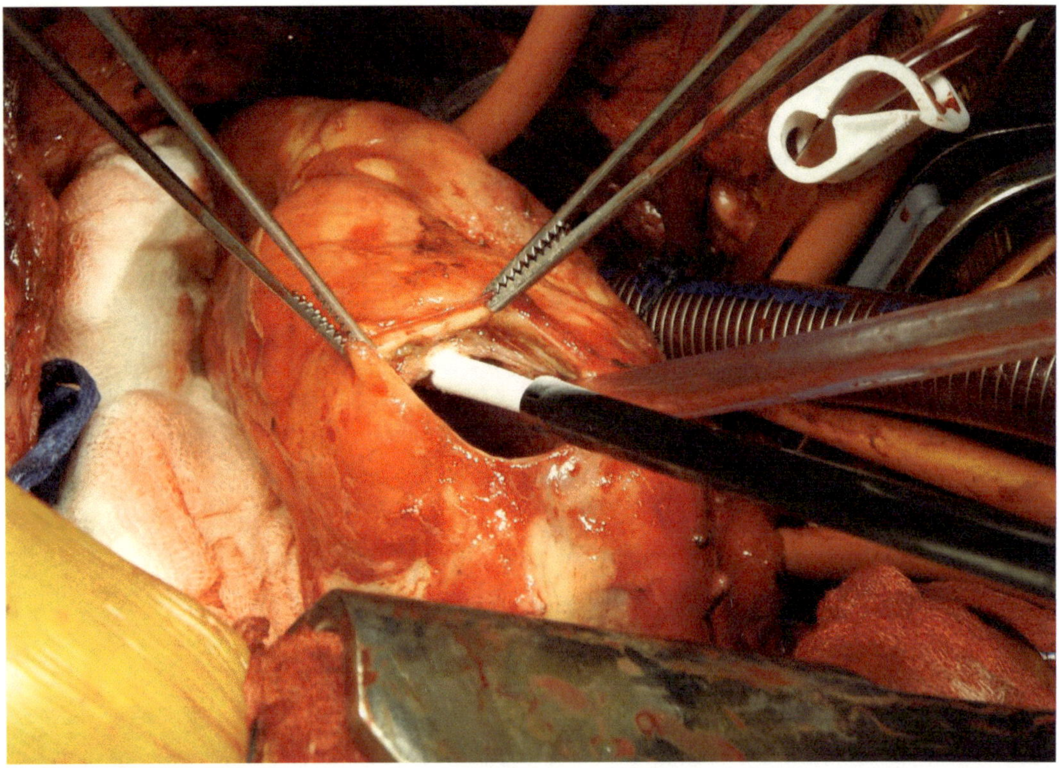

Fig. 6. Endocardial Ablation

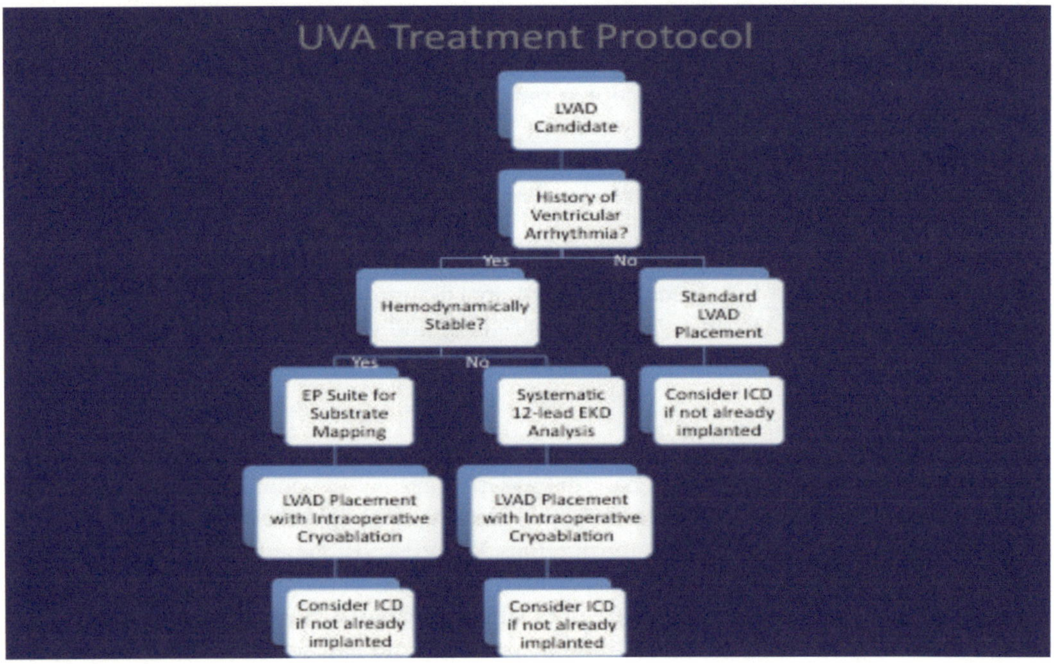

Fig. 7. Treatment Protocol

patients were asymptomatic, the arrhythmias were easily controlled with medical therapy, were not recurrent, and did not require additional intervention. None of the 28 patients required additional catheter-based interventions for arrhythmia control. Prior to instituting this protocol for intra-operative cryoablation, 8 of 23 patients (34.7%) required intervention for recurrent post-operative ventricular tachyarrhythmias. After initiating the protocol 0 of 28 patients required further intervention. It is still too early to know whether and how this procedure has impacted other results; however, it is clear that directed intra-operative cryoablation is useful in decreasing the rates of post-operative ventricular tachyarrhythmias following HeartMate II LVAD implantation.

8. Future direction

The protocol, technique, and results presented above show promise toward the goal of eliminating ventricular tachyarrhythmias following LVAD placement. Admittedly, our experience with this technique is in its infant status and we will develop further refinements as we implant more devices and gain clinical experience managing patients with LVADs and with ventricular tachyarrhythmias. The first question we will have to address is whether to ablate all patients at the time of LVAD implantation, not just those with a prior history of ventricular tachyarrhythmias. Previous studies had demonstrated that the patients who experience problems with post-operative ventricular arrhythmias are not necessarily the same patients with a history of ventricular tachyarrhythmias pre-operatively (Ziv et al., 2005);(Oswald et al., 2010). In the only prospective study to date, Oswald et al. demonstrated that patients with no previous arrhythmia history had an estimated 1-year risk of 24% for appropriate ICD treatment for sustained VT or VF following continuous flow LVAD placement. Other studies have shown similar rates of new ventricular arrhythmias following LVAD placement.

In our experience, although limited, we have not seen any patients with clinically significant VT or VF requiring additional catheter-based therapy in either group. Only time will tell whether this is a sustained finding with our methodology. Notably in the Dor experience, the incidence of post-operative ventricular arrhythmias is less than 2% (Dor et al., 1994). Similar to our approach to cryoablation, in the Dor procedure for ventricular reconstruction for ischemic heart failure, only those patients who have a history of previous sustained VT or VF undergo cryoablation of the border zone surrounding the resected myocardium. In 1994, Dor and colleagues reported on 287 who patients underwent programmed ventricular stimulation prior to subtotal endocardiectomy with surgical ventricular reconstruction. 106 patients were found to have inducible (57) or spontaneous (49) ventricular tachycardia pre-operatively; however, ventricular tachycardia was no longer inducible in 92% of patients after operation and only two patients had spontaneous ventricular tachycardia after the operation (Dor et al., 1994). Subsequent studies have replicated this result (Sartipy et al., 2005). It is unclear exactly why the Dor procedure is so successful in limiting the prevalence of post-operative arrhythmias. Logic suggest that the reconstructed ventricle experiences less wall stress and with that, the neurohormonal, mechanical, and hemodynamic conditions which predispose to arrhythmia generation are eliminated. In addition, cryoablation destroys the border-zone ischemic tissue where monomorphic VT may be generated. If this is the case for the Dor procedure, our approach to HeartMate II LVAD implantation with cryoablation may replicate the same results.

Regardless of whether these results bear out over the long term, this chapter should demonstrate that the management and treatment of ventricular arrhythmias in the LVAD population will be an important topic for the heart failure specialist, electrophysiologist, and cardiac surgeon to understand over the coming decades. Destination therapy is here to stay. With over half a million Americans suffering from heart failure, and over 100,000 in NYHA class IIIb or IV heart failure, the pool of patients who may benefit from ventricular assists devices is large. In addition, with over 550,000 people newly diagnosed with heart failure each year and an aging population, all of these numbers stand to expand over the coming years. The benefit of LVAD implantation is clear with large trials now showing two-year HeartMate II survival rates of almost 60% in a population which only ten years ago had a survival rate of 8% with optimal medical therapy (Slaughter et al., 2009);(Rose et al., 2001). With third-generation non-contact bearing devices now approved in Europe and on the horizon in the U.S., LVAD survival and quality of life may soon eclipse the gold standard for heart failure treatment: heart transplant. In order for this to happen, issues such as post-operative ventricular arrhythmias need to be worked out. We believe that following our approach will significantly limit the prevalence of post-operative ventricular tachyarrhythmias, but the nuances of patient selection and procedure performance have room for development. Only with multi-institutional prospective trials will the true answers be known: who to treat, how to map, and where and how to ablate. We hope definitive answers will be known soon and that ventricular arrhythmias in patients with ventricular assist devices will become only a historical footnote. Until then, we push on.

9. References

Aaronson KD, Eppinger MJ, Dyke DB, Wright S, Pagani FD. Left ventricular assist device therapy improves utilization of donor hearts. *J Am Coll Cardiol* 2002;39:1247–1254.

Aliot EM, Stevenson WG, Almendral-Garrote JM, Bogun F, Calkins CH, Delacretaz E, Bella PD, Hindricks G, Jaïs P, Josephson ME, Kautzner J, Kay GN, Kuck KH, Lerman BB, Marchlinski F, Reddy V, Schalij MJ, Schilling R, Soejima K, Wilber D; European Heart Rhythm Association; European Society of Cardiology; Heart Rhythm Society. "EHRA/HRS Expert Consensus on Catheter Ablation of Ventricular Arrhythmias: developed in a partnership with the European Heart Rhythm Association (EHRA), a Registered Branch of the European Society of Cardiology (ESC), and the Heart Rhythm Society (HRS); in collaboration with the American College of Cardiology (ACC) and the American Heart Association (AHA)." *Europace.* 2009 Jun;11(6):771-817.

American Heart Association. Heart Disease and Stroke Facts, 2006 Update. Dallas, Texas; AHA, 2006.

Andersen M, Videbaek R, Boesgaard S, Sander K, Hansen PB, Gustafsson F. Incidence of ventricular arrhythmias in patients on long-term support with a continuous-flow assist device (HeartMate II). *J Heart Lung Transplant* 2009;28:733–735.

Arai H, Swartz MT, Penninton DG, et al. Importance of ventricular arrhythmias in bridge patients with ventricular assist devices. *ASAIO Trans* 1991;37:M427–8.

Bedi M, Kormos R,Winowich S, McNamara DM, Mathier MA, Murali S. Ventricular arrhythmias during left ventricular assist device support. *Am J Cardiol* 2007;99:1151–1153.

Boineau JP, Cox JL: Slow ventricular activation in acute myocardial infarction. A source of re-entrant premature ventricular contractions. *Circulation* 1973;48:702.

Chaudhary KW, Rossman EI, Piacentino V 3rd, Kenessey A, Weber C, Gaughan JP, Ojamaa K, Klein I, Bers DM, Houser SR, Margulies KB. Altered myocardial Ca2+ cycling after left ventricular assist device support in the failing human heart. *J Am Coll Cardiol* 2004;44:837–845.

Chaudhary KW, Rossman EI, Piacentino V 3rd, Kenessey A, Weber C, Gaughan JP, Ojamaa K, Klein I, Bers DM, Houser SR, Margulies KB. Altered myocardial Ca2+ cycling after left ventricular assist device support in the failing human heart. *J Am Coll Cardiol* 2004;44:837–845.

Cox JL. Cardiac Surgery for Arrhythmias. *J Cardiovasc Electrophysiol* 2004; 15:250-262.

Damiano JR, Tripp HF, Small KW, Asano T, Jones RH, Lowe JE. The functional consequences of prolonged supraventricular tachycardia. *J Am Coll Cardiol* 1985;5:541–547.

Doenst T, Faerber G, Grandina S, Kuntze T, Menicanti L, Border MA, Mohr FW. Surgical Therapy of Ventricular Arrhythmias. *Herzchr Elektrophys* 2007; 18:62-67

Dor V, Saab M, Coste P, Kornaszewska M, Montiglio F. Left ventricular aneurysm: a new surgical approach. *Thorac Cardiovasc Surg*. 1989 Feb; 37(1): 11-19

Dor V, Sabatier M, Montiglio F, Rossi P, Toso A, Di Donato M. Results of nonguided subtotal endocardiectomy associated with left ventricular reconstruction in patients with ischemic ventricular arrhythmias. *J Thorac Cardiovasc Surg* 1994; 107:1301- 8.

El-Banayosy A, Arusoglu L, Kizner L, et al. Novacor left ventricular assist system versus HeartMate vented electric left ventricular assist system as a long-term mechanical circulatory support device in bridging patients: a prospective study. *J Thorac Cardiovasc Surg*. 2000; 119:581–587.

Frazier OH, Rose EA, Oz MC, et al. Multicenter clinical evaluation of the HeartMate vented electric left ventricular assist system in patients awaiting heart transplantation. *J Thorac Cardiovasc Surg*. 2001;122:1186–1195.

Frazier OH. Advanced heart failure treated with continuous-flow left ventricular assist device. *N Engl J Med* 2009;361:2241–2251.

Grzywacz FW, Piacentino V 3rd, Marble J, Bozorgnia B, Gaughan JP, Rothman SA, Margulies KB. Effect of acute unloading via head-up tilt on QTc prolongation in patients with ischemic or non-ischemic cardiomyopathy. *Am J Cardiol* 2006;97:412-415.

Guido J, Bues Genis A, Dominquez de Rozas JM, Fiol M, Vinolas X, Bayes de Luna A. Sudden Death in Heart Failure. *Heart Failure Reviews* 1997;1:249-260

Han J, Gael BG, Hansen CS: Re-entrant beats induced in the ventricle during coronary occlusion. *Am Heart J* 1970;80:778.

Harding JD, Piacentino V 3rd, Gaughan JP, Houser SR, Margulies KB. Electrophysiologica alterations after mechanical circulatory support in patients with advanced cardiac failure. *Circulation* 2001;104:1241–1247.

Harding JD, Piacentino V 3rd, Rothman S, Chambers S, Jessup M, Margulies KB. Prolonged repolarization after ventricular assist device support is associated with arrhythmias in humans with congestive heart failure. *J Card Fail* 2005;11:227–232.

Hawkins NM, Petrie MC, Burgess MI, McMurray JJ. Selecting patients for cardiac resynchronization therapy. *J Am Coll Cardiol* 2009;53:1944-1959.

Jauhar S, M.D., Ph.D. "The Artificial Heart." *New England Journal of Medicine* (2004): 542-544.

Jones RH, Velazquez EJ, Michler RE, et al. Coronary bypass surgery with or without surgical ventricular reconstruction. *N Engl J Med* 2009;390:1709-1717.

Josephson ME, Harken AH, Horowitz LN: Endocardial excision: A new surgical technique for the treatment of recurrent ventricular tachycardia. *Circulation* 1979;60:1430.

Kaiser GA,Waldo AL, Harris PD, Bowman FO Jr, Hoffman BF, Malm JR: New method to delineate myocardial damage at surgery. *Circulation* 1969;39(Suppl 1):83.

Koilpillai C, Quinones MA, Greenberg B, et al. Relation of ventricular size and function to heart failure status and ventricular dysrhythmia in patients with severe left ventricular dysfunction. *Am J Cardiol* 1996; 77:606 –11.

Kokolis S.; Clark L.; Kokolis, R.; Kassotis, J. (2006). Ventricular Arrhythmias and Sudden Cardiac Death. *Progress in Cardiovascular Diseases*, Vol. 48, No. 6, (May/June 2006) pp 426-444.

Lall SC, Damiano RJ. Surgical Ablation Devices for Atrial Fibrillation. *J Interv Card Electrophysiology* 2007; 20:73-82.

Mahapatra S, Tucker-Schwartz J, Wiggins D, Gillies GT, Mason PK, McDaniel G, Lapar DJ, Stemland C, Sosa E, Ferguson JD, Bunch TJ, Ailawadi G, Scanavacca M. Pressure frequency characteristics of the pericardial space and thorax during subxiphoid access for epicardial ventricular tachycardia ablation. *Heart Rhythm.* 2010 May;7(5):604-9.

Mann DL, Acker MA, Jessup M, et al. Clinical evaluation of the CorCap Cardiac Support Device in patients with dilated cardiomyopathy. *Ann Thorac Surg* 2007;84:1226-1235.

McMurray JJ, Pfeffer MA. Heart Failure. *Lancet* 2005; 365: 1877-89.

Miller LW, Pagani FD, Russell SD, et al. Use of a continuous-flow device in patients awaiting heart transplantation. *N Engl J Med.* 2007;357:885- 896.

Myerburg RJ, Interian A Jr, Mitrani RM, Kessler KM, Castellanos A. Frequency of Sudden Cardiac Death and Profiles of Risk. *Am J Cardiol.* Sept, 1997.

Nguyen D, Thourani V. Third-Generation Continuous Flow Left Ventricular Assist Devices. *Innovations* 2010; Vol. 5, No. 4 (July/August 2010) pp 250-258.

O'Connell J, HeartMate II: A Reliable Destination. *American Heart Association: Heart Failure Clinical Updates.* March, 2009.

O'Rourke RA. Role of myocardial revascularization in sudden cardiac death. *Circulation* 1992; 85(Suppl 1):I112–7

Oswald H, Klein G, Struber M, Gardiwal A. Implantable defibrillator with left ventricular assist device compatibility. *Interact Cardiovasc Thorac Surg* 2009;8:579–580.

Oz MC, Rose EA, Slater J, Kuiper JJ, Catanese KA, Levin HR. Malignant ventricular arrhythmias are well tolerated in patients receiving long-term left ventricular assist devices. *J Am Coll Cardiol* 1994;24:1688 -91.

Oz MC, Rose EA, Slater J, Kuiper JJ, Catanese KA, Levin HR. Malignant ventricular arrhythmias are well tolerated in patients receiving long-term left ventricular assist devices. *J Am Coll Cardiol* 1994;24:1688–1691.

Refaat M, Chemaly E, Lebeche D, Gwathmey JK, Hajjar RJ. Ventricular arrhythmias after left ventricular assist device implantation. *Pacing Clin Electrophysiol* 2008;31:1246–1252.

Rodrigue-Way A, Burkhoff D, Geesaman BJ, Golden S, Xu J, Pollman MJ, Donoghue M, Jeyaseelan R, Houser S, Breitbart RE, Marks A, Acton S. Sarcomericgenes involved in reverse remodeling of the heart during left ventricular assist device support. *J Heart Lung Transplant* 2005;24:73–80.

Roger VL, Weston SA, Redfield MM et al. Trends in heart failure incidence and survival in a community-based population. *JAMA*, 2004; 292: 344-350.

Rose EA, Gelijns AC, Moskowitz AJ, Heitjan DF, Stevenson LW, Dembitsky W, Long JW, Ascheim DD, Tierney AR, Levitan RG, Watson JT, Meier P, Ronan NS, Shapiro PA, Lazar RM, Miller LW, Gupta L, Frazier OH, Desvigne-Nickens P, Oz MC, Poirier VL. Long-term mechanical left ventricular assistance for end-stage heart failure. *N Engl J Med 2001;*345:1435–1443.

Sacher F MP, Nault I, Wright M, Lellouche N, Derval N, Pioux S, Hocini M, Bordachar P, Deplange A, RitterP, Clementy J, Haissguerre M, Jais P. Prevelance of epicardial scar in patients referred for ventricular tachycardia ablation. *Heart Rhythm.* 2009;6:S175

Sartipy U, Albåge A, Lindblom D. The Dor procedure for left ventricular reconstruction. Ten-year clinical experience. *Eur J Cardiothorac Surg*. 2005 June;27(6); 1005-10.

Singh BN, D.Phil, Significance and Control of Cardiac Arrhythmias in Patients with Congestive Cardiac Failure. *Heart Failure Reviews* 2002;7:285-300.

Skinner JL, Bourge RC, Shepard RB, Epstein AE, Holman WL. Simultaneous use of an implanted defibrillator and ventricular assist device. *Ann Thorac Surg* 1997;64:1156–1158.

Slaughter MS, Rogers JG, Milano CA, Russell SD, Conte JV, Feldman D, Sun B, Tatooles AJ, Delgado RM 3rd, Long JW, Wozniak TC, Ghumman W, Farrar DJ. Advanced heart failure treated with continuous-flow left ventricular assist device. *N Engl J Med.* 2009; 361:2241–2251.

Stevenson WG, Kyoko S. Catheter Ablation for Ventricular Tacchycardia. *Circulation* 2007; 115:2750-2760.

Taylor DO, Stehlik J, Edwards LB, et al. Registry of the international society for heart and lung transplantation: twenty-sixth official adult heart transplant report-2009. *J Heart Lung Transplant* 2009;28:1007-1022.

Vollkron M, Voitl P, Ta J, Wieselthaler G, Schima H. Suction Events During Left Ventricular Support and Ventricular Arrhythmias. *J Heart Lung Transplant* 2007;26:819-25

Westaby S, Frazier OH, Banning A. Six years of continuous mechanical circulatory support. *N Engl J Med.* 2006;355:325–327.

Wetstein L, Mark R, Kaplan A. Nonarrhythmogenicity of therapeutic cryothermic lesions of the myocardium. *Journal of Surgical Research* 1985; 39: 543-554

Ziv O, Dizon J, Thosani A, Naka Y, Magnano AR, Garan H. Effects of left ventricular assist device therapy on ventricular arrhythmias. *J Am Coll Cardiol* 2005;45:1428–1434.

9

Ventricular Assist Device-Specific Infections

Sunil Pauwaa, MD and Geetha Bhat, PhD, MD
Center for Heart Transplant and Assist Devices
Advocate Christ Medical Center
United States of America

1. Introduction

Ventricular assist devices (VADs) have been shown to offer a significant survival benefit over medical therapy in patients with advanced heart failure. Despite significant advances in device technology and surgical technique, VAD-specific infections still remain among the most common causes of morbidity and mortality in patients with VADs. VAD-specific infections may involve the driveline exit site, the VAD pocket, or the device pump/cannula. The incidence of infection after VAD implantation depends on the type of device implanted, the location of the device, pre-operative patient characteristics, and post-operative driveline/device management. This chapter provides a summary of the various characteristics that may contribute to a patient's risk of VAD-specific infection and describes pre-, peri-, and postoperative management to aid in limiting the risk of VAD-specific infection. The chapter also includes definitions of the various types of VAD-specific infections and outlines a general guideline for the treatment of these different infections. This guide builds upon current literature available on VAD-specific infection (Chinn et al., 2005; Slaughter et al., 2010).

2. Definition and types of VAD infection

In 2010 the International Society for Heart and Lung Transplantation (ISHLT) drafted an expert opinion paper regarding the standardization of definitions of infection in patients with VADs (ISHLT, 2010). This document outlines a classification system to organize and delineate different types of VAD-related infections. The first level of classification calls for the differentiation of VAD-*specific* infections, VAD-*related* infections, and Non VAD-related infections. The VAD-specific infection category contains three distinct subcategories of infection, percutaneous driveline infections, pocket infections, and pump and/or cannula infections.

VAD-related infections refer to infections not directly involving the VAD itself but possibly occurring as a result of VAD placement. These include infective endocarditis (IE), bloodstream infections (BSIs) and mediastinitis. Further details regarding these infections can be found in the ISHLT document.

2.1 Types of VAD-specific infection

2.1.1 Driveline infection

Infection of the percutaneous driveline can be divided into three clinical situations, minor exit site erythema, superficial infection or cellulitis, and deep infection.

Minor erythema is defined as involving only the superficial layer of skin and should involve an area of less than 2cm radius around the margin of the incision/exit site. The patient should have no evidence of purulent discharge coming from the exit site and should not have any systemic symptoms or increase in temperature around the driveline site. Erythema at the exit site may represent irritation from mobility of the driveline or it could signal the early stages of cellulitis.

A superficial infection involves tissues superficial to the fascia and muscle layers of the incision. The patient should have either purulent drainage from the incision site or cellulitis spreading from around the exit site in a greater than 1cm radius from the margin of incision with erythema and increased local temperature. Fever, drainage, warmth, tenderness at the site, and leukocytosis would all suggest cellulitis over minor erythema.

Deep infection of the driveline involves the deep soft issues such as the fascial and muscle layers of the incision. The patient should have purulent discharge from the site, spontaneous dehiscence along the driveline, and/or an abscess or other evidence of infection involving the deep incision.

Defining the characteristics of any particular percutaneous driveline infection is crucial as each clinical situation demands a different therapeutic strategy.

2.1.2 Pocket Infection

In VADS where the device is kept inside the body cavity, pocket infections refer to infections that occur in the space that holds the pump device. In most cases the pocket is either intra-abdominal or intra-thoracic. In order to diagnose a pocket infection there must either be positive cultures obtained from the pocket space, either surgically or by needle sampling, or radiographic evidence of infection in the pocket area. There should also be systemic signs of infection including fever, nausea, vomiting, or pain at the site of the pocket.

According to the ISHLT document on infections in VAD patients pocket infections must meet at least one of the following criteria: 1) The patient must have organisms cultured from the pocket space obtained during a surgical operation or needle sampling, 2) Isolation of indistinguishable organisms from either 2 exterior aspects of the VAD, or 1 exterior aspect and one pocket space culture, 3) Abscess or other evidence of infection seen in the pocket during a surgical operation or histopathologic examination, or 4) At least two of the following signs or symptoms with no other recognized cause: fever, nausea, vomiting, pain in the pocket area, or jaundice <u>and</u> organisms seen or cultured from aspirated fluid or pocket area. (ISHLT, 2010)

2.1.3 Pump and/or Cannula infections

The portion of the VAD referred to as the 'pump' is the part of the device involved in the propulsion of blood and includes both continuous and/or pulsatile flow devices either intra- or para-corporeal. The cannula is the part of the VAD connecting the pump device to the patient's cardiovascular system. According to the ISHLT, a pump and/or cannula infection may either be diagnosed by microbiological, histopathological, or clinical criteria. Although some of these require exploration or explantation of the device itself, a diagnostic criterion based on the modified Duke's criteria has been used to clinically diagnose pump and/or cannula infection.

If the VAD is not actively explanted, a set of criteria adapted from the modified Duke's criteria have been formulated to diagnose pump and/or cannula infection. Within this system a clinical diagnosis requires either 2 major criteria, 1 major and 3 minor criteria, or 4 minor criteria. Major criteria include 1) The recovery of an indistinguishable organism recovered from 2 or more sets of peripheral blood cultures obtained over a 4-week period, with no other focus of infection, 2) Blood cultures from a central venous catheter (CVC) turning positive ≤2 hours after blood cultures drawn from peripheral blood, and 3) positive echocardiogram showing oscillating mass that is adherent to the VAD. Minor criteria include 1) Fever ≥ 38°Celsius, 2) Vascular phenomena such as major arterial emboli, septic pulmonary infarcts, mycotic aneurysm, intracranial hemorrhage, conjunctival hemorrhage, or Janeway's lesions, 3) Immunological phenomena such as glomerulonephritis, Osler's nodes, or Roth spots, or 4) Microbiological evidence such as positive blood cultures that do not meet criteria as noted above.

3. Epidemiology of VAD-specific infection

Infection is a relatively common complication after mechanical circulatory support (MCS). The exact incidence of infection in mechanical device patients has varied over time mostly due to a lack of uniformity in the definition of VAD-specific infection. In 2003, Holman et al. published an article reviewing the prevalence/incidence of VAD infection in 15 prior studies from 1998 to 2001 (Holman et al., 2003). The prevalence of infection in this series ranged from 21% to 89% depending on the type of infection and the VAD used. The original REMATCH study from 2001 demonstrated an incidence of 0.6 infectious events per patient year with sepsis accounting for 41% of deaths in the mechanical support arm (Rose et al.,2001). The follow-up 2007 HeartMate II bridge-to-transplant pivotal trial demonstrated that 14% of the 133 study patients developed percutaneous lead infections however a total of 20% of the total population developed sepsis (Miller et al., 2007). In the 2009 HeartMate II destination therapy pivotal trial, 35% of patients undergoing HeartMate II continuous flow left ventricular assist device (LVAD) implantation developed LVAD-related infections versus 36% in the pulsatile HeartMate XVE group (Slaughter et al. 2009). The incidence of LVAD-related infection in these two groups was .48 infectious events per patient year in the continuous flow group versus .90 infectious events per patient year in the pulsatile flow group.

Although there is some variation among incidence and prevalence of infection depending on the type of infection and the type of mechanical circulatory support being employed it is clear that infection is a major cause of morbidity and mortality in patients supported by MCS. In a recent series reviewing 81 patients receiving continuous-flow LVADs, patients who had an infection on VAD had a significantly prolonged hospital stay with a trend toward increased mortality in comparison with patients who did not have infection (Topkara et al., 2010). Sepsis has also been shown to significantly decrease survival in VAD patients with both continuous and pulsatile-flow devices (Topkara et al., 2010; Holman et al., 2004). Prevention, diagnosis and treatment of these infections is therefore paramount in proper VAD management.

4. Common organisms

While VAD infection could theoretically involve any organism there are particular organisms that are more common than others. Bio-film producing organisms, especially gram positive bacteria and fungi such as staphylococcus species (sp.) and candida are among the most common organisms causing VAD-specific infections. Gram negative bacteria such as pseudomonas and enterococcus are also bio-film producing organisms commonly implicated in VAD-specific infection (Holman et al., 2003). Pre-operative prophylactic antibiotics are therefore tailored against these organisms. Likewise, empiric therapy for VAD patients presenting with fever or other signs or symptoms of infection usually include antimicrobial therapy directed against these organisms.

5. Pre-operative considerations

Prevention of VAD-specific infection begins even before surgical implantation of the device. To this end, patient selection plays an important role in successful surgical outcomes. At the center of this issue is the immune status of the patient. While it is well accepted that heart failure itself causes some amount of immunodeficiency, one must ensure that a VAD candidate's immune status is not so compromised as to negatively affect outcome after VAD. Although VAD implantation has been carried out even in a patient with human immunodeficiency virus, immunodeficiency could increase risk of infection after surgery (Fieno et al, 2009). Patients on immunosuppression for comorbid conditions (i.e. rheumatology or transplant patients) should also be thoroughly evaluated prior to proceeding for VAD. Comorbid conditions that may themselves alter a patient's immune status such as hyperglycemia in diabetes should also be optimized prior to surgery. Nutritional status also contributes to a patient's overall immune status and a thorough nutritional evaluation should be undertaken in any patient being considered for VAD.

In addition to intrinsic patient characteristics, a thorough evaluation for active or occult infection should also be undertaken in every candidate. Any elevation in the white blood cell (WBC) count should be investigated and possibly treated pre-operatively. Any known active infection should also be treated to completion to ensure a sterile surgical implantation and to prevent hematogenous seeding of the device by any active infection. Dental hygiene should be evaluated by an oral surgeon/dentist and x-rays of the teeth should be obtained to rule out occult dental infections. Each patient should be screened for decubitus ulcers as these may also be a source of infection. Immediately prior to surgery, central venous catheters (CVCs), urinary catheters, peripherally inserted central catheters (PICC lines) and any other non-implanted devices should be removed and if necessary replaced peri-operatively.

From a provider standpoint, CVC implantation peri-operatively should be carried out in sterile fashion according to the general principles for prevention of catheter-specific bloodstream infection (CRBSI) from the Centers for Disease Control and Prevention (CDC) (O'Grady et al., 2002).

6. Preoperative management

The night before surgery the patient should be bathed in an antiseptic agent such as chlorhexidine. Pre- and perioperative prophylactic antibiotic strategies are commonly employed in cardiovascular surgery as well as surgeries involving implantation of hardware (i.e. orthopedic surgery) (Raymond et al., 2002; Martorell et al., 2004). While there is no VAD-specific data that clearly favors a particular perioperative antibiotic strategy, data from the cardiovascular and orthopedic literature has been extrapolated to guide therapy during VAD implantation.

The primary pathogens of concern are gram-positive organisms, specifically staphylococcal sp. since this is the most common group of organisms causing device infections (Holman et al., 2003). Vancomycin, 15mg/kg, intravenously (IV) 1 hour preoperatively, then every 12 hours for 48 hours along with Rifampin, 600mg IV 1-2 hours preoperatively, then daily for 48 hours, is usually an acceptable strategy for perioperative antibiotic coverage. Some studies have also suggested that nasal colonization by staphylococcus aureus (S. aureus) may predict S. aureus bacteremia and surgical site infection after cardiac surgery and that treatment of this colonization might actually help prevent infection (Raymond et al., 2002; Martorell et al., 2004). The evidence to support this strategy is not entirely confirmatory however for those with a nasal culture positive for S. aureus preoperatively, it may be beneficial to treat with mupirocin 2% nasal ointment the evening before surgery and then twice daily for 5 days afterward.(Perl et al., 2003;Bratzler et al., 2004).

Gram negative coverage should be tailored to the patient and/or the institutional patterns of colonization and susceptibility. There is no definitive recommended agent for prophylaxis against gram negative organisms, however at some centers fluoroquinolones such as ciprofloxacin are also used peri-operatively. Although doses should be adjusted for renal clearance, Ciprofloxacin 400mg IV before surgery and every 12 hours for 48 hours after surgery is a generally acceptable strategy.

Another virulent infection that may cause significant device related infection are fungal organisms (Bagdasarian et al., 2009). Fungal VAD infections are associated with high morbidity and mortality and prophylactic agents should be employed to prevent their development. The most commonly employed agent is Fluconazole, 400mg IV preoperatively, then every 24 hours for 48 hours afterward.

The use of prophylactic antibiotics beyond 48 hours after surgery does not seem to be beneficial and may actually be harmful in that it may increase antimicrobial resistance patterns. The practice of continuing prophylactic antibiotics beyond 48 hours is therefore not recommended.

7. Intraoperative management

An elevated level of precaution in the operating room (OR) can also help prevent VAD-related infection. As with any sterile procedure proper hand and arm washing with an antimicrobial agent for a minimum of 3 minutes is essential (Mangram et al., 1999). Caps, masks, gloves, and sterile gowns should be worn by all OR staff and OR traffic should be limited. The patient should be prepared using a solution of broad spectrum antimicrobials, alcohol and iodophor such as DuraPrep (3M Corporation) and sterile drapes. The device itself should also be opened under sterile conditions and only immediately before use.

7.1 The Percutaneous Driveline/Tube

The percutaneous driveline/tubing is among the most important channels for infection with VADs. Proper tunneling and positioning are therefore imperative for infection prevention.

When positioning the percutaneous driveline one should consider body habitus, angle between costal margins, and thickness of subcutaneous tissue. The driveline should begin at the VAD and tunnel to the right upper quadrant where it should exit near the midclavicular line, 4-6cm below the costal margin. The distance between the exit site and pump pocket should be maximized so as to prevent the transmission of infection from the exit site to the pocket itself. The length of the percutaneous pathway should be maximized (10-12cm) and should enter the muscle within 4-8cm of the VAD. The velour portion of the percutaneous driveline should not extend more than 1-2cm outside the body (Chinn et al., 2005; Slaughter et al., 2010). Some centers have even begun fully implanting the velour portion however this has not yet been supported with any large-scale studies.

7.2 Hemostasis and drainage

Fluid and blood collections within the patient can potentially become infected and should therefore be avoided. It is often helpful to place bilateral chest tubes and mediastinal or pocket drains to prevent fluid from accumulating. Likewise, patients should be monitored for bleeding post-operatively and potentially re-explored if there is evidence of excessive or persistent fluid or blood output from any of a patient's drains or tubes.

8. Postoperative management

The post-operative period is the most important time for infection prevention with VADs. Prophylactic systemic antibiotics are usually discontinued after 48 hours postoperatively. After discontinuation of post-operative antibiotics prevention of infection depends primarily on proper exit site management and nutritional support.

8.1 Driveline exit site management

The percutaneous driveline exit site should be carefully managed post-operatively in order to prevent the introduction of pathogens. Dressings should be changed starting 24-48 hours after surgery and earlier if the dressing becomes saturated with blood or drainage. Dressings should be changed under sterile conditions using sterile technique with a sterile drape, and sterile gown and gloves as well as cap and mask. Using sterile gloves, the old dressing should be removed and discarded. At this point a new set of sterile gloves should be put on and the exit site should be inspected for signs of infection, tissue breakdown, and drainage. Deep probing should generally be avoided. Any drainage should be swabbed and sent for culture. The wound should then be cleaned with an antiseptic agent such as 1% chlorhexidine and rinsed with 0.9% normal saline solution. The area should then be dried to completion using sterile gauze and then dressed with sterile gauze with enough gauze placed to cover and protect the entire exit site. After completion of all these steps the abdominal binder should be reapplied.

Over time there should be incorporation of the driveline at the site of the exit site with good tissue in-growth around the driveline itself. This may take weeks to months to occur and need not fully occur prior to discharge, however it is imperative that good hygiene and sterile technique be exercised at all times. It is generally advised that patients avoid showering until after adequate tissue in-growth into the velour has occurred and until there is no drainage or signs of infection at the exit site. Even when sponge bathing, the exit site should be kept dry. Ultimately it will be the responsibility of the patient's caregiver to maintain and change driveline dressings therefore, the caregiver should be carefully and thoroughly educated in proper sterile technique and should demonstrate competency in this task prior to discharge.

8.2 Nutrition

Post-operative nutritional status is critical to patient success and is known to influence morbidity and mortality in surgical patients (Holdy et al., 2005). Nutritional supplementation, either oral or parenteral, should be instituted as soon as possible after surgery. Oral or nasogastric supplementation is preferable given the increased risk of infection with parenteral feeding. Supplementation should be done under the supervision of a clinical dietician/nutritional specialist to ensure that the patient receives appropriate protein and caloric intake to ensure proper recovery and wound healing. This will also help prevent infection. Blood sugar control is also imperative post-operatively and endocrine consultation may be of assistance in maintaining a blood sugar as close to 110mg/dl as possible (Van Den Berghe et al. 2001)

9. Diagnosis of VAD-specific infection

VAD-specific infections include infections occurring at the cutaneous exit site, in the device pocket, or infections of the internal surface of the device or valves. VAD specific infections are commenced in many ways: a) inoculation at the time of surgery b) from percutaneous driveline exit site onto the device; or c) hematogenous spread from a blood stream infection. Post-operative VAD infections can result from hematogenous spread from line related blood stream infections or bacteremia from open wound infection, urinary tract infection or pneumonia.

9.1 Driveline Infection

Driveline exit site infections should be diagnosed by thorough physical examination at the driveline exit site. Erythema and poor wound healing can be suggestive of driveline infection. Associated signs of systemic infection such as fever, tachycardia and leukocytosis may or may not be present with driveline exit site infection. In the case of a suspected driveline infection, cultures and gram stain of the driveline exit site should be obtained without deep probing. This may not be always helpful because of skin colonization by variety of microorganisms and may be positive in absence of true infection. Ultrasonography, computed tomography, or localizing abscess scan (gallium, indium) may also be helpful in detecting the driveline infection. Findings suggestive of infection include inflammation or fluid collection along the driveline pathway.

9.2 Pump pocket Infection

Pump pocket infections present with local inflammation and can be associated with signs of sepsis. It may present as a local abscess which can be diagnosed by palpation and by the imaging studies. If the suspicion of abscess is high on imaging, incision and drainage should be performed. Persistent drainage from the driveline exit site can be another presentation of underlying pocket infection. In patients with signs of systemic infection complete blood count and multiple blood cultures should be obtained.

9.3 Device Infection

Intravascular device infections occur during the implantation procedure or by hematogenous spread when a biofilm forming bacteria is introduced onto the external and/or internal surfaces of the device. The most common pathogens causing blood stream infection in patients with VAD related infection are coagulase negative staphylococci, staphylococcus aureus, Candida spp., and gram negative infections like Pseudomonas aeruginosa. Infections with multidrug-resistant pathogens result from prolonged hospitalization and increased antibiotic exposure.

A VAD related blood stream infection is difficult to differentiate from a non-VAD-related blood stream infection. Diagnosis of VAD related blood stream infection is typically made when: 1) the same organism is isolated from drainage around the exit site or obtained through a percutaneous aspiration of a fluid collection; 2) no other source of bacteremia is identified 3) the bacteremia is sustained despite appropriate antibiotic therapy or despite adequate drainage of an identified source. Positive cultures of the device (valves, internal pump surface, pump pocket) in presence of bacteremia is the gold standard but it is rare for patients with permanently implanted VAD to undergo explantation of the device. Clinical manifestations of infected intravascular devices are fever, leukocytosis, new incompetence of the pump inflow or outflow valves, and septic embolization in absence of vegetation on the native cardiac valves. For the diagnosis of device infections, exclude other device infection from pacemakers and automatic implantable cardiac defibrillators and line related infections. Multiple blood cultures from peripheral line and central venous catheter should be obtained in suspected line related infection. Intradevice echocardiography can be very helpful to evaluate device valves and function.

10. Treatment of VAD infection

Prior to initiating treatment for a VAD infection blood cultures, drainage culture, and if possible, aspirates should be obtained in order to identify the offending pathogen. Broad-spectrum antibiotics may be initiated early but therapy should be tailored to the particular organism once speciation and susceptibilities have been completed. Infectious disease consultation should be obtained for antibiotic selection as well as dosing and timing of therapy.

Therapy for VAD-specific infection is based on the type of VAD infection (Driveline, Pocket, or Device) as well as the patient's infection history. A more invasive infection or a history of recurrent or resistant infection may prompt a more aggressive therapeutic approach.

10.1 Driveline infection

Therapy for driveline exit site infections typically begins with oral antibiotics targeted against gram-positive organisms. Blood and drainage cultures should be drawn and evaluated for possible organism identification and susceptibility. If an organism is identified therapy can be targeted toward that organism; if not, empiric therapy directed toward cutaneous flora such as staphylococcus aureus should be initiated. Aggressive wound care is also important. The driveline exit site and dressing should be kept clean and should be immobilized to prevent disruption of the area surrounding the driveline itself.

If the infection appears to be more extensive or invasive, surgical incision and debridement may be necessary. This should be done in the OR under sterile conditions.

Over time, driveline infections have a tendency to become recurrent (Vilchez et al., 2001). In the case of recurrent driveline infections intravenous antibiotics may become necessary. Infectious disease consultation can be helpful to guide such therapy. Ultimately long-term antibiotic therapy may be helpful to suppress and prevent recurrence of infection. The need for this type of therapy must be weighed against the risk of developing resistant organisms and antibiotic side effects (Tayama et al., 2006)

10.2 Pocket Infection

The initial steps in treating a pocket infection are similar to those with a driveline infection. After cultures have been obtained, broad spectrum antibiotics should be initiated with narrowing of therapy once species and susceptibilities have been identified.

If an abscess or fluid collection is identified either on exam or radiologically it should be aggressively drained, either percutaneously or by surgical incision and drainage. Any fluid obtained from a pocket should be sent immediately for culture.

If antibiotics and percutaneous or surgical drainage are unsuccessful and the patient continues to exhibit signs and symptoms of an active infection, a device pocket revision may be necessary. This approach may also be indicated if cultures grow particularly virulent organisms such as gram negative bacilli or yeast.

Another approach to pocket infections that is still under investigation is the implantation of polymethylmethacrylate (PMMA) beads that are impregnated with vancomycin, tobramycin, and possibly other antibiotic agents. These can be surgically placed to coat the external surface of the VAD. These beads are currently approved for use with chronic osteomyelitis and infected orthopedic implants and their use with VADs is still experimental and requires further research as to optimum size, shape, and positioning of the beads. A potential risk of using these beads is that they may breed more resistant organisms (Chinn et al., 2005; Slaughter et al., 2010).

After either percutaneous or surgical incision and drainage, aggressive wound care is critical to successful treatment of an infected VAD pocket. Patients should undergo sterile daily dressing changes and monitoring for signs of continued infection. Antibiotics should be used and patients may be discharged home on intravenous treatment via a PICC line for prolonged antibiotic therapy. This should be done under the supervision of an infectious disease specialist.

Vacuum assisted closure (V.A.C., KCI USA, Inc. San Antonio, TX, USA) of a pocket wound may assist with wound healing after surgical incision and drainage and should be considered (Baradarian et al., 2006).

10.3 Pump and/or Cannula infection

Infection of the actual pump or device cannulae is a very serious complication of VAD therapy. Although difficult to establish a concrete diagnosis there are a number of factors that may make pump or cannulae infection more likely. These are described in more detail in the definition and diagnosis sections of this chapter but include persistent bacteremia or fungemia, especially in the case of gram negative bacilli or yeast. Also suggestive of a pump or cannula infection is the presence of a vegetation or interruption in the flow through the VAD cannulae on echocardiogram. Alterations in pump parameters such as low flow states, spikes in power or in the rotations per minute demonstrated by the VAD may also suggest infection.

If a pump or cannula infection is suspected then device replacement should be considered. The natural history of this type of infection portends a poor prognosis and early rather than late replacement is preferable. If VAD replacement is not an option then aggressive intravenous antibiotic therapy should be pursued and continued for a prolonged period of time. This should be guided by an infectious disease specialist based on the organism involved and the history of the infection. Many patients with persistent pump or cannula infection will ultimately require lifelong oral suppressive therapy.

11. Additional considerations in VAD patients

11.1 Immune function after VAD

Immune function in VAD patients is an area of active research and early studies have shown an alteration in immune function in comparison to heart failure controls. This is an important finding as it suggests that patients with VADs may inherently be at increased risk for infection. Temporary alterations in T-cell function and quantity have been observed early after VAD implantation (Deng et al., 1999; Itescu et al., 2000; Clark et al., 2001; Itescu et al., 2003; Rothenberger et al., 2001; Ankersmit et al., 1999). Cellular immunity has also been shown to remain impaired at 6 months after VAD implantation (Kimball et al., 2008). Among the indices found to be altered at 6 months were a decrease in proliferative response to an immune challenge, a decrease in expression of interleukin 2 and tumor necrosis factor-α, an increase in interleukin 10, and an increased prevalence of suppressive T-regulatory cells. These all suggest a compromise in cellular immunity among long-term VAD recipients secondary to a downregulatory cytokine imbalance and an increase in suppressive T-regulatory cells.

11.2 VAD Infection and transplantation

Given that VADs are commonly used as a bridge to transplantation it is important to understand the effect of VAD-related infections on post-transplant outcomes. A retrospective review from Columbia University in 2009 reported that pre-transplant device-related infection of any kind had no effect on post-transplant 1-year survival rates, but was associated with an increased rate of post-transplant infection. In particular, a driveline infection during VAD support predisposed to infection of the former VAD pocket and driveline site after cardiac transplantation (Schulman et al,. 2009). No other VAD-related infections including pocket infection, wound infection, or sepsis were associated with post-transplant infection.

The primary concern with VAD-related infection in patient's awaiting transplantation is that these infections can have a significant effect on survival to transplantation. For this reason, VAD-related infection can actually be used as a reason to upgrade a patient's priority on the transplant list in order to expedite the course to transplantation.

12. Future implications

VAD implantation represents a major development in the treatment of advanced heart failure. Despite major advances in the size, durability and portability of VADs, infection remains a significant cause of morbidity and mortality after VAD implantation. Improving outcomes in the future will require better infection prevention through developments in device and driveline technology. Among the ultimate goals is total implantability of the VAD which would eliminate the need for a driveline and thereby eliminate one of the most important pathways for infection . The clinical utility baseline study (CUBS) trial from 2007 compared the totally implantable LionHeart to the REMATCH data and demonstrated decreased incidence of infection with the totally implantable device suggesting that total implantability may improve infectious outcomes after VAD (Pae et al., 2007)

13. Conclusion

At the present time infection prevention depends upon thorough pre-operative evaluation and treatment to improve modifiable risk factors such as nutrition, glycemic control, and infectious and immune status. Peri-operatively, attention to sterile technique and appropriate prophylactic antibiotics can help prevent infection around the time of implantation. After surgery, immobilization of the driveline along with sterile driveline wound care and patient education are key to long-term success with VADs.

14. Acknowledgements

We would like to acknowledge the team at the Center for Heart Transplant and Assist Devices at Advocate Christ Medical Center in Oak Lawn, Illinois. This includes our surgeons, Pat Pappas, MD, Antone Tatooles, MD, Michael Bresticker, MD, as well as our VAD/advanced heart failure nurses.

15. References

Ankersmit, HJ, Tugulea, S, Spanier T, Weinberg, AD, Artrip, JH, Burke EM, Flannery, M, Mancini, D, Rose, EA, Edwards, NM, Oz, MC & Itescu, S. (1999). Activation-induced T-cell death and immune dysfunction after implantation of left-ventricular assist device. Lancet. 354, 9178 (Aug 1999), pp. (550-555), ISSN: 0140-6736.

Ankersmit, HJ, Edwards, NM, Schuster, M, John R, Kocher, A, Rose EA, Oz, M & Itescu, S. (1999). Quantitative changes in T cell populations after left ventricular assist device implantation. *Circulation*, 100, Suppl II, (1999), pp. (II-211–II-215), ISSN: 0009-7322.

Bagdasarian NG, Malani AN, Pagani FD & Malani PN. (2009). Fungemia associated with left ventricular assist device support. *J Card Surg*. 24, 6, (Nov-Dec, 2009), pp. (763-5), ISSN: 0886-0440.

Baradarian, S, Stahovich M, Krause S, Adamson, R & Dembitsky, W. (2006). Case series: clinical management of persistent mechanical assist device driveline drainage using vacuum-assisted closure therapy. *ASAIO J*., 52, 3, (May/Jun 2006), pp. (354-356), ISSN: 1058-2916.

Bratzler DW & Houck PM, for the Surgical Infection Prevention Guidelines Writers Workgroup: Oklahoma Foundation for Medical Quality, Oklahoma City, Oklahoma; and Centers for Medicare and Medicaid Services, (2004). Antimicrobial prophylaxis for surgery: An advisory statement from the National Surgical Infection Prevention Project, *Clin Infect Dis*, 38, pp. (1706-1715), ISSN: 1058-4838.

Chinn R., Dembitsky W., Eaton L., Chillcott, S, Stahovich, M, Rasmusson, B & Pagani, F. (2005). Multicenter experience: Prevention and management of left ventricular assist device infections. *ASAIO J*, 51,4, (July/August 2005) pp. (461-470), ISSN: 1058-2916.

Clark, AL, Loebe, M, Potapov, EV, Egerer, K, Knosalla, C, Hetzer, R & Anker, SD. (2001). Ventricular assist device in severe heart failure. Effects on cytokines, complement and body weight. *Eur Heart J*, 22, 24, (March 2001), pp. (2275- 2283), ISSN: 0195-668X.

Deng, MC, Erren, M, Tjan, TD, Tamminga, N, Werntze, B, Zimmermann, P, Weyand, M, Schmidt, C & Scheld, HH. (1999). Left ventricular assist system support is associated with persistent inflammation and temporary immunosuppression. *Thorac Cardiovasc Surg*, 47, Suppl 2, (Feb 1999), pp. (326-331), ISSN: 1341-1098.

Fieno, DS, Czer, LS, Schwarz, ER & Simsir S. (2009). Left ventricular assist device placement in a patient with end-stage heart failure and human immunodeficiency virus. *Interact Cardiovasc Thorac Surg*. 9, 5, (Nov 2009), pp. (919-920), ISSN: 1569-9293.

Holdy, K, Dembitsky, W, Eaton, LL, Chillcott, S, Stahovich, M, Rasmusson & Pagani F. (2005). Nutrition assessment and management of left ventricular assist device patients, *J Heart Lung Transplant*, 24, 10, (Oct 2005), pp. 1690-1696, ISSN: 1053-2498.

Holman, WL, Park, SJ, Long, JW, Weinberg, A, Gupta, L, Tierney, AR, Adamson, RM, Watson, JD, Raines, EP, Couper, GS, Pagani, FD, Burton, NA, Miller, LW & Naka, Y for the REMATCH Investigators. (2004). Infection in permanent circulatory support: experience from the REMATCH Trial. *J Heart Lung Transplant*, 23, 12, (Dec 2004), pp. (1359-1365), ISSN: 1053-2498.

Holman, WL, Rayburn, BK, McGiffin, DC, Foley, BA, Benza RL, Bourge, RC, Pinderski, LJ & Kirklin, JK. (2003). Infection in ventricular assist devices: prevention and treatment. *Ann Thorac Surg* 75, Suppl 6, (June 2003), pp. (S48-S57), ISSN: 0003-4975.

ISHLT Working Group, A 2010 Working Formulation For The Standardization Of Definitions Of Infections In Patients Using Ventricular Assist Devices (Vads). *J Heart Lung Transplant* in press.

Itescu S, John R. (2003) Interactions between the recipient immune system and the left ventricular assist device surface: immunological and clinical implications. *Ann Thorac Surg* 75, Suppl 6, (June 2003) pp. (S58–S65). ISSN: 0003-4975.

Itescu, S, Ankersmit, JH, Kocher, AA & Schuster, MD. (2000). Immunobiology of left ventricular assist devices. *Prog Cardiovasc Dis* 43, 1, (Jul-Aug 2000), pp. (67– 80), ISSN: 0033-0620.

Kimball, PM, Flattery, M, McDougan, F & Kasirajan, V. (2008). Cellular immunity impaired among patients on left ventricular assist device for 6 months. *Ann Thorac Surg*, 85, 5, (May 2008), pp. 1656-1661, ISSN: 0003-4975.

Mangram, AJ, Horan, TC, Pearson, ML, Silver, LC & Jarvis, WR. (1999). Guideline for prevention of surgical site infection, 1999. Hospital Infection Control Practices Advisory Committee. *Infect Control Hosp Epidemiol* 20, 4, (Apr 1999), pp. (250-280), ISSN: 0899-823X.

Martorell, C, Engelman, R, Corl, A & Brown, RB. (2004). Surgical site infections in cardiac surgery: An 11-year perspective. *Am J Infect Control* 32, 2, (Apr 2004), pp. (63-68), ISSN: 0196-6553.

Miller, LW, Pagani, FD, Russell, SD, John, R, Boyle, AJ, Aaronson, KD, Cont, JV, Naka, Y, Mancini, D, Delgado, RM, MacGillivray, TE, Farrar, DJ, Frazier, OH; HeartMate II Clinical Investigators. (2007). Use of a continuous-flow device in patients awaiting heart transplantation. *N Engl J Med*, 357, 9, (Aug 2007), pp. (885-896), ISSN: 0028-4793.

O'Grady, NP, Alexander, M, Dellinger, EP, Gerberding, JL, Heard, SO, Maki, DG, Masur, H, McCormick, RD, Mermel, LA, Pearson, ML, Raad II, Radolph, A & Weinstein, RA. (2002). Guidelines for the prevention of intravascular catheter-related infections. Centers for Disease Control and Prevention. (2002). *MMWR Recomm Rep*, 51, RR-10, (Aug 2002), pp. (1-29), ISSN: 1057-5987.

Pae , WE, Connell, JM, Adelowo, A, Boehmer, JP, Korfer, R, El-Banayosy, A, Hetzer, R, Vigano, M, Pavie, A; Clinical Utility Baseline Study (CUBS) Group. (2007). Does total implantability reduce infection with the use of a left ventricular assist device?

The LionHeart Experience in Europe. (2007). *J Heart Lung Transplant* 26, 3, (Mar 2007), pp.(219-229), ISSN: 1053-2498.

Perl, TM. (2003). Prevention of sstaphylococcus aureus infections among surgical patients: Beyond traditional perioperative prophylaxis. *Surgery*, 134, Suppl 5, (Nov 2003), pp. (S10-S17), ISSN: 0039-6060.

Raymond, DP, Kuehnert, MJ & Sawyer, RG. (2002). Preventing antimicrobial-resistant bacterial infections in surgical patients. *Surg Infect (Larchmt)*, 3, 4, (Winter 2002) pp. (375-385), ISSN: 1096-2964.

Rose, EA, Gelijns, AC, Moskowitz, AJ, Heitjan, DF, Stevenson, LW, Dembitsky, W, Long, JW, Ascheim, DD, Tierney, AR, Levitan, RG, Watson, JT, Meier, P, Ronan, NS, Shapiro, PA, Lazar, RM, Miller, LW, Gupta, L, Frazier, OH, Desvigne-Nickens, P, Oz & MC, Poirier, VL; Randomized Evaluation of mechanical Assistance for the Treatment of Congestive Heart Failure (REMATCH) Study Group. (2001). Long-term use of a left ventricular assist device for end-stage heart failure. *N Engl J Med* 345, 20, (Nov 2001), pp. (1435-1443), ISSN: 0028-4793.

Rothenburger, M, Wilhelm, M, Hammel, D, Schmid, C, Plenz, G, Tijan, TD, Baba, H, Schluter, B, Scheld, HH & Deng, MC. Immune response in the early postoperative period after implantation of a left-ventricular assist device system. *Transplant Proc* 33, 1-2, (Feb-Mar, 2001) pp. (1955–1957), ISSN: 0041-1345.

Schulman, AR, Martens, TP, Russo MJ, Christos, PJ, Gordon, RJ, Lowy, FD, Oz, MC & Naka, Y. (2009) Effect of left ventricular assist device infection on post-transplant outcomes. *J Heart Lung Transplant*, 28, 3, (Mar 2009), pp. (237-242), ISSN: 1053-2498.

Slaughter, MS, Pagani, FD, Rogers, JG, Miller, LW, Sun, B, russell, SD, Starling, RC, Chen, L, Boyle, AJ, Chillcott, S, Adamson, RM, Blood, MS, Camacho, MT, Idrissi, KA, Petty, M, Sobieski, M, Wright, S, Myers, TJ & Farrar, DJ; HeartMate II Clinical Investigators. (2010) Clinical management of continuous-flow left ventricular assist devices in advanced heart failure. *J Heart Lung Transplant*. 29, Suppl 4, (Apr 2010), pp. (S1-S39), ISSN: 1053-2498.

Slaughter, MS, Rogers, JG, Milano, CA, Russell, SD, Conte, JV, Feldman, D, Sun, B, Tatooles, AJ, Delgado, RM III, Long, JW, Wozniak, TC, Ghumman, W, Farrar, DJ & Frazier, OH; HeartMate II Investigators. (2009) Advanced heart failure treated with continuous-flow left ventricular assist device. *N Engl J Med* 361, 23, (Dec 2009), pp. (2241-2251), ISSN: 0028-4793.

Tayama, E, Arinaga, K, Shojima, T, Takagi, K, Yokokura, Y, Yoshikawa, K, Hori, H, Fukunaga, S, Akashi, H & Aoyagi, S.. (2006) Infection management in a patient with a left ventricular assist device: a case report of long-term cefazolin sodium hydrate administration. *J Artif Organs*. 9, 2, (2006), pp. (118-121), ISSN: 1434-7229.

Topkara, VK, Kondareddy, S, Malik, F, Wang, I, Mann, DL, Ewald, GA & Moazami, N. (2010). Infectious complications in patients with left ventricular assist device: etiology and outcomes in the continuous-flow era, *Ann Thorac Surg*, 90, (April 2010), pp. (1270-1277), ISSN: 0003-4975.

Van Den Berghe G, Wouters P, Weekers F, Verwaest, C, Bruyninckx, F, Schetz, M, Vlasselaers, D, Ferdinande, P, Lauwers, P & Bouillon, R. (2001). Intensive insulin therapy in critically ill patients. *N Engl J Med* 345, 19, (Nov 2001), pp. (1359-1367), ISSN: 0028-4793.

Vilchez, RA, McEllistrem, MC, Harrison LH, McCurry, KR, Kormos, RL & Kusne, S. (2001). Relapsing bacteremia in patients with ventricular assist device: an emergent complication of extended circulatory support. *Ann Thorac Surg*, 72, 1, (April 2001), pp. (96-101), ISSN: 0003-4975.

Part 6

Management of Venrtricular Assist Device Out-patients

10

Community Based Management of Ventricular Assist Devices

Marnie Rodger RN MN and Vivek Rao MD PhD
University Health Network
Canada

1. Introduction

Heart failure is a progressive disease associated with high mortality and poor quality of life. It is an increasingly common condition that affects over 5 million Americans with 670 000 new cases diagnosed each year (Lloyd-Jones et al., 2010). Patients with end stage heart failure have a grave prognosis even with maximal medical therapy. Hershberger and colleagues reported that the survival of inotrope dependent patients with end stage heart failure was 51 %, 26% and 6 % at 3, 6, 12 months respectively (Hershberger et al., 2003). Ventricular assist devices (VADs) have been in use for over two decades as a treatment option for patients with advanced heart failure. These mechanical pumps provide hemodynamic support to patients as bridges to cardiac transplantation or destination therapy for transplant ineligible patients. Development of VAD technology and improvements in medical management have allowed individuals with VADs to be discharged from hospitals to their communities. As the number of patients on VAD support continues to rise and more patients are discharged from hospital, outpatient management of VAD patients has become a critical component of mechanical circulatory support programs. This chapter will examine the literature on outpatient VAD support. The fundamental elements of a safe and effective discharge process will be summarized. VAD outpatient outcomes and community based management of device related complications will be discussed.

The Randomized Evaluation of Mechanical Assistance for the Treatment of Congestive Heart Failure (REMATCH) trial was a landmark clinical trial that demonstrated that the use of left ventricular assist devices (LVADs) in patients with advanced heart failure resulted in a 48% reduction in the risk of death as compared to optimal medical management. The REMATCH trial randomized patients with end stage heart failure who were ineligible for cardiac transplantation to either LVAD therapy or optimal medical management. One year survival was 52% in the LVAD group and 25% in the medical therapy group and 2 year survival was 23 and 8 % respectively. The quality of life was significantly improved at one year in the device group. However, the frequency of serious adverse events in the device group was 2.35 times that in the medical therapy group (Rose et el., 2001). Despite substantial survival benefit and significant better quality of life, the study revealed that morbidity and mortality associated with the use of LVADs is considerable.

2. Device designs

A variety of long term VADs have been developed to benefit patients with end stage heart failure. Devices are classified based on a number of characteristics including device location and the method by which the device supports circulation. There are three generations of VADs currently available for use. First generation pumps use pulsatile action with volume displacement. Pulsatile VADs have multiple moving components that are vulnerable to failure over time. Second generation VADs are designed to address some of the problems seen with the first generation VADs. Developed over the past decade, second generation VADs are rotary pumps that provide continuous blood flow. Nonpulsatile flow allows for smaller and quieter devices with less mechanical parts. Continuous axial blood flow is generated by an impeller rotating at high speeds on mechanical bearings. The newest version, third generation VADs are continuous axial or centrifugal flow devices with bearingless impellers or rotors that are magnetically or hydrodynamically levitated (Visouli & Pitsis, 2008). There exist a number of different VADs and a complete review of all the devices is beyond the scope of this chapter. Table 1 briefly reviews some of the long term devices, their mode of action and current status.

Device	Manufacturer	Position	Type	Status
Novacor®	WorldHeart Corporation, Salt Lake City, UT, USA	Intracorporeal	Pulsatile	No longer in use since 2008
HeartMate® XVE	Thoratec Corporation, Pleasanton, Ca, USA	Intracorporeal	Pulsatile	CE mark approval 2003 FDA approval for BTT 2001 for DT 2003
HeartMate II®	Thoratec Corporation, Pleasanton, Ca, USA	Intracorporeal	Continuous Axial flow with blood-immersed bearings	CE mark approval 2005 FDA approval for BTT 2008 for DT 2010
Jarvik 2000	Jarvik Heart Inc. New York, NY, USA	Intracorporeal	Continuous Axial flow with blood-immersed bearings	CE mark approval 2005 USA trial BTT in progress
HeartWare® HVAD	HeartWare International Inc. Framingham, MA, USA	Intracorporeal	Centrifugal Continuous flow Hydromagnetic rotor suspension	CE mark approval 2009 USA BTT and DT trial in progress
DuraHeart®	Terumo Heart Inc. Ann Arbor, MI, USA	Intracorporeal	Centrifugal Continuous flow Magnetically levitated impeller	CE mark approval 2007 USA trial BTT in progress

BTT (Bridge to transplantation); DT (Destination therapy); FDA (Food and Drug Administration); CE (European Conformity)

Table 1. Long term implantable left ventricular assist devices

Many VAD centers use a variety of different types of LVADs in their mechanical circulatory support programs. Therefore, managing LVAD outpatients with different types of systems is not uncommon. Clinicians need to be familiar with the specifics of each device to minimize complications. While each device may have its own unique challenges, many of the issues are universal to all devices.

3. Preparing for hospital discharge

A review of the literature reveals that most mechanical circulatory support programs have similar criteria for discharging patients from hospital on LVAD support. See Table 2 for general criteria for discharging LVAD patients home.

1.	Stable vital signs, LVAD hemodynamics and pump function
2.	Stable hemoglobin and end organ function
3.	Native heart able to support patient in the case of serious VAD malfunction.
4.	Adequate wound healing
5.	Patient is ambulatory-approved for discharge by physiotherapist
6.	Patient able to perform activities of daily living (ADLs) with minimal assistance-approved for discharge by occupational therapist
7.	Patient and caregiver complete LVAD training and demonstrate proficiency in LVAD management
8.	Patient and caregiver have completed out of hospital excursions
9.	Notification of emergency medical services, local emergency room staff and electric company
10.	List of emergency contacts given to LVAD patient
11.	Outpatient appointment scheduled

Table 2. Criteria for discharging left ventricular assist device patients home

The LVAD patient's medical condition must be determined to be stable before discharge. This includes patient's volume status, LVAD function, medication regime and laboratory results. The LVAD patient must be physically capable of managing his or her self care. Self care activities include monitoring daily weights, administration of medication, device management and exit site care. Completion of a physical and occupational therapy program permits LVAD patients to be independent and perform their activities of daily living (ADLs) with minimal assistance. Maintaining a stable international normalized ratio (INR) in the therapeutic range ensures the risk of bleeding or thromboembolism after discharge is minimized.

Although patient's medical readiness for discharge is critical, patient and caregiver must be knowledgeable on all aspects of the care and operation of the LVAD prior to discharge. Patient and caregiver must complete a comprehensive LVAD educational program that encompasses routine care to trouble shooting device problems. Both patient and caregiver must be able to respond appropriately to LVAD system alarms and emergency situations. Proficiency with changing LVAD batteries and power sources must be demonstrated by patient and caregiver. Following extensive training, competency evaluation and skill demonstration must be performed by patient and caregiver before discharge. Since meticulous care of the LVAD exit site is critical, education emphasizing proper exit site care is essential. Patient or caregiver must be able to perform independent LVAD exit site dressing changes using aseptic technique. Patient and caregiver must be able to monitor the device for proper function, identify alarm conditions and know when to contact the VAD team for support and assistance. Once the patient and caregiver demonstrate competence with their device, it is important for the LVAD patient and caregiver to go on out of hospital excursions to foster independence and promote confidence prior to formal discharge.

4. Community support

Discharge preparation involves notification of the LVAD patient's community resources. Methods of informing local care providers include providing written material, a training CD or LVAD education presentations. VAD coordinators play an important role in coordinating the care between local care providers and the VAD team. As LVAD patients may present to their local emergency room with urgent LVAD related problems such as arrhythmias, device malfunction or stroke, communication between local care providers and the VAD team is vital. Instructing local Emergency Medical Services (EMS) personnel and emergency room (ER) staff on LVAD emergency measures may be considered. However, ensuring the training of all EMS and ER personnel may be difficult. Therefore training the patient and their family to direct the actions of EMS and ER personnel in collaboration with the personnel at the VAD center may be at better approach (Holman et al., 2001). LVAD patients that live a considerable distance from the VAD center may require routine follow up with their local cardiologist and primary care physician. Therefore, it is important that local physicians are familiar with the device and have access to the VAD team at any time. Emergency contact numbers for the patient's VAD center should be with the LVAD patient at all times. Also, community dentists must be informed that VAD patients should receive bacterial endocarditis prophylaxis prior to dental procedures. The electric company should be notified of the LVAD patient's dependence on electrical power and need for priority status for power restoration should a power failure occur. And lastly, local cardiac rehabilitation centers must be given information to safely exercise the VAD patient. Patient and community education and support are key elements of a successful outpatient program.

5. Outpatient follow up

Follow up in the clinic is an essential component of the care and management of outpatient LVADs. See Table 3 for routine outpatient follow up care. The frequency of clinic visits

- Weekly clinic visits that include a physical exam, interrogation of the device, laboratory testing, optimization of medical therapy and discussion of patient concerns.
- All LVAD patients are re-started on heart failure medications. Up titration of ace inhibitor and beta blocker is assessed during clinic visits.
- Routine echocardiograms every month or when clinically indicated to evaluate left and right ventricular function, valvular function and estimation of right ventricular systolic pressure (RVSP). Echo based adjustments to VAD speed may be required.
- Clinic visits are decreased to bi-weekly or monthly when LVAD patients are on optimal medical therapy and there are no active issues.

Table 3. Outpatient LVAD follow up care

depends on the patient's condition, medical issues or concerns with device function. Once discharged from hospital, LVAD patients usually return to the outpatient clinic weekly until the VAD team determines less frequent visits are warranted. However, an outpatient should be assessed whenever there is a significant change in the patient's medical status, LVAD pump readings or any alarm condition occurs. It is critical that the outpatient has access to the VAD team at all times for any emergencies or for technical support. Emergency procedures should be reviewed in clinic with patient and caregiver on a regular basis.

6. Discharge rates

Although LVADs have been in use for nearly two decades, the Food and Drug Administration (FDA) only allowed LVAD bridge to transplantation patients to be discharged to their home environment as of 1996 (Park et al., 2005). In 2001, a review of outpatient VAD programs revealed that only 40-60% of patients with LVADs awaiting cardiac transplantation were discharged (Holman et al., 2001). However as mechanical circulatory support programs become more comfortable with discharging patients on LVAD support, the number of patients discharged from hospital is increasing. Lietz and colleagues reported 71% of destination therapy LVAD patients were discharged home or to a nursing facility (Lietz et al., 2007). In a study with bridge to transplantation LVAD patients, 75 % of patients with HeartMate II (Thoratec, Pleasanton, CA, USA) continuous flow LVAD were discharged from hospital. The median hospital stay after surgery was 25 days. 54% of discharged patients required rehospitalization for complications (Miller et al., 2007). Similar results were reported by Pagani and associates. In this study with bridge to transplantation patients, 78% of patients with HeartMate II LVAD were discharged from hospital with a medium hospital stay after surgery of 25 days. 68% of discharged patients required rehospitalization (Pagani et al., 2009). In a recent clinical trial of patients who were ineligible for cardiac transplantation, 86% of patients with a continuous flow LVAD and 76% of patients with a pulsatile LVAD were discharged from hospital. The median length of stay after surgery was 27 days with continuous flow device and 28 days with pulsatile device (Slaughter et al., 2009). MacIver and colleagues reported that 71% of LVAD patients were discharged home and that complications occurring in the community were low. This study found that patients supported for more than 3 months spent 70% of their support time at home and this increased to 94 % for patients supported for more than 1 year (MacIver et al., 2009). As demonstrated in the literature, an increasing number of patients on VAD support are discharged from hospitals and outpatient management is crucial to successful LVAD outcomes.

7. Results of long term VAD support

Management of LVAD patients requires a thorough understanding of the risks and potential complications associated with LVAD therapy. Reviewing the literature on mechanical circulatory support allows clinicians to identify and manage common LVAD issues and adverse events in order to improve patient outcomes and survival. HeartMate VE and XVE (Thoratec, Pleasanton, CA, USA) and Novacor (World Heart, Oakland, CA, USA) have been the most widely used and studied long term implantable LVADs. The HeartMate VE LVAD was the device used in the REMATCH trial. The 1 and 2 year survival rates of LVAD patients in the REMATCH trial was 52% and 23 % respectively. The most common causes of death in the LVAD group were sepsis (41%), failure of the device (17%) and ischemic stroke (10%) (Rose et al., 2001). Extended follow-up of the REMATCH trial patients confirmed survival rates at 1 year and 2 year for patients receiving LVADs was 52% and 29% respectively (Park et al., 2005). Outcomes of LVAD destination therapy in the post REMATCH era described by Leitz and associates showed relatively no change in the overall survival after HeartMate XVE LVAD implantation. Survival was 56 % and 30.9% at 1 year and 2 years respectively. The leading causes of overall mortality included sepsis (29.5%), multiorgan failure (12.8%) and right heart failure (8.4%). LVAD failure accounted for 6% of deaths (Lietz et al., 2007). However, a more recent study of patients undergoing destination therapy with HeartMate XVE demonstrated that long term LVAD destination therapy can be improved. Long and his colleagues reported a 2 year survival of 77 % for the LVAD destination therapy group as compared with the REMATCH trial rate of 23%. This study also had a 38% reduction of adverse events as compared with the REMATCH trial results. Causes of death long term were related to LVAD failure (8.7%), infection (8.7%) and malignancy (4.3%). Therefore, relative to the REMATCH trial results, the rate of death after discharge was decreased by a factor of 2.5 (Long et al., 2008). Although the study was a single center experience and not a randomized controlled trial, the results suggest that patient selection and advances in LVAD patient management have the potential for improving destination therapy outcomes.

The prospective, non randomized Investigation of Nontransplant-Eligible Patients Who Are Inotrope Dependent (INTrEPID) trial compared the outcomes of patients supported on the Novacor LVAD with patients treated with optimal medical therapy. The study demonstrated that patients with a Novacor LVAD had superior survival rates at 1 year as compared to the medical therapy group (27 % vs. 11%). This trial found that stroke (34%) and infection (24%) accounted for the majority of deaths in the LVAD group. While 62 % of the LVAD patients experienced a stroke or transient ischemic attack during the study, there was no mortality attributable to LVAD malfunction (Rogers et al., 2007). Although the REMATCH and the INTrEPID trials demonstrated that patients treated with LVAD destination therapy had significant improvement in survival compared with optimal medical therapy, morbidity due to sepsis, stroke and device failure is common with the first generation pulsatile devices.

Over the past 2 years a rapid growth in the use of continuous flow LVADs and a decline in pulsatile LVADs have been observed (Kirklin et al., 2010). In a prospective study, Miller and associates reported the survival rate of LVAD patients implanted with HeartMate II LVAD as a bridge to cardiac transplantation was 75% at 6 months and 68% at 12 months. The use of a continuous flow pump was not without complications. At 6 months, 19% of patients had died while on device support, 4 % had medical complications that precluded transplantation and 2 % had their devices replaced. Causes of death included sepsis (4%), ischemic stroke (4%) multisystem organ failure (3%) hemorrhagic stroke (2%) anoxic brain injury (1.5%), and right heart failure (1.5%). This study also reported that percutaneous lead infection occurred in 14% of patients but no pump pocket infection was observed (Miller et al., 2007).

A retrospective European study of LVAD patients who had received a HeartMate II LVAD reported a 1 year survival of 69% in the destination therapy group and 63% in the bridge to transplant group. Main causes of death were multiple organ failure, in most instances due to septic complications, and cerebrovascular accidents (CVA). One third of adverse events occurred within the first week post LVAD implant and only one cerebrovascular accident occurred after the first 9 days after surgery. There was no mechanical failure of the device. Sepsis remained the leading cause of death overall (Strűber et al., 2008).

In a recent prospective study by Pagani and associates, the overall survival for patients with a HeartMate II LVAD as bridge to transplant was 73% at 1 year and 72% at 18 months. The primary causes of death were sepsis (4%), stroke (4% ischemic and 2% hemorrhagic), right heart failure (3%) and device related deaths (3%). Only 4.6 % of deaths occurred after 6 months of device support and included sepsis, LVAD power loss and withdrawal of support. Although LVAD replacement occurred in 4% of patients due to device thrombosis (1.4%), percutaneous lead wire damage (1.4%) or for device infection (0.3%), there were no failures of the mechanical pumping mechanism. Also reported were significant improvements in LVAD patients' functional status, 6-minute walk test and quality of life (Pagani et al., 2009).

Slaughter and colleagues reported their results of a randomized controlled trial comparing outcomes in patients with advanced heart failure who were ineligible for transplantation and received either a pulsatile flow HeartMate XVE LVAD or a continuous flow HeartMate II LVAD. Estimates of the 1 and 2 year survival rates were 68% and 58 % respectively with the continuous flow device and 55% and 24 % with the pulsatile device. The leading causes of death in patients with continuous flow device were hemorrhagic stroke (9%), right heart failure (5%), sepsis (4%) and external power interruption (4%) while the leading cause of death in patients with a pulsatile device were hemorrhagic stroke (10%), right heart failure (8%), multiorgan failure (7%) and ischemic stroke (5%). Continuous flow LVAD significantly improved the probability of survival free from stroke and reoperation for device repair or replacement at 2 years (Slaughter et al., 2009). While both devices significantly improved patients' quality of life and functional capacity, the 2 year survival rate with the continuous flow device was more than twice the rate with pulsatile device.

The Interagency Registry for Mechanically Assisted Circulatory Support (INTERMACS) database first annual report found that cardiovascular causes (including right ventricular failure and fatal arrhythmias) and multiorgan failure predominated as early causes of death whereas central nervous system events and infection were the most common causes of death after the first month of LVAD implantation. Bleeding and infection were the most common adverse events both early and later (Kirklin et al., 2008). While pulsatile VADS were the only available devices in the first INTERMACS report, the second INTERMACS report included data on continuous flow devices. The report demonstrated that continuous flow devices have become the preferred choice for bridge to transplantation therapy as 85% of LVADs implanted between July 2008 and January 2009 were continuous flow VADS. In general, adverse events were reduced in patients with continuous flow devices for device malfunction, infection, hepatic dysfunction and neurologic events (Kirklin et al., 2010). A review of the studies with HeartMate II LVAD, a second generation device, provides evidence of improved outcomes and reduced morbidity with continuous flow pumps as compared with pulsatile pumps. Overall there was significant reduction of adverse events including percutaneous lead infection and neurological events with the non pulsatile device.

8. Outpatient LVAD outcomes

A review of the literature reveals that there is limited research on outpatient outcomes. The literature consists mostly of single center reports that are based on small numbers of outpatients. Also, the majority of studies describe outpatient outcomes while on pulsatile VAD support with very few studies that include non pulsatile VADs. See Table 3 for a review of the literature on LVAD outpatient outcomes.

Authors	Study period	Number of discharged patients	Device	Results
Myers et al., 1996	Unknown	21	HeartMate VE	15 readmissions to the hospital: 9 for medical reasons and 6 for device related problems. No deaths occurred outside of the hospital. Two patients returned to full-time employment
Schmid et al., 1999	1995-1998	16	HeartMate VE, Novacor	Reasons for readmission included systemic or driveline infections, suspected or true thromboembolic events, suspected malfunction of LVAD, 1 death due to cerebral bleed, 1 death due to ventricular fibrillation
Morales et al., 2000	1993-1998	44	HeartMate VE	None of the outpatients died. No strokes occurred. 46% minor device malfunctions and 6.8 % major device malfunctions occurred. 18% device related infections
El-Banayosy et al., 2001	1994-2000	66	HeartMate VE, Novacor	29 patients were not readmitted. Primary reasons for readmission were neurologic disorders and infection complications. 24% died on LVAD support (15% multiorgan failure and/or sepsis, 4.5% cerebral infarction, 3% cerebral bleed, 1.5% brain death)
Richenbacher & Seemuth, 2001	1999-2001	13	HeartMate VE	1 death due to fungal sepsis with embolic event. 62% required readmission (2 patients with device related infections, 2 patients with neurologic events, 1 device malfunction requiring pump replacement, 3 non VAD related admissions)

Authors	Study period	Number of discharged patients	Device	Results
Holman et al., 2002	1997-2001	20	Thoratec VAD (Thoratec Corp., Pleasanton, CA), HeartMate VE	5 deaths after hospital readmission (1 sepsis, 1 conduit tear, 3 neurologic events) 4 device infections, 3 device malfunctions that required pump replacement
Drews et al., 2003	1996-2001	38	Novacor, Berlin Heart (Berlin Heart GmbH, Germany)	Total mortality 16%. 2 deaths due to cerebral embolism, 1 death due to cerebral hemorrhage, 2 deaths due to systemic infection, 1 death due to multiorgan failure. 84 % patients required readmission for cerebral embolism (9%), bleeding (1%), wound infection (24%), coagulation disorder (14%), non VAD related (46%)
Frazier et al., 2007	2003-2007	35	HeartMate II	No device malfunctions in outpatient setting. 1 device removed due to pump pocket infection. 1 death due to hemorrhagic stroke. 2 patients had sudden death at home.
Potapov et al., 2008	1996-2006	114	Berlin Heart, Novacor, MicroMed DeBakey (MicroMed Cardiovascular Inc. Houston, Tx, USA), HeartMate VE, DuraHeart, Incor (Berlin Heart, Germany) LionHeart (Arrow International, Inc. Reading, PA, USA)	Outpatients spent 67% time at home. 56% readmission unrelated to VAD, 20.9% wound infection, 10.9% coagulation disorders, 7.7% cerebral embolism

Authors	Study period	Number of discharged patients	Device	Results
MacIver et al., 2009	2001-2006	17	HeartMate XVE, Novacor, HeartMate II	88% outpatients survived until transplant or explant. 1 death due to cerebral vascular accident. 1 subarachnoid hemorrhage (patient survived to transplant). 29% incidence of driveline or pocket infection. 29% had device malfunction. 1 patient remained on support at end of study period

Table 3. Literature on LVAD outpatient outcomes

Allen and associates published a retrospective review of patients supported more than 1 year on a Heartmate I or HeartMate II LVAD from 2000 to 2009 which revealed that although LVAD support is not without complications, LVAD patients spend the majority of time (87%) out of hospital enjoying a good quality of life. Causes of readmission included infection (43.2%), anticoagulation complications (11.5%), gastrointestinal bleeding (8.8%), LVAD malfunction (8.1%), neurologic (7.4%). There were 10% of patients that were never readmitted while on LVAD support with HeartMate II LVAD. However, 26.7% of patients required LVAD exchange for mechanical failure, electrical failure and thrombosis. While there was a trend toward higher exchange rates and shorter exchange times with HeartMate I, the differences were not statistically significant. While 77% of LVAD patients required additional operations, 57% were related to percutaneous lead or LVAD pocket infections (Allen et al., 2010). This study found that device related infections are common no matter which generation of device and that they are detrimental to the LVAD patient's quality of life.

9. Quality of life

An important aspect to consider for outpatient support is the impact of LVAD therapy on quality of life. A majority of patients with advanced heart failure express a strong desire for improvements in quality of life and functionality even at the expense of longevity (Rogers et al., 2010). The REMATCH trial provided evidence that LVADs improved the quality of life for end stage heart failure patients ineligible for transplantation (Rose et al., 2001). A review of the literature reveals there is strong evidence that demonstrates the positive effect of long term mechanical support on functional capacity. In a study with patients who received a Heartmate VE LVAD, 30% of outpatients were able to return to work or school, 33 % to sexual activity and 44% to driving (Morales et al., 2000). Data from advanced heart failure patients enrolled in the HeartMate II LVAD trials were analyzed by Rogers and colleagues to assess the impact of continuous flow LVADs on functional capacity and heart failure-related quality of life. The study found that LVAD patients demonstrated early and sustained improvement in functional status and quality of life. Following implantation with HeartMate II LVAD, 82% bridge to transplantation and 80% destination therapy patients at 6 months and 79 % destination therapy patients at 24 months improved to New York Heart Association (NYHA) functional class I or II. Mean 6 minute walk distance in destination therapy patients was 204 meters in patients able to ambulate at baseline, which improved to 350 and 360 meters at 6 and 24 months. There were significant and sustained improvements from baseline in both bridge to transplantation and destination therapy patients in median Minnesota Living With Heart Failure and Kansas City Cardiomyopathy Questionnaires overall summary scores (Rogers et al., 2010). Pagani and his colleagues reported similar findings with patients who underwent HeartMate II LVAD implantation as bridge to transplantation. At 6 months, there were significant improvements in functional status and 6-minute walk test (from 0% to 83 % of patients in New York Heart Association functional class I or II and from 13% to 89% of patients completing a 6 -minute walk test) and in quality of life (mean value improved 41% with Minnesota Living With Heart Failure and 75% with Kansas City Cardiomyopathy Questionnaires) (Pagani et al., 2009). While the literature shows there is substantial survival benefit and significant improvement in quality of life, clinicians must manage and reduce the complications associated with LVAD therapy.

10. Outpatient medical management

The literature reveals that device related infection is a major cause of morbidity and mortality in LVAD patients. Infection prevention and management is an important aspect of LVAD outpatient care. The percutaneous driveline exit site remains the major source of device related infections in LVAD patients. It is vital to treat percutaneous driveline infections in order to prevent pump pocket infections. The usual organisms cultured are Staphylococcus and other biofilm forming organisms such as Pseudomonas, Enterococcus and Candida (Holman et al., 2003). Patients must be taught strict adherence to aseptic technique for LVAD exit site care. Another critical component of infection prevention is immobilization of the percutaneous driveline to promote tissue ingrowth and reduce infection risk. Patients must monitor for signs and symptoms of infections such as fever, chills, erythema or tenderness at exit site or along driveline or purulent drainage from exit site and notify the VAD team immediately should signs of infection develop. If infection is suspected, the clinician should initiate broad spectrum antibiotics once a culture of exit site has been obtained. After the organism is identified the patient should be started on the most appropriate antibiotic therapy as per culture and sensitivity results. Consultation with Infectious Diseases Service may be necessary to optimize antibiotic therapy.

Advanced practice guidelines for HeartMate destination therapy is an excellent resource for clinicians and contains care guidelines for infection prevention, management and treatment that can be applied to all devices. General recommendations include performing an ultrasound or computed tomography (CT) scan to detect presence of fluid accumulation or infection (Chinn et al., 2004). If LVAD patient experiences systemic symptoms such as fever, chills, leukocytosis, blood cultures should be obtained to exclude bacteremia. Bacteremia must be treated aggressively as it may lead to endocarditis of the pump. If LVAD pocket infection is suspected, incision and drainage may be necessary to obtain cultures. Increasing the LVAD patient's status on the transplant list may be indicated if patient develops LVAD exit site infection. Fungal infections have been associated with vegetative growth on LVADs and persistent systemic fungal infection may require LVAD replacement (Thoratec Corporation, 2008). While it is possible to treat some patients on an outpatient basis, many LVAD patients require rehospitalization for intravenous antibiotic administration for driveline exit site infections. MacIver and colleagues reported that 75% of driveline infections in outpatient LVADs were managed in the outpatient clinic with a single course of oral antibiotics (MacIver et al., 2009).

Research demonstrates that LVAD patients may experience a neurological event during LVAD support. LVAD patients are routinely placed on anticoagulation and antiplatelet therapy to decrease the risk of thromboembolic complications during LVAD support. Antiplatelet therapy for LVAD patients usually consists of enteric coated aspirin 81 to 325 mg daily. Some VAD centers add dipyridamole to the antiplatelet regime. For patients who have an allergy to aspirin, clopidogrel may be used in its place. Thromboelastography can be performed to assess antiplatelet effect. The HeartMate II clinical trial found that pump thrombosis was rare with 4% occurring in destination therapy patients and 1.4% in bridge to transplantation patients (Slaughter et al., 2010). However, as there is a potential for a neurologic event to occur while on LVAD support, it is prudent for clinicians to order a computed tomography (CT) scan for any change in the mental status of a LVAD patient to assess for subdural hematoma, thromboembolism or intracerebral hemorrhage. It is important to maintain adequate pump flows to avoid transient ischemic attacks (TIA) or ischemic strokes. Likewise it is critical not to be too aggressive with anticoagulation in order to avoid hemorrhagic strokes. A recent study by Boyle and associates found that while thrombotic event rates in patients discharged with HeartMate II was 3.3%, hemorrhagic event rates were 22%. The gastrointestinal system was identified as the most frequent site of bleeding in outpatients. In Boyle's analysis of outpatient anticoagulation, 9.4% of patients discharged from hospital on HeartMate II support required blood transfusions due to gastrointestinal bleeding (Boyle et al., 2009). Outpatient LVAD management must include regular testing of anticoagulation and complete blood counts. Anticoagulation and antiplatelet therapy must be carefully monitored to avoid adverse events and may need to be adjusted to minimize risks of thromboembolism or hemorrhage.

Device malfunction is a potential complication that can occur in the outpatient setting. Diagnosing device malfunctions can be accomplished by interrogating the device on a routine basis. LVAD malfunctions can include controller failure, LVAD motor issues or percutaneous lead problems. LVAD patients must notify the VAD team whenever an alarm condition occurs. Teaching the LVAD patient to monitor for changes in pump readings enables patients to notify the VAD team whenever there are significant changes. Technical support from VAD manufacturers is available to assist clinicians and waveforms can be down loaded and sent for analysis. It is important for clinicians to accurately diagnose and manage LVAD malfunctions to prevent serious adverse events. Patients must be trained to recognize and respond to device problems.

Arrhythmias may occur in patients on LVAD support. Ambardeker and associates reported that 24% of LVAD patients in their study received an appropriate implantable cardioverter-defibrillator (ICD) shock for a ventricular arrhythmia (Ambardeker et al., 2010). In order to avoid potential arrhythmias, it is important for clinicians to closely monitor and correct electrolyte imbalances. LVAD patients should be considered for placement of an ICD as prophylactic treatment for ventricular arrhythmias. Anti-arrhythmics or beta blockers may also be used to suppress ventricular arrhythmias. For patients supported on a continuous flow device, it is important to avoid setting the pump speed too high as this may result in a suction induced arrhythmia.

11. Conclusion

LVAD support has become an accepted standard of care for patients with advanced heart failure. The literature demonstrates that LVAD patients can be safely and effectively managed as outpatients in the community. Minor LVAD complications can be managed in an outpatient LVAD clinic and most LVAD outpatients spend the majority of their time out of hospital. However, serious adverse events may require LVAD outpatients to be readmitted to hospital for care. In general, driveline infection is the most common complication reported in the outpatient setting with both pulsatile and continuous flow devices. The literature reveals that due to the limited durability of pulsatile VADs, there has been an increase in the number of patients implanted with continuous flow LVADs. A review of recent clinical studies demonstrates that there are fewer device related complications with continuous flow LVADs. However, the development of continuous flow LVADs has resulted in the creation of new clinical problems. Frazier and colleagues found that continuous flow introduces physiologic phenomena such as arteriovenous malformation leading to gastrointestinal bleeding, septal shift with resultant right heart failure, thrombosis of the aortic valve non coronary sinus, aortic valve fusion and aortic valve insufficiency (Frazier et al., 2007). Further research is required to determine the durability and potential long term problems that may arise with long term use of continuous flow LVADs. Longer duration follow up of destination therapy patients on continuous flow LVAD support may reveal new issues with non pulsatile devices.

12. References

Allen, J.G., Weiss, E.S., Schaffer, J.M., Patel, N.D. Ullrich, S.L. et al. (2010). Quality of life and functional status in patients surviving 12 months after left ventricular assist device implantation. *J Heart Lung Transplant* Vol. 29(No. 3): 278-85.

Ambardekar, A.V., Allen, L.A., Lindenfeld, J., Lowery, C.M., Cannon, A.P. et al. (2010). Implantable cardioverter-defibrillator shocks in patients with a left ventricular assist device. *J Heart Lung Transplant*. Vol. 29(No. 7): 771-6.

Boyle, A.J., Russell, S.D., Teuteberg, J.J., Slaughter, M.S., Moazami, N. et al. (2009). Low thromboembolism and pump thrombosis with the HeartMate II left ventricular assist device: Analysis of outpatient anti-coagulation. *J Heart Lung Transplant*. Vol. 28(No. 9): 881-7.

Chinn, R., Dembitsky, W., Rasmusson, B., Chillcot, S., Stahovich, M. et al. (2004). *Advanced practice guidelines for HeartMate destination therapy*. Vol 1. Pleasanton, CA: Thoratec Corporation.

Drews, T.N., Loebe, M., Jurmann, M.J., Weng, Y., Wendelmuth, C. et al. (2003). Outpatients on mechanical circulatory support. *Ann Thorac Surg*. Vol. 75(No. 3): 780-5.

El-Banayosy, A., Fey, O., Sarnowski, P., Arusoglu, L., Boethig, D., et al. (2001). Midterm follow-up of patients discharged from hospital under left ventricular assistance. *J Heart Lung Transplant*. Vol. 20(No. 1): 53-58.

Frazier, O.H., Gemmato, C., Myers, T.J., Gregoric, I.D., Radovancevic, B. et al. (2007). Initial clinical experience with the HeartMate II Axial-Flow Left Ventricular Assist Device. *Texas Heart Institute Journal*. Vol. 34(No. 3): 275-281.

Hershberger, R.E., Nauman, D. & Walker, T.L. (2003). Care processes and clinical outcomes of Continuous Outpatient Support with Inotropes (COSI) in patients with refractory endstage heart failure. *J Card Fail*. Vol. 9(No. 3): 180-187.

Holman, W.L., Ormaza, S., Seemuth, K., Boehmer, J.P., Richenbacher, W.E. (2001). How to run an outpatient VAD program: Overview. *ASAIO Journal*. Vol. 47 (No. 6): 588-589.

Holman, W.L., Davies, J.E., Rayburn, B.K., McGiffin, D.C., Foley, B.A. et al. (2002). Treatment of end-stage heart disease with outpatient ventricular assist devices. *Ann Thorac Surg*. Vol. 73 (No. 5): 1489-94.

Holman, W.L., Rayburn, B.K., McGiffin, D.C., Foley, B.A., Benza, R.L. et al. (2003). Infection in ventricular assist devices: Prevention and treatment. *Ann Thorac Surg*. Vol.75 (No. 6): S48-57.

Kirklin, J.K., Naftel, D.C., Stevenson, L. W., Kormos, R.L., Pagani, F.D., Miller, M.A., Ulisney, K. & Young, J.B. (2008). INTERMACS Database for Durable Devices for Circulatory Support: First Annual Report. *Journal of Heart and Lung Transplantation*. Vol. 27 (No. 10): 1065-1072.

Kirklin, J.K., Naftel, D.C., Kormos, R.L., Stevenson, L.W., Pagani, F. D., Miller, M.A., Ulisney, K.L., & Young, J.B. (2010). Second INTERMACS annual report: More than 1000 primary left ventricular assist device implants. *Journal of Heart and Lung Transplantation*. Vol. 29 (No. 1): 1-10.

Lietz, K., Long, J.W., Kfoury, A.G., Slaughter, M.S., Silver, M.A., Milano, C.A., Rogers, J.G., Naka, Y., Mancini, D. & Miller, L.W. (2007). Outcomes of Left Ventricular Assist Device Implantation as Destination Therapy in the Post -REMATCH era. *Circulation* Vol. 116(No. 5): 497-505.

Lloyd-Jones, D., Adams, R.J., Brown, T.M., Carnethon, M., Dai, S., De Simone, G., Ferguson, T.B., et al., on behalf of the American Heart Association Statistics Committee and Stroke Statistics Subcommittee. (2010). Heart Disease and Stroke Statistics 2010 update: A Report From the American Heart Association. *Circulation* Vol. 121(No. 7): e46-e215.

Long, J.W., Healy, A.H., Rasmusson, B.Y., Cowley, C.G., Nelson, K.E., et al. (2008). Improving outcomes with long-term "destination" therapy using left ventricular assist devices. *J Thorac Cardiovasc Surg*. Vol. 135(No. 6): 1353-61.

MacIver, J., Ross, H.J., Delgado, D.H., Cusimano, R.J., Yau, T.M., et al. (2009). Community support of patients with a left ventricular assist device: The Toronto General Hospital experience. *Can J Cardiol*. Vol.25 (No. 11): e377-381.

Miller, L.W., Pagani, F.D., Russell, S.D., John, R., Boyle, A.J. et al. for the HeartMate II clinical Investigators. (2007). Use of a Continuous-Flow Device in Patients Awaiting Heart Transplantation. *N Engl J Med.* Vol. 357(No. 9): 885-96.

Morales, D.L., Catanese, K.A., Helman, D.N., Williams, M.R., Weinberg, A., et al. (2000). Six-year experience of caring for forty-four patients with a left ventricular assist device at home: safe, economical, necessary. *J Thorac Cardio-vasc Surg.* Vol. 119 (No. 2): 251-9.

Myers, T.J., Catanese, K.A., Vargo, R.L., & Dressler, D.R. (1996). Extended cardiac support with a portable left ventricular assist system in the home. *ASAIO Journal.* Vol. 42 (No. 5): m576-579.

Pagani, F.D., Miller, L.W., Russell, S.D., Aaronson, K.D., John, R., et al. for the HeartMate II Investigators. (2009). Extended Mechanical Circulatory Support With a Continuous-Flow Rotary Left Ventricular Assist Device. *J Am Coll Cardio.* Vol.54 (No. 4): 312-21.

Park, S.J., Tector, A., Piccioni, W., Raines, E., Gelijns, A. et al. (2005). Left ventricular assist device as destination therapy: A new look at survival. *J Thorac cardiovasc Surg.* Vol. 129(No. 1): 9-17.

Potapov, E.V., Loforte, A., Weng, Y., Jurmann, M., Pasic, M., et al. (2008). Experience with over 1000 implanted ventricular assist devices. *J Card Surg.* Vol. 23 (No.3): 185-194.

Richenbacher, W.E & Seemuth, S.C. (2001). Hospital discharge for the ventricular assist device patient: Historical perspective and description of a successful program. *ASAIO Journal.* Vol. 47(No. 6): 590-595.

Rogers, J.G., Butler, J., Lansman, S.L., Gass, A., Portner, P.M., et al. for the INTrEPID Investigators. (2007). Chronic Mechanical Circulatory Support for Inotrope-Dependent Heart Failure Patients Who Are Not Transplant Candidates. *J Am Coll Cardiol.* Vol. 50(No. 8): 741-7.

Rogers, J.G., Aaronson, K.D., Boyle, A.J., Russell, S.D., Milano, C.A., et al. for the HeartMate II Investigators. (2010). Continuous Flow Left Ventricular Assist Device Improves Functional Capacity and Quality of Life of Advanced Heart Failure Patients. *J Am Coll Cardiol.* Vol. 55(No. 17): 1826-34.

Rose, E.A., Gelijns, A.C., Moskowitz, A.J., Heitjan, D.F., Stevenson, L.W., et al. for the Randomized Evaluation of Mechanical Assistance for the Treatment of Congestive Heart Failure (REMATCH) Study Group. (2001). Long-Term use of a Left Ventricular Assist Device for end-stage heart failure. *N Engl J Med.* Vol. 345 (No. 20): 1435-1443.

Schmid, C., Hammel, D., Deng, M.C., Weyand, M., Baba, H. et al. (1999). Ambulatory care of patients with left ventricular assist devices. *Circulation.* Vol. 100 (supp II): II-224-II-228.

Slaughter, M.S., Rogers, J.G., Milano, C.A., Russell, S.D., Conte, J.V. et al. for the HeartMate II Investigators. (2009). Advanced Heart Failure Treated with Continuous-Flow Left Ventricular Assist Device. *N Engl J. Med.* Vol. 361(No. 23): 2241-2251.

Strüber, M., Sander, K., Lahpor, J., Ahn, H., Litzler, P., et al. (2008). HeartMate II left ventricular assist device; early European experience. *European Journal of Cardio-thoracic Surgery*. Vol. 34(No. 2): 289-294.

Thoratec Corporation. (2008). HeartMate II left ventricular assist system. Instructions for use. Pleasanton, CA: Thoratec Corporation.

Visouli, A.N. & Pitsis, A.A. (2008). Will modern miniaturized left ventricular assist devices offer a viable alternative to heart transplantation? *Hellenic J Cardio.*Vol. 49 (No. 5): 335-348.

Part 7

Long Term Outcomes Following Ventricular Assist Device

11

Long-Term Management of Pulsatile Extracorporeal Left Ventricular Assist Device

Tomoko Sugiyama Kato, MD. PhD, Kazuo Komamura MD. PhD,
Noboru Oda, MD. PhD, Taro Sasaoka, MD, Ikutaro Nakajima, MD,
Ayako Tkakahashi, MD and Masafumi Kitakaze, MD, PhD
National Cerebral and Cardiovascular Center, Osaka, Japan

1. Introduction

Heart transplantation provides considerable survival benefits for patients with end-stage heart failure, but it is available for only a small fraction of such patients all over the world due to donor shortage. Therefore, many heart transplant candidates require long-term support by a left ventricular assist device (LVAD) while they await transplantation. However, the long-term LVAD support can result in serious complications such as cerebrovascular accident (CVA) and infection, which are the leading cause of death and the primary reason for elimination from transplant eligibility in patients supported by LVAD **(Rose EA et al., 2001; Holman WL et al., 2009)**.

In Japan, only less than 100 organ transplants from brain-dead donors have been performed over the past 10 years. The mean waiting period for heart transplant candidates after LVAD surgery frequently exceeds 2 years. In addition, the only available LVAD covered by the National Health Insurance System in Japan is pulsatile extracorporeal LVAD (Toyobo-LVAS®; Nipro, Tokyo, Japan). Implantable LVADs have not yet been approved and are still under clinical trials, awaiting approval by the Ministry of Health, Labour and Welfare as of October 2010.

Toyobo-LVAS® was primarily designed for short-term support, but it is used in Japan over the long term as a 'bridge-to-transplant' device **(Figure 1)**. Patients supported by pulsatile extracorporeal LVAD cannot be discharged from the hospital, and cannot leave the intensive care ward without attendant medical doctors. Some patients required to be supported by such device for 4 years until being transplanted.

Given these circumstances, the long-term management skills of Japanese cardiologists for overcoming "extracorporeal pulsatile" LVAD-related complications have improved over time, with the 1-year survival now being 82% **(Sasaoka T et al., 2010)**.

The extracorporeal pulsatile LVAD is the devise that is not utilized in a first line anymore in a world except for Japan. However, CVA and infection, on which we have paid considerable attention during long-term management of extracorporeal pulsatile LVAD, still remain to be important complication even in the era of new generation continuous flow devises. Therefore, we believe that our delicate care for such complication to accomplish long-term survival in patients supported by extracorporeal pulsatile LVAD is worthwhile information even today.

In this chapter, we focused on the management strategies of CVA and infection in patients with extracorporeal pulsatile LVAD according to our past 10 years experience.

2. Survival rate and frequency of complications after extracorporeal pulsatile LVAD

Recently, the survival rate and transplant rate of patients supported by pulsatile extracorporeal LVAD (Toyobo-LVAS®) in Japan have improved considerably.
The National Cerebral and Cardiovascular Center (NCVC) (Osaka, Japan) is one of the main heart transplant institution in Japan, which underwent nearly half of the all heart transplant cases performed in Japan. The technology of Toyobo-LVAS® was initially developed based on the basic research conducted by Takano et al at NCVC in 1982, with collaboration with Toyobo Co., Ltd. in Japan. Accordingly, the NCVC has most experience in Toyobo-LVAS® surgeries and has been mostly familiar with this devise management in Japan. Thus, as a representative data of clinical outcome after Toyobo-LVAS® surgery, we introduced the papers regarding Toyobo-LVAS®, which were recently published by our NCVC group (**Takahashi A et al., 2010; Sasaoka T et al, 2010**).
In order to describe how the survival after Toyobo-LVAS® improved over the years, the retrospectively review of 69 consecutive patients with Toyobo-VAS® as a bridge to heart transplantation between 1994 and 2007 at NCVC were shown. Thirty patients who had LVAD surgery between 1994 and 2000 were assigned to group A, and 39 patients who underwent surgery between 2001 and 2007 were assigned to group B.

2.1 Outcome after extracorporeal pulsatile LVAD surgery over the years

The demographics of patients and the severity of heart failure as indicated by laboratory and hemodynamic examination before LVAD surgeries were not significantly different between the groups. However, the duration of LVAD support was significantly longer in the recent era (group B) than that in the initial era (group A). Mortality was significantly higher in the initial era (group A) than in the recent era (group B). **Table 1** and **Figure 2** summarizes the outcomes of patients.
Figure 3 shows Kaplan-Meier survival curves of these patients. Survival after LVAD surgery was significantly lower in the initial era (group A) than that in the recent era (group B). **Figure 4** shows the causes of death in both groups of patients. The proportion of deaths due to CVA was significantly higher in the initial era (group A) than that in the recent era (group B) (50% vs. 13%, $p < 0.0001$), whereas that of infection did not differ significantly between two groups. The proportion of deaths due to right ventricular failure, defined as fatal liver or renal insufficiency under LVAD support and requirement of inotropic agents, was higher in the recent era (group B).

2.2 CVA after pulsatile extracorporeal LVAD

Among the 69 patients studied, 37 patients developed CVA after pulsatile extracorporeal LVAD. The incidence and outcome after CVA in the patients are summarized in Table 2. Rapid reversal of warfarin-induced anticoagulation was attempted in all patients who developed intracerebral hemorrhage (**Takahashi A et al., 2010**). Vitamin K was never used after the events. Prothrombin complex concentrate (PCC), which contains a high level of vitamin K-dependent coagulation factors II, VII, IX and X, rapidly and effectively reverses warfarin-induced anticoagulation. This product (PPSB-HT®; Nihon Pharmaceuticals, Tokyo, Japan) has become available since 2001, and it has been used for emergency reversal of warfarin-induced anticoagulation in cases of intracranial bleeding, intra-abdominal hemorrhage and cardiac tamponade.

Neither the incidence of CVA nor the proportion of CVA that required succeeding neurosurgery differs significantly between two groups. However, the proportion of patients in which CVA led to death was significantly higher in the initial era (group A) than that in the recent era (group B). The proportion of patients treated with PCC after CVA was significantly higher in the recent era (group B) than that in the initial era (group A). **Figure 5** shows the Kaplan-Meier survival curves of patients who developed CVA. The survival rates of patients with CVA episodes were significantly lower in the initial era (group A) than that in the recent era (group B).

2.2 Infection after pulsatile extracorporeal LVAD

Among the 69 patients studied, 53 patients developed systemic infection (SI) after pulsatile extracorporeal LVAD. SI was defined as a positive blood culture when patients developed any symptom of infection. **Table 3** summarizes the incidence of SI among the patients studied. Neither the incidence of patients who developed SI nor the proportion of SI leading to death differed significantly between two groups. In addition, the cumulative number of SI episodes and the number of SI episodes per year per patient were not significantly different between two groups. However, although SI itself was not a direct cause of death, a subgroup analysis of patients with a history of SI revealed that the proportion of patients who were alive, including those who received transplant and those who remained on LVAD support, was significantly lower in the initial era (group A) than that in the recent era (group B). The proportion of patients with a history of SI who could undergo transplantation was significantly lower in the initial era (group A) than in the recent era (group B). The duration from infection to death in patients with a history of SI after LVAD surgery was significantly shorter in initial era (group A) than that in the recent era (group B) (256.0 ± 203.1 vs. 749.7 ± 328.8 days, $p < 0.01$).

The proportion of methicillin-susceptible Staphylococcus aureus (MSSA) or/and methicillin-resistant Staphylococcus aureus (MRSA) was significantly higher in the recent era (group B) than in the initial era (group A). Linezolid is a powerful synthetic oxazolidinone antibiotic against Gram-positive pathogens that produce toxins **(Stevens DL et al., 2007).** It is commonly used to combat severe infection with staphylococci including MRSA. Linezolid has been available at our institution since 2001, and has been administered to patients with recurrent refractory MRSA or MSSA infection under all treatment modalities. We decide to use lineszolid under diagnosis of refractory staphylococcal infection.

3. Management of CVA after pulsatile extracorporeal LVAD

In spite of the recent progression of ventricular devises, CVA still remains the leading cause of death and the primary reason for elimination from transplant eligibility in patients supported by LVAD. In addition, transplant recipients with a history of CVA face tremendous difficulties in being reintegrated into society due to neurological after-effects, often for years after transplant.

Patients supported by LVAD require extensive oral anticoagulant therapy. Therefore, rapid reversal of warfarin-induced anticoagulation to prevent hematoma growth and facilitate hematoma evacuation (**Hanley JP. 2004**) has a decisive impact on prognosis in such patients. The anticoagulation effect of warfarin is related to its ability to inhibit synthesis of the vitamin K-dependent clotting factors II, VII, IX, and X. The appropriate way to reverse the anticoagulation effect of warfarin depends on the clinical situation. Minor or asymptomatic bleeding needs a less aggressive reversal, whereas serious bleeding requires rapid reversal to avoid succeeding fatal events, regardless of the reason for anticoagulation. For major bleeding, guidelines recommend the administration of vitamin K (5 mg i.v. or oral), and/or PCC (50 U/kg), and/or FFP (15 ml/kg) (**British Committee for Standards in Haematology. 1998; Ansell J et al., 2001**).

The PCC contains a high level of the vitamin K-dependent coagulation factors II, VII, IX, and X. The PCC promotes a much more rapid reversal of INR than FFP or/and vitamin K, which is explained by its higher concentration of coagulation factors than FFP. A large volume of FFP is required to achieve adequate INR reversal (**Aguilar MI et al., 2007**) because vitamin K-dependent coagulation factors vary considerably in FFP, which is not adequate for patients with heart failure. Reversing anticoagulation with vitamin K requires 4 to 24 hours (**Aguilar MI et al., 2007**) then might cause a fatal situation after CVA events, and also its persistent effect may promote clot formation. Thus, vitamin K administration is not an adequate treatment for patients with CVA as well as any major hemorrhage supported by LVAD, either.

Several studies demonstrated the effect of recombinant activated factor VII on warfarin reversal and reported successful results treating CVH events (**Deveras RAE et al., 2002**). Although recombinant activated factor VII does reverse the INR, it does not lead to complete reversal of all aspects of warfarin associated coagulopathy. Further studies are required to establish the difference of the effect of warfarin reversal between PCCs and recombinant activated factor VII.

4. Management of Infection after pulsatile extracorporeal LVAD

The REMATCH study showed that sepsis is the leading cause of death (29.5%) after LVAD surgery while cerebrovascular accidents (CVA) are the third cause of death (9.0%) (**Rose EA et al, 2001**). Coagulase negative staphylococci and staphylococcus aureus have been reported to be the most common pathogens in LVAD-related infections (**Malani PN et al., 2002; Nurozler F et al., 2001**).

Although a high frequency of side effects has limited its use, linezolid is reported to be superior to vancomycin for treating MRSA infection. In addition, linezolid is a powerful drug to treat severe infections by not only MRSA but also other Gram-positive bacteria, even in peculiar anatomical sites in which therapeutic levels of antibiotics cannot be achieved (**Bassetti M et al., 2004**). The effectiveness of linezolid for endocarditis due to multidrug-resistant Gram-positive cocci has also been reported. Indeed, most of the patients who had systemic infection described in our observation were infected by Gram-positive pathogens. Therefore, linezolid might be a useful antibiotic agent for treating the most common responsible pathogens in LVAD patients.

Linezolid should be used only in patients with refractory staphylococcal infection. Linezolid-resistant staphylococcus is becoming a recent concern in severe systemic infection, which requires careful observation.

It would be sometimes difficult to identify the causes of infections, which vary depending on the duration after LVAD implantation. In the acute phase, infectious complications may be related to preoperative condition, and/or surgical intervention. In the chronic phase, they are mostly due to infection of exit sites of inflow and/or outflow cannula. Driveline infections may require surgical debridement. LVAD-associated endocarditis and bacteremia may relapse after prolonged courses of antibiotics. Heart transplantation could cure LVAD-related endocarditis by removal of the infected heart; which require careful administration of immunosuppressant under monitoring infection even after transplant.

5. Conclusion

The donor shortage in Japan has been extremely severe compared to other countries. The cardiac donation rate per million population in Japan is only 0.08, whereas it is 7.3 in the United States. The mean duration of LVAD support for transplant candidates was 1220 days. As the duration of support increases, patients are placed at more risk for LVAD-related complications. In addition, only one type of pulsatile extracorporeal LVAD (Toyobo-LVAS®) is available in Japan. This unique situation surrounding LVAD issues in Japan may be quite different from that in Europe or United Stats.

However, under such circumstances Japanese cardiologists have made a considerable effort to accomplish long-term survival of patients supported by such LVAD.

Delicate and timely treatment of LVAD-related complications, such as CVA and infection would play an important role in long-term LVAD support. The recent improvement of survival after pulsatile extracorporeal LVAD surgery is associated with prompt warfarin reversal for CVA and well-selected administration of antibiotics for staphylococcus-related systemic infection.

We believe that the LVAD-management strategies described in this chapter could provide worthwhile information even in the era of new generation devises.

6. Tables and figures

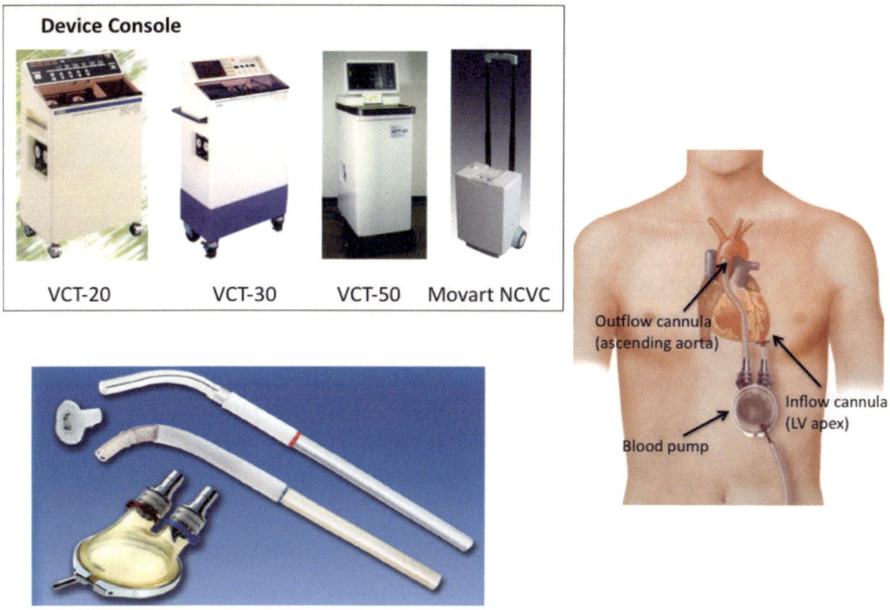

Fig. 1. Toyobo-LVAS® system.

Different types of devise console (**left upper panel**); blood pumps and inflow/outflow cannula (**left lower panel**); and the chart of LVAD system (**right panel**). The blood pump was consisted of diaphragm with pulsatile flow through two mechanical valves, operated by pneumatic driven system. The maximum stroke volume was 70 mL per bear under testing with water. Material of blood contacting surface is covered by segmented-polyurethane for medical use.

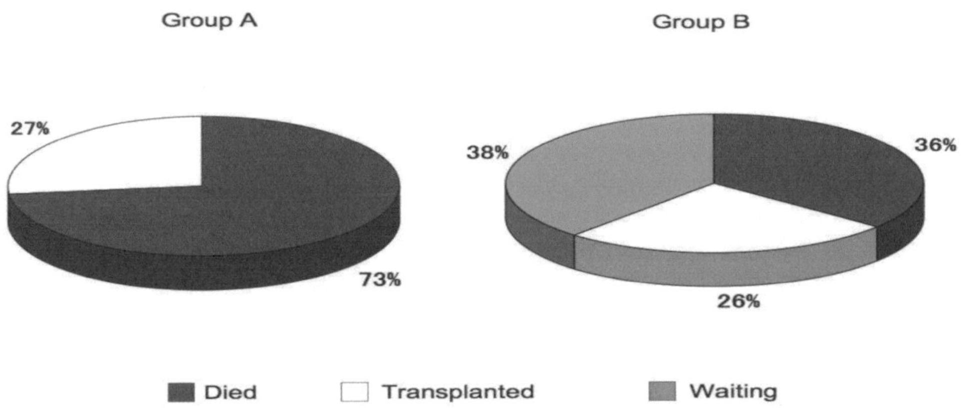

Fig. 2. Outcome of transplant candidates after LVAD surgery.
The initial era (patients in group A) **(left panel)** and the recent era (patients in group B) **(right panel).** (Adopted from Sasaoka T, et al. J Cardiol. 2010; 56:220-8)

Parameter	Group A (n = 30)	Group B (n = 39)	*p* value
Duration of LVAD support (days)	369.3±337.2	674.6±321.3	*0.00029*
Outcome (no. of patients, %)			
Transplanted in Japan	6 (20.0%)	11 (28.2%)	*0.615*
Transferred and transplanted abroad *	2 (6.6%)	4 (10.2%)	*0.925*
Died	22 (73.3%)	14 (35.9%)	*0.0045*
Remaining on waiting list	0 (0%)	10 (25.6%)	*0.0069*

Table 1. Outcome after LVAD surgery
* A number of transplant candidates who were transferred and underwent heart transplantation abroad, due to extreme donor shortage and legal constraints in Japan. Japanese organ transplant law did not have criteria for the diagnosis of brain death for those aged under 15 years as of July 2010, thus, pediatric patients had no chance of receiving heart transplant surgery in Japan. (Adopted from Sasaoka T, et al. J Cardiol. 2010; 56:220-8)

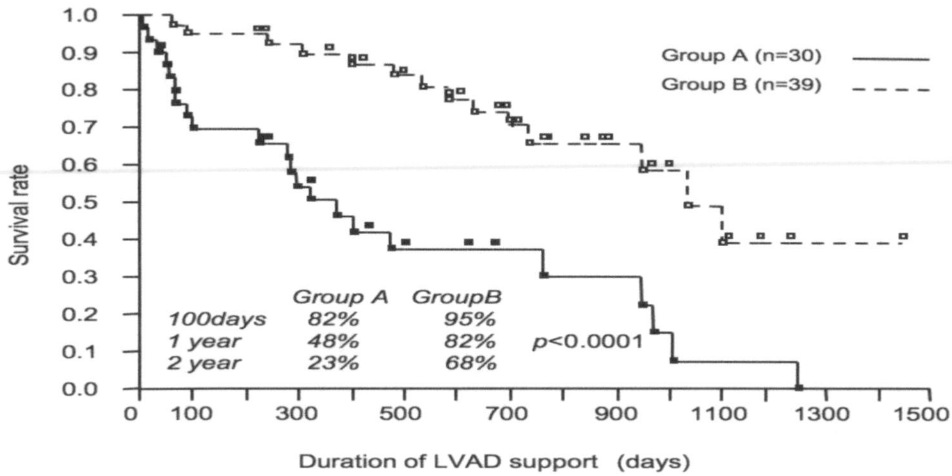

Fig. 3. Kaplan-Meier survival curves of patients supported by extracorporeal pulsatile LVAD.
Survival rates of groups A and B at 100 days, 1 and 2 years after LVAD surgery. Solid line and closed squares, group A; dotted line and open squares, group B. (Adopted from Sasaoka T, et al. J Cardiol. 2010; 56:220-8)

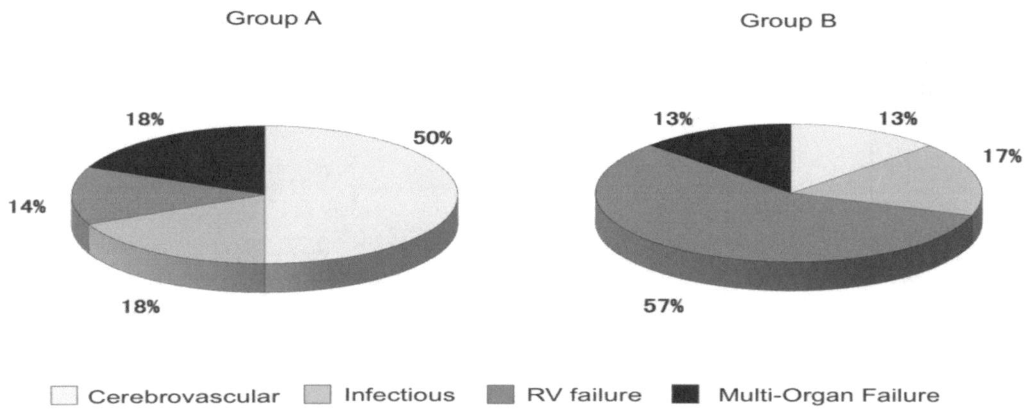

Fig. 4. Causes of death after extracorporeal pulsatile LVAD surgery.
The initial era (patients in group A) (left panel) and the recent era (patients in group B) (right panel). (Adopted from Sasaoka T, et al. J Cardiol. 2010; 56:220-8)

Parameter	Group A (n = 30)	Group B (n = 39)	*p* value
Incidence of CVA (no. of pts, %)	17 (56.7%)	20 (51.2%)	0.841
Intracranial hemorrhage (no. of pts, %)	16 (53.3%)	18 (46.1%)	0.727
Intracranial infarction (no. of pts, %)	13 (43.3%)	12 (30.7%)	0.410
Anticoagulant status			
Baseline INR at stable situation	3.2 ± 1.5	3.3 ± 1.2	0.759
INR on the day of CVA even	3.8 ± 2.1	3.2 ± 1.3	0.149
Among patients developed CVA			
Proportion of CVA requiring neurosurgery (no. of pts, %)	12/17(70.6%)	8/20 (40.0%)	0.062
Proportion of CVA leading to death (no. of pts, %)	11/17(64.7%)	3/20 (15.0%)	0.0057
Proportion of patients given PCC (no. of pts, %)	3/17 (17.6%)	12/20 (60.0%)	0.023

Table 2. Incidence of cardiovascular accidents
Pts, patients; PCC, prothrombin complex concentrate. (Adopted from Sasaoka T, et al. J Cardiol. 2010; 56:220-8)

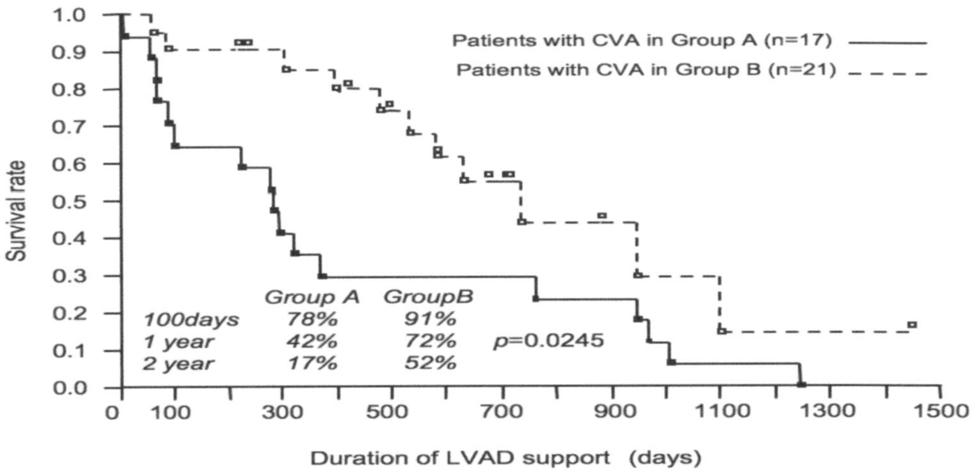

Fig. 5. Subgroup analysis of Kaplan-Meier survival curves of patients who developed CVA (group A, n = 17 vs. group B, n = 21) after extracorporeal pulsatile LVAD surgery. Survival rates at 100 days, 1 and 2 years after LVAD surgery, of patients in groups A and B who developed CVA. Solid line and closed squares, patients in group A; dotted line and open squares, patients in group B. (Adopted from Sasaoka T, et al. J Cardiol. 2010; 56:220-8)

Parameter	Group A (n = 30)	Group B (n = 39)	p value
Incidence of SI (no. of pts, %)	22 (73.3%)	31 (79.5%)	0.754
Among patients developed SI			
Proportion of SI leading to death (no. of pts, %)	4/22 (18.2%)	5/31 (16.1%)	0.861
Proportion of patients presently alive (no. of pts, %)	3/22 (13.6%)	17/31 (54.8%)	0.0058
Proportion of patients undergoing transplants (no. of pts, %)	3/22 (13.6%)	11/31 (35.5%)	0.049
Cumulative number of SI episodes (cumulative no. of episodes)	76	102	-
Number of episodes per year per pts	1.18±0.33	1.26±0.23	0.240

Table 3. Incidence of systemic infection.
SI, systemic infection defined as positive blood culture when patients developed any symptoms of infection. (Adopted from Sasaoka T, et al. J Cardiol. 2010; 56:220-8)

7. References

Aguilar MI, Hart RG, Kase CS, et al. Treatment of warfarin-associated intracerebral hemorrhage: literature review and expert opinion. Mayo Clin Proc 2007; 82:82–92.

Ansell J, Hirsh J, Dalen J, Bussey H, et al. Managing Oral Anticoagulant Therapy. Chest 2001; 119:22S–38S

Bassetti M, Di Biagio A, Del Bono V, Cenderello G, Bassetti D. Successful treatment of methicillin-resistant Staphylococcus aureus endocarditis with linezolid. Int J Antimicrob Agents. 2004; 24:83-4.

British Committee for Standards in Haematology. Guidelines on oral anticoagulation: third edition. Br J Haematol 1998; 101:374–87.

Deveras RAE, Kessler CM. Reversal of Warfarin-Induced Excessive Anticoagulation with Recombinant Human Factor VIIa Concentrate. Ann Intern Med. 2002. 137: 884-888.

Hanley JP. Warfarin Reversal. J Clin Pathol 2004; 57:1132–39.

Holman WL, Kormos RL, Naftel DC, Miller MA, Pagani FD, Blume E, Cleeton T, Koenig SC, Edwards L, Kirklin JK. Predictors of death and transplant in patients with a mechanical circulatory support device: a multi-institutional study. J Heart Lung Transplant 2009; 28:44-50

Malani PN, Dyke DBS, Pagani FD, Chenoweth CE. Nosocomial infections in left ventricular assist devices. Clin Infect Dis 2002,34:1295-1300.

Nurozler F, Argenziano M, Oz MC, Naka Y. Fungal left ventricular assist device endocarditis. Ann Thorac Surg 2001, 71:614-618.

Rose EA, Gelijns AC, Moskowitz AJ, Heitjan DF, Stevenson LW, Dembitsky W, et al.; Randomized Evaluation of Mechanical Assistance for the Treatment of Congestive Heart Failure (REMATCH) Study Group. Long-term mechanical left ventricular assistance for end-stage heart failure. N Engl J Med 2001; 15; 345:1435-43

Sasaoka T, Kato TS, Komamura K, Takahashi A, Nakajima I, Oda N, Hanatani A, Mano A, Asakura M, Hashimura K, Niwaya K, Funatsu T, Kobayashi J, Kitamura S, Shishido T, Wada K, Miyata S, Nakatani T, Isobe M, Kitakaze M. Improved long-term performance of pulsatile extracorporeal left ventricular assist device. J Cardiol. 2010; 56:220-8

Stevens DL, Ma Y, Salmi DB, McIndoo E, Wallace RJ, Bryant AE. Impact of antibiotics on expression of virulence-associated exotoxin genes in methicillin-sensitive and methicillin-resistant Staphylococcus aureus. J Infect Dis. 2007; 195: 202-11.

Takahashi A, Kato TS, Oda N, Komamura K, Asakura M, Hashimura K, et al. Prothrombin Complex Concentrate for Rapid Reversal of Warfarin-Induced Anticoagulation in Patients with Intracerebral Hemorrhages Supported by Left Ventricular Assist Device. Int J of Gerontol. 2010; 4: 143-147

12

Outcomes Following Heart Transplantation among Those Bridged with VAD

Jeffrey H. Shuhaiber MD
Department of Surgery
University of Cincinnati and Cincinnati Children Hospital, Cincinnati, Ohio. 45229
USA

1. Introduction

Clinical assessment of outcome for post heart transplant recipients who were bridged with ventricular assist device is essential for service evaluation, device evaluation and audit. This chapter will provide a summary assessment of clinical studies and reviews. While most of the data available is retrospective, important aspects of this assessment relies on the quality of assessment and timely re-evaluation of strategy used in the assessment.

We will review the clinical outcomes measured so far in the field of heart transplant recipients who were bridged with VAD. In this chapter we will review the ongoing methods of assessment of outcomes for transplant recipients bridged by VAD and discuss the potential challenges facing the clinicians. We will finalize with brief conclusions and future directions.

2. Survival following heart transplantation: Does VAD Type matter?

There have been many clinical studies comparing outcomes following heart transplantation. Only one has been done in a multicenter fashion with clinically relevant as well as a robust risk-adjustment.

In 2006 we asked the question- does survival differ between those who did and did not receive the left ventricular assist device (LVAD) following heart transplantation?

And in summary we found that survival following heart transplantation for patients who received an LVAD prior to transplantation was comparable to those who did not receive an LVAD. The results of this study were published as lead research article in the British Medical Journal earlier this year (Shuhaiber).

We reviewed all patients above 18 years of age who received heart transplants registered in the United Network for Organ Sharing (UNOS) Registry from 1996 to 2004. The study included 2786 status 1/1A/1B heart transplant patients. We used the entry data for all patients who received LVAD pulsatile device. Our study design included a prospective cohort study in which post-transplant survival between patients who received an LVAD and those who did not receive an LVAD was compared.

Patients were assigned to one of five strata based on the propensity score analysis where the first stratum consists of patients most similar to those that had a heart transplant with no prior bridging of an LVAD and the last stratum consists of patients most similar to those patients that had an LVAD device prior to heart transplantation. As a sensitivity analysis, a

1:1 propensity score matching analysis was also performed. Comparisons of survival distributions were made using the Kaplan-Meier method and the risk ratios were estimated using Cox proportional model.
Our primary outcomes as well as risks and exposures included survival following heart transplantation in heart transplant recipients who did or did not receive ventricular assist device.
The strength of the study was in adopting a robust statistical methodology that can adequately control for confounding variables. A *stratified propensity score analysis* of data revealed that the risk of death following heart transplantation in an LVAD patient was not significantly different from those who did not have an LVAD within each stratum (see table for estimated hazard ratios and their 95% confidence intervals). A 1:1 propensity score matching analysis also revealed no significant difference in post heart transplant survival between the two groups (hazard ratio = 1.18, 95% CIs=0.75 to1.86).
The propensity score matching was performed in order to control potential selection biases that can lead to a false association (or false lack of association) between LVAD and survival. Although we attempted to minimize bias through propensity score matching, hidden bias could potentially remain because of other relevant known as well as unknown covariates not available in the UNOS database. Nonetheless, the work provided an application of robust statistical methodology and provided a good signal to noise ratio, that VAD support is safe and is not detrimental to outcomes following heart transplantation.
The other studies published in specialized surgical journals, reflected mainly single center experiences. Nonetheless, they supplement the growing interest in the areas of post heart transplant outcomes in patients with VAD insertion.
In a study from Utah (Bull), patients with idiopathic dilated cardiomyopathy (IDC) that had placement of a Heart mate I (Thoratec Corp, Pleasanton, Calif) ventricular assist device as a bridge to a cardiac transplant were reviewed. The authors studied both alloimmunization as well as survival. They found that the VAD group was associated with elevation in pretransplantation panel reactive antibody sensitization and a decrease in 1- and 5 year survivals after cardiac transplantation. Over the time period from 1993 to 2009, a total of 525 cardiac transplants were performed. VADs were placed as a bridge to transplant in 110 patients. The focus of the study was IDC (n=201) and coronary artery disease (n=213). The authors used variables including gender, age, date of transplant, cause of heart failure, prior heart transplant, placement of a ventricular assist device, type of ventricular assist device, and panel-reactive antibody sensitization. Analysis was performed by Kaplan-Meier survival probabilities and multivariable Cox regression models.
Interestingly, the authors found that the patients who had idiopathic dilated cardiopmyopathy- VAD group had a decreased survival at 1 year (P=0.008) and 5 years (P-.019) but not at 10 years post transplant. The number of patients was small and it was not adjusted according to other important donor variables and use of other life support measures such as ventilation or use of intra-aortic balloon pump. The extrapolation to and extension of the results to more than 1 year becomes both conceptually and clinically difficult to comprehed. Moreover, the hazard related death is more early at the time of transplantation due to re-entry and cardiac injury, or VAD related injury mainly at the inflow or outflow conduits.
In a separate multicenter study of post transplant survival after support with a continuous – flow left ventricular assist device, the authors followed 468 patients that underwent heart

transplantation (John 2010). 53% underwent cardiac transplant after a median duration of LVAD support of 151 days (longest:3.2 years) of which 23% died, 2.6% recovered ventricular function and the device was removed successfully. 21% were still receiving LVAD support. The overall 30-day and 1 year post-transplant survival was 97% and 87%. Patients requiring more than 2 units of packed red blood cells in 24 hours during LVAD support had a statistically significant inferior 1- year survival than those who did not.
Implantation of the VAD with its associated risk factors both perioperatively and postoperatively is important to appreciate as long as the device is in place. After heart transplantation, the device is removed and the patient continues to survive based on the context of graft function, immune suppression and overall patient management assuming that that no serious transplant-surgery related events occurred.
A list of contemporary studies reviewing post VAD heart transplant outcomes is detailed in table 1. While there are studies that demonstrate superior survival among those who received VADs, other studies did not show that. The single most robust study from our group showed that VAD placement really does not have any influence on post-heart transplant outcomes.
Finally, optimal timing of cardiac transplantation after ventricular device implantation is an important variable that can directly or indirectly influence outcome. Although intuitively the transplantation around the time of VAD placement has been associated with far worse outcomes due to patient illness as well as VAD related complications. In a study based on the UNOS registry of 2692 heart transplantations performed between 1999 and 2001, 17% received a VAD (Gammie). Almost half of patients with VAD undergoing transplantation were upgraded to status 1 A as a result of VAD related complications. Creatinine and total bilirubin levels were less in patients undergoing transplantation after 2-4 weeks of mechanical support. One-year survival was higher in the non-ventricular assist device than in the VAD group. Within the VAD, survival was lowest for patients who received a heart within 2 weeks of VAD implantation. Multivariate analysis demonstrated a significant effect of time interval from VAD implantation to transplantation on post heart transplantation mortality. The plausible explanation underlying this finding is when a patient requires a VAD usually they are in decompensated state of heart failure. In this state, there often maintain a similar degree of other end-organ injury mainly renal dysfunction. Weeks of hemodynamic support are required to achieve normalization of end-organ function and are concordant with prior reports that have demonstrated improvement of both hepatic and renal function during long-term VAD support (Gammie). Therefore the general rule is to wait a few weeks between time of VAD insertion and before heart transplantation.

3. VAD induced alloimmunization and post heart transplant rejection

Insertion of VAD is associated with relatively increased risk for blood transfusion. Blood contains a large number of antigen load for which the body mounts selective and non-selective antibodies. These antibodies are naturally formed and can be measured by a test called panel reactive assay. A high PRA has been shown to reduce cardiac graft survival because it increases the absolute risk for rejection both in early and late post transplant stages. We review contemporary studies regarding the role of alloimmunization and post-transplant outcomes.
Also a device such as VAD is placed in circulation, the textured surface of the device results in the formation of pseudointima that contains an abundance of T cells, macrophages, and

Author	Type	LVAD number	Median/Mean Age	1 year survival	Post Transplant Survival Bias
Shuhaiber 2010	Thoratec	1354 LVAD	50.6	no significant difference in survival between the two groups	No difference VAD or no VAD
John 2010	Heart Mate II	468	54	87%	No difference VAD or no VAD
Bull 2010	Heartmate I	110	54 CAD 42 IDC	90 % 77%	VAD Bridge to TX inferior survival
Russo 2009	Implantable Para-& extracorporal	Intra-1680 Para-514 Extra-128	Intra-50 Para-46 Extra-49	1 year Intra-87% Para-81% Extra-57%	No difference
Pal 2009	Authors did not specify type of implantable device	86	49	84% 1 yr 72% 5 yr	No difference
Paltolla 2009	Authors did not specify type of implantable or extracorporal device	1433 Intracorporeal 448 extracorporal	Intra-50 Extra-47	IntraCorp 85% 1 yr 70% 5 yr Extracorp 75% 1 yr 66% 5 yr	Higher with extracorporal
Klotz 2006	Micromed DeBakey,	50	44	68%	No difference

Table 1. List of Contemporary studies detailing survival outcome following VAD bridge to heart transplantation

monocytes as a result of the continuous dynamic interaction of the blood with the device. Aberrant T Cell proliferation and polyclonal B cell hyper-reactivity with CD 40 ligand interaction has all been reported in association with the use of the Hearmate I device. The interaction between the blood constituents and biomaterials of the VAD, specifically the textured chamber surface found in the Heartmate I, may be the responsible for the increased immunologic and inflammatory response seen in this group of patients.

A study from Utah (Drakos 2007), showed that patients with IDC receiving VADs as a bridge to transplant were more likely to have a PRA greater than 10% than the precardiac transplant population without VADs. In a study by Bull et al, patients who received a VAD as a bridge to transplant, the pretransplant PRA was elevated to 35% versus only 5% in the patients without VADs. Interestingly, the incidence and severity of acute cellular and humoral rejection, immunosuppressive agents, immnosuppression protocols, and cardiac allograft vasculopathy did not differ between those with and without VADs in the IDC and CAD groups.

HLA antibodies are present around 3 months following VAD insertion (Kumpati). PRA greater than 10% is considered positive for anti-HLA antibodies. Sensitisation has been found to be more prevalent with increasing length of support. Patient factors determine the temporal pattern of sensitisation and while some argue that the type of device influences allosensitization, others do not (Kumpati). Table 2 reviews the level of sensitization following VAD.

Author	Type	LVAD number	Allosensitization
George 2008	Heartmate I v.s. Heartmate II (1999-2006)	24 36	Heartmate II and DeBakey device produced less sensitization Heart mate I. There were fewer rejection episodes but did not reach Statistical significance.
Drakos 2007	Heart Mate I	71	Leuokfilration in 54 patients and fresh frozen plasma in 17 patients. There were significant trends for less sensitization and lower peak PA with greater blood transfusion.

Table 2. Contemporary studies

The type of VAD as a bridge to transplant does not seem to influence the incidence of posttransplant rejection or survival at 1 year post transplant, but can at 5 years post transplant. In addition, the rate and severity of postransplant rejection has been noted to be higher in LVAD recipients with continous flow devices than in patients with pulsatile devices. However, further studies need to be conducted to determine if these observations are consistent

For example, in a recent study by Bull et al, implantation of the Heartmate II device was not associated with an increase in the PRA (Bull).

We also reviewed the UNOS registry from October 1991 and June 1994 to determine the influence of the type of left ventricular assisted device as predictor of hospitalizations due to rejection following heart transpalntation to delineate any further predictors of such outcome. Patients who received a left ventricular assist device (HeartMate [Thoratec Corp.,

Pleasanton, CA, USA] or Novacor [World Heart Corporation, Ottawa, Canada]) prior to heart transplantation were evaluated. Rejection rates between the two devices were analyzed using multivariable logistic regression model. We reviewed 1255 patients with HeartMate I and 154 patients with Novacor. All-time posttransplant hospitalizations due to rejection were similar between HeartMate and Novacor recipients after adjusting for patient case mix. Interestingly, although the PRA was higher in the HeartMate than the Novacor, this did not reach statistical difference.

While there have been several attempts in reducing PRA levels prior to transplantation, none have shown consistent benefit in reducing absolute rejection episodes post transplantation. Even when leukofiltration has been shown to in reducing sensitization, there is no consistent evidence that it would reduce the burden of acute rejection. Further plasmapheresis can reduce the antibody burden, however the process and hospital-dependent protocols in which it has been developed varies from one to the other. This variation of practice and protocols provides some uncertainty as to what is the best method for managing allosensitization.

4. Infections and infection-related complications following heart VAD support in heart transplant recipients.

Infection is one of the leading causes of mortality during ventricular assist device (VAD) observed during the randomized evaluation of mechanical assistance in chronic heart failure (i.e., REMATCH) Trial (Rose 2001). While the REMATCH was not directed towards heart transplantation, its findings are relevant. Bloodstream infection (BSI) during VAD support is a unique clinical problem whose management is one of three options 1) local remedy of the infected VAD directly affecting the pocket or infected VAD valves 2) explant the VAD 3) replace the VAD 4) cardiac transplantation. In a sub-set of patients with VADs, the BSI clears after appropriately treating the source. In others, the BSI persists without an identifiable extra-device source, strongly implicating device-related infection. A conservative approach to these patients, using long-term suppressive antibiotics, leads to 40% to 50% mortality. Further, two reports have demonstrated infection rate of 50% after heart transplants in patients who had a LVAD. The reasons for this increased infection rate was likely due to many factors including the presence of foreign objects in the blood circulation, in addition to patient comorbidities and immune suppression (Omoto, Messner)

In a study by the Pittsburgh group VAD patients who underwent heart transplantation from 1987 to 2001 and who had BSI during VAD support, and who had positive cultures at VAD explant (device-related BSI, n = 10) were compared with those with negative cultures at explant (non-device-related BSI, n = 11) (Poston). Of the 123 patients who underwent VAD implantation at the University of Pittsburgh Medical Center from 1987 to 2001, a total of 65 (53%) remained free of infection for the entire duration of support. The length of time that patients received VAD support was nearly 3 times longer in those with infection compared with those with no infection during VAD support (132 vs 48 days, $p < 0.0001$). The variables that were significant predictors of infection in univariate analysis (age, BMI, length of hospitalization pre- and post-VAD implantation, length of ICU stay, and history of alcohol abuse) all lost their significance when controlling for the length of VAD support. Only young age showed a trend for predicting infection ($p = 0.06$). Of the patients with devices who underwent heart transplantation during this time (88/123), infection of any type (i.e., BSI or non-BSI) during VAD support was associated with significantly decreased survival after heart transplantation ($p = 0.01$). In the multivariate analysis, the only significant predictors of post-transplant mortality were any infection during device support ($p < 0.01$) and device-related BSI ($p < 0.02$).

In this study, device-related BSI was a significant risk factor for pre-transplant mortality and showed a strong trend for adverse effects on post-transplant survival. Compared with those with no previous history of VAD support, 1-year post-transplant mortality in those with a history of device-related BSI nearly tripled (10% to 26%). After transplantation, these patients had significantly longer intubation requirements and worse renal function. Combined with heightened concerns of sepsis, a greater forced reduction in nephrotoxic immunosuppression was seen in those with former device-related BSI. Some of the limitations in this study, were that inability to prospectively differentiate BSI as originating from a device vs a non-device source. A history of re-operation after initial VAD implantation and of prolonged ICU stay were also significant predictors in multivariate analysis that highlight the need for meticulous attention to hemostasis and the broad benefit of aprotinin. The latter unfortunately no longer exists given its side effects.

Further in a similar study publishd in the Journal of Cardiac Surgery, we reviewed 1255 patients with HeartMate I and 154 patients with Novacor. All-time posttransplant hospitalizations due to infection were similar between HeartMate and Novacor recipients after adjusting for patient case mix (Shuhaiber 2008).

Overall, while infections have decreased in general due to several quality improvement initiatives both during surgery as well as postoperatively, an episode of infection during VAD can have direct implications on the post-transplant patient. Our group documented a case of pseudoaneurysm of the ascending aorta in a patient who had biventricular assist device for refractory ventricular fibrillation. Aortic aneurysms after heart transplantation are rare. Although this condition is associated with a history of infection, causality remains to be fully explained. The marked difference in compliance between donor and recipient aorta has been presented as a potential mechanism of pseudoaneurysm formation. However, other causes, such as suture dehiscence or aortic wall tissue necrosis, cannot be excluded. Resection of residual aortic tissue harboring pathogenic organisms associated with the aortic cannulation site of the VAD should be considered to avoid future aortic complications in this immunosuppressed group (Shuhaiber 2008).

5. Neurocognitive following following VAD insertion

With more than 5 million people sustaining heart failure and more than 550000 newly diagnosed each year. The number of VAD placements will only increase. While this occurs, there has been more interest in understanding quality of life for VAD patiens. One aspect regarding this involves neurocognitive changes (NC) in heart failure patients receiving left ventricular assist devices. While concerns have been raised about functional and nuerobehavioural changes during mechanical support, there are few studies objectively assessing this.

One interesting study details neurocognitive function in heart failure patients receiving left ventricular assist devices. While the study did not review NC outcomes following heart transplantation, the findings are relevant in this review. A protocol designed to evaluate patient performance at 1, 3, 6 months after LVAD implantation at 11 centers was carried out.

A total of 239 sessions were complete in 93 patients including paired evaluations in 51 to 57 patients from 1 to 3 months, and in 20 to 28 patients with results from 1,3 and 6 months. Five NC domains were assessed, including visual spatial perception, auditory and visual memory, executive functions, language and processing speed. The devices included continuous-flow HeartMate II LVAD as a bridge to transplant.

Overall there were no statistical significant differences but limited improvements between 1,3 and 6 months in NC domain performances as seen in visual memory, executive functions and visual spatial perception and processing speed. Interestingly, there were no significant declines in any neurocognitive test in any domain over these time periods.

The cognitive performance of advanced heart failure patients remained stable or showed slight improvments from month 1 to Month 6 of continuous-blood flow support with the HeartMate II LVAD.

Patients who received a VAD and survived heart transplantation will have a recollection of the events surrounding both the time to VAD implantation, explantation and heart transplantation. Such recollections can have an effect on their cognition, psychological feelings and thoughts. There has been much interest in the role of psychology, as well as behavioural responses following cardiac surgery in the adult population. For example, a proportion of patients with depression following heart surgery are associated with poor outcomes. Patients following transplantation particularly with prior VAD implantation may have different psychological profile that is different from those with heart transplanation only. Further studies in understanding these differences may help in changing the outlook of such patients.

Finally, when a VAD is implanted, there is subclinical thromboemboli formed systemically. This may surface clinically with direct injury to vital organs. The burden of thromboembolic disease can present with worsening end-organ function following heart transplantation. For example, if the kidney injury fails later, renal failure ensues and the survival of heart transplant recipient decreases. Or if there are unwitnessed decline in mental status from silent thromboemboli to the brain, neurocognitive impairment ensues. To provide some more quantitative numbers regarding thromboemboli complications following VAD, we reviewed autopsy findings of patients who had a temporary mechanical device placed (Levitronix). Although we clinically witnessed 3 patients with cerebrovascular infarcts, autopsy revealed far more thromboembolic events (Shuhaiber 2009). Among the 18 patients who did not survive after Levitronix implantation, autopsy was obtained in 11 and the results show that 6 (54%) had evidence of thromboembolism, including pulmonary thromboembolism, and 3 had cerebrovascular infarcts. The autopsy findings of the non-survivors demonstrated a bedside underestimation of the thromboembolic burden of VADs. The underlying etiology for thromboembolism was complex and related to cerebrovascular disease, calcification of the aorta, repeat operative procedures, recent myocardial infarction and mural thrombosis, as well as terminal low flow states with secondary venous and arterial thrombosis. Furthermore, 2 patients developed retroperitoneal hemorrhage from unknown causes contributing to significant blood loss, which were not clinically apparent.

The next decade will begin to appreciate these intricate areas further as the methods of diagnosis and assessment of bleeding as well thromboembolic disease during VAD support become more sophisticated and reliable.

6. Future directions and follow up of patients following VAD bridged to heart transplantation

The future has been rewarding since the introduction of VADs into surgery. Its role in prolonging the lives of patients who would not otherwise be candidates or live long enough for heart transplantation has been astounding. The current state of affairs in VAD technology is continuous evolution of myriad of devices for various diagnostic cardiomyopathy patients. Quality outcome research and assessment of small series for different patient cohortsdifferent patient cohort is not the best way to study the device at hand especially since not all patients survive VAD implantation and or heart transplantation. Standardized clinical assessment and management protocols for designated safe VAD in qualified institutions is essential before we can fully appreciate the impact of VAD on post heart transplant outcomes. While certain devices may suit some patients, others may not benefit from this. The next challenge is to begin stratifying those patients who will benefit them the most.

7. References

Shuhaiber JH, Hur K, Gibbons R. The influence of preoperative use of ventricular assist devices on survival after heart transplantation: propensity score matched analysis. BMJ. 2010 Feb 10;340:c392.

Bull DA, Reid BB, Selzman CH, Mesley R, Drakos S, Clayson S, Stoddard G, Gilbert E, Stehlik J, Bader F, Kfoury A, Budge D, Eckels DD, Fuller A, Renlund D, Patel AN. The impact of bridge-to-transplant ventricular assist device support onsurvival after cardiac transplantation. J Thorac Cardiovasc Surg. 2010Jul;140(1):169-73

John R, Pagani FD, Naka Y, Boyle A, Conte JV, Russell SD, Klodell CT, MilanoCA, Rogers J, Farrar DJ, Frazier OH. Post-cardiac transplant survival aftersupport with a continuous-flow left ventricular assist device: impact of duration of left ventricular assist device support and other variables. J ThoracCardiovasc Surg. 2010 Jul;140(1):174-81

Russo MJ, Hong KN, Davies RR, Chen JM, Sorabella RA, Ascheim DD, Williams MR, Gelijns AC, Stewart AS, Argenziano M, Naka Y. Posttransplant survival is not diminished in heart transplant recipients bridged with implantable left ventricular assist devices. J Thorac Cardiovasc Surg. 2009 Dec;138(6):1425-32.e1-3

Patlolla V, Patten RD, Denofrio D, Konstam MA, Krishnamani R. The effect of ventricular assist devices on post-transplant mortality an analysis of the United network for organ sharing thoracic registry. J Am Coll Cardiol. 2009 Jan 20;53(3):264-71

Pal JD, Piacentino V, Cuevas AD, et al. Impact of Left Ventricular Assist Device Bridging on Posttransplant Outcomes. Ann Thorac Surg. 2009;88:1457-1461.

Klotz S, Stypmann J, Welp H, Schmid C, Drees G, Rukosujew A, Scheld HH. Does continuous flow left ventricular assist device technology have a positive impact on outcome pretransplant and posttransplant? Ann Thorac Surg. 2006Nov;82(5):1774-8

Drakos SG, Kfoury AG, Long JW, Stringham JC, Fuller TC, Nelson KE, Campbell BK, Gilbert EM, Renlund DG. Low-dose prophylactic intravenous immunoglobulin does not prevent HLA sensitization in left ventricular assist device recipients. Ann Thorac Surg. 2006 Sep;82(3):889-93

Drakos SG, Stringham JC, Long JW, Gilbert EM, Fuller TC, Campbell BK, Horne BD, Hagan ME, Nelson KE, Lindblom JM, Meldrum PA, Carlson JF, Moore SA, Kfoury AG, Renlund DG. Prevalence and risks of allosensitization in HeartMate left ventricular assist device recipients: the impact of leukofiltered cellular blood product transfusions. J Thorac Cardiovasc Surg. 2007 Jun;133(6):1612-9.

Kumpati GS, Cook DJ, Blackstone EH, Rajeswaran J, Abdo AS, Young JB, Starling RC, Smedira NG, McCarthy PM. HLA sensitization in ventricular assist device recipients: does type of device make a difference? J Thorac Cardiovasc Surg. 2004 Jun;127(6):1800-7.

George I, Colley P, Russo MJ, Martens TP, Burke E, Oz MC, Deng MC, Mancini DM,Naka Y. Association of device surface and biomaterials with immunologic sensitization after mechanical support. J Thorac Cardiovasc Surg. 2008 Jun;135(6):1372-9

Rose EA, Gelijns AC, Moskowitz AJ, Heitjan DF, Stevenson LW, Dembitsky W, Long JW, Ascheim DD, Tierney AR, Levitan RG, Watson JT, Meier P, Ronan NS, Shapiro PA, Lazar RM, Miller LW, Gupta L, Frazier OH, Desvigne-Nickens P, Oz MC, Poirier VL; Randomized Evaluation of Mechanical Assistance for the Treatment of Congestive Heart Failure (REMATCH) Study Group. Long-term use of a left ventricular assist device for end-stage heart failure. N Engl J Med. 2001 Nov 15;345(20):1435-43

Poston RS, Husain S, Sorce D, Stanford E, Kusne S, Wagener M, Griffith BP, Kormos RL. LVAD bloodstream infections: therapeutic rationale for transplantation after LVAD infection. J Heart Lung Transplant. 2003 Aug;22(8):914-21.

Shuhaiber J, Hur K, Gibbons R. Does the type of ventricular assisted device influence survival, infection, and rejection rates following heart transplantation? J Card Surg. 2009 May-Jun;24(3):250-5

Messner GN, Vatcharasiritham C, Gregoric I, Radovancevic B, Odegaard P, Flamm SD, Frazier OH. Prosthetic graft remnant-related pseudoaneurysm after leftventricular assist device explantation: a case report. J Thorac Cardiovasc Surg. 2004 Jan;127(1):259-61.

Gammie JS, Edwards LB, Griffith BP, Pierson RN 3rd, Tsao L. Optimal timing ofcardiac transplantation after ventricular assist device implantation. J Thorac Cardiovasc Surg. 2004 Jun;127(6):1789-99.

Omoto T, Minami K, Muramatsu T, Kyo S, Körfer R. Pseudoaneurysm after heart transplantation with history of LVAD driveline infection. Ann Thorac Surg. 2001 Jul;72(1):263-4.

Shuhaiber J, Nemeh H, Schwartz J. Pseudoaneurysm of ascending aorta after biventricular assist device support. J Heart Lung Transplant. 2008 Dec;27(12):1348-9

Blumenthal JA, Lett HS, Babyak MA, White W, Smith PK, Mark DB, Jones R, MathewJP, Newman MF; NORG Investigators. Depression as a risk factor for mortality after coronary artery bypass surgery. Lancet. 2003 Aug 23;362(9384):604-9.

Shuhaiber JH, Jenkins D, Berman M, Parameshwar J, Dhital K, Tsui S, Large SR. The Papworth experience with the Levitronix CentriMag ventricular assist device. J Heart Lung Transplant. 2008 Feb;27(2):158